Using Computers in the Medical Office

Microsoft® Word | Excel PowerPoint

2016

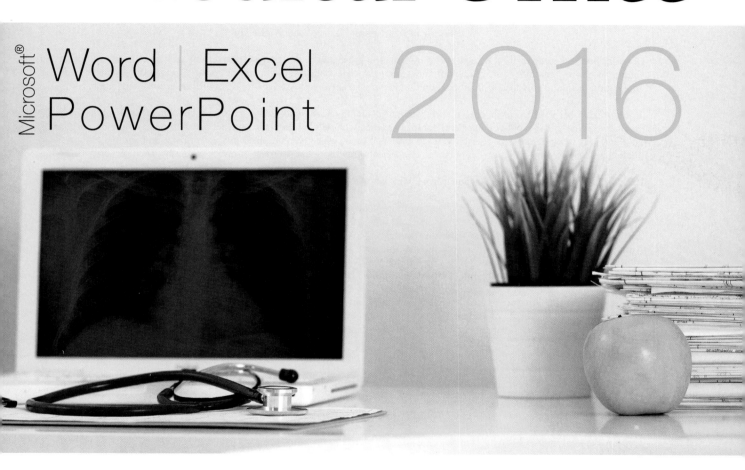

Audrey Roggenkamp
Pierce College Puyallup
Puyallup, Washington

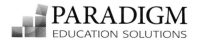

PARADIGM
EDUCATION SOLUTIONS

St. Paul

Division President	Linda Hein
Vice President, Content Strategy	Christine Hurney
Managing Editor	Cheryl Drivdahl
Developmental Editor	Jennifer Gehlhar
Assistant Developmental Editor	Mamie Clark
Tester	Janet Blum
Director of Production	Timothy W. Larson
Production Editor	Jen Weaverling
Senior Design and Production Specialist	Jaana Bykonich
Copy Editor	Sarah Kearin
Proofreader	Shannon Kottke
Indexer	Terry Casey
Vice President, Digital Solutions	Chuck Bratton
Digital Projects Manager	Tom Modl
Digital Production Manager	Aaron Esnough
Vice President Sales and Marketing	Scott Burns
Director of Marketing	Lara Weber McLellan

Care has been taken to verify the accuracy of information presented in this book. However, the authors, editors, and publisher cannot accept responsibility for web, email, newsgroup, or chat room subject matter or content, or for consequences from the application of the information in this book, and make no warranty, expressed or implied, with respect to its content.

Trademarks: Microsoft is a trademark or registered trademark of Microsoft Corporation in the United States and/or other countries. Some of the product names and company names included in this book have been used for identification purposes only and may be trademarks or registered trade names of their respective manufacturers and sellers. The authors, editors, and publisher disclaim any affiliation, association, or connection with, or sponsorship or endorsement by, such owners.

Paradigm Publishing, Inc., is independent from Microsoft Corporation and not affiliated with Microsoft in any manner.

Photo Credits: © Dutko/iStock.com, © yumiyum/iStock.com; **Information Technology Essentials Photo Credits:** Page ITE-1: Image 1, © Photobank/Shutterstock.com and Image 2, © iStockphoto.com/Whitehoune, page 8 (header); Page ITE-2: (top) © iStockphoto.com/Andrew Parfenov, (middle) © iStockphoto.com/Neustockimages, (bottom) courtesy of Epson America, Inc.; Page ITE-3: (top) © iStockphoto.com/darren wise, (bottom left) © iStockphoto.com/Oleksiy Mark, (bottom right) courtesy of Motorola; Page ITE-4: (top) courtesy of McKesson Provider Technologies, (middle) courtesy of SanDisk Corporation, (bottom) courtesy of Intel Corporation; Page ITE-5: (top) courtesy of ASUSTeK Computer Inc., (bottom) © Alexey Rotanov / Shutterstock; Page ITE-6: (top) courtesy of Logitech, (middle) courtesy of Western Digital Corp., (bottom) courtesy of Verbatim Americas LLC.; Page ITE-8: (top) used with permission from Microsoft Corporation; Page ITE-11: (bottom left) © iStockphoto.com/killerb10, (bottom right) courtesy of Intuit Inc.; Page ITE-12: (top) courtesy of Opera Software APA; Page ITE-16 (middle) © iStockphoto.com/nolimitpictures, (bottom) © iStockphoto.com/Sebastien Cote; Page ITE-25 (top) © iStockphoto.com/MHJ.

We have made every effort to trace the ownership of all copyrighted material and to secure permission from copyright holders. In the event of any question arising as to the use of any material, we will be pleased to make the necessary corrections in future printings.

ISBN 978-0-76387-833-7 (print)
ISBN 978-0-76387-834-4 (digital)

© 2018 by Paradigm Publishing, Inc.
875 Montreal Way
St. Paul, MN 55102
Email: CustomerService@ParadigmEducation.com
Website: ParadigmEducation.com

Printed in the United States of America

26 25 24 23 22 21 20 19 18 17   1 2 3 4 5 6 7 8 9 10

Contents

Preface

Using Computers in the Medical Office: Microsoft Word, Excel, and PowerPoint 2016 prepares students to work with Microsoft Office 2016 in medical office settings. Incorporating an accelerated, step-by-step, project-based approach, this text builds student competency in Word, Excel, and PowerPoint 2016. Medical offices are fast-paced environments that require employees to manage a variety of tasks. Many of these tasks require proficiency in the Microsoft Office suite. This text teaches the key computer competencies needed to use Microsoft Office and provides practice in applying the skills in realistic healthcare scenarios.

Throughout *Using Computers in the Medical Office*, authentic medical documents provide the context for learning essential computer tasks performed in the medical office. Students prepare documents, reports, and presentations for two medical clinics and a hospital. Cascade View Pediatrics is a full-service pediatric clinic that provides comprehensive primary pediatric care to infants, children, and adolescents. North Shore Medical Clinic is an internal medicine clinic, and the healthcare providers in this clinic specialize in a number of fields including internal medicine, family practice, cardiology, and dermatology. Columbia River General Hospital is an independent, not-for-profit hospital providing high-quality, comprehensive care. All of the computer skills are taught in the context of preparing materials to support the services provided by these three healthcare settings.

Student Textbook Features

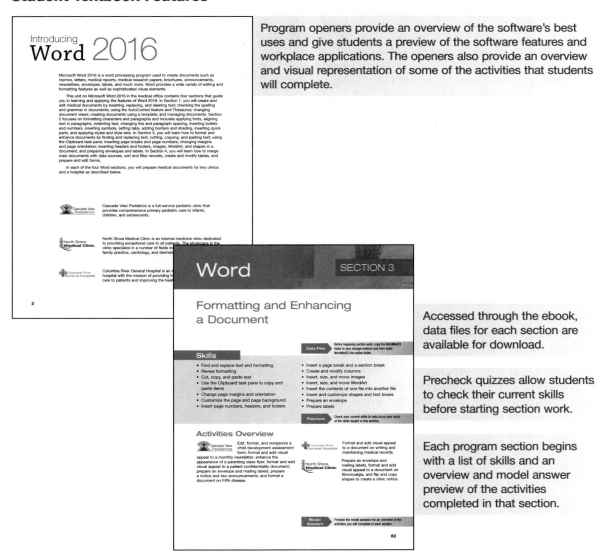

Program openers provide an overview of the software's best uses and give students a preview of the software features and workplace applications. The openers also provide an overview and visual representation of some of the activities that students will complete.

Accessed through the ebook, data files for each section are available for download.

Precheck quizzes allow students to check their current skills before starting section work.

Each program section begins with a list of skills and an overview and model answer preview of the activities completed in that section.

Activities begin with a short explanation of the application's features followed by streamlined, point-and-click instruction that pares reading to a minimum.

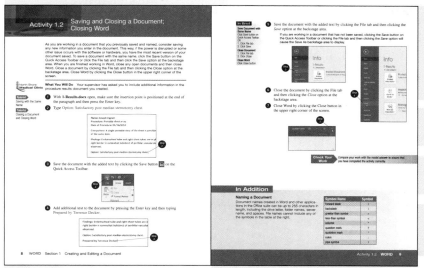

In Brief—Bare-bones summaries of major commands and features provide instant review and a quick reference of the steps required to accomplish a task.

Magenta color highlights text to be typed.

Screen captures visually reinforce activity steps.

In Addition—Sidebars offer extra information on key features and subfeatures.

Interactive tutorials provide guided training and measured practice.

Check Your Work—Accessed through the ebook, locked PDFs allow students to confirm that they have completed the activity correctly.

Integrating Programs—Activities devoted to integrating information among Microsoft Office 2016 programs highlight the benefits of using the Office suite. Activities include copying, exporting, linking, and embedding data. Students learn how to manage data efficiently in the medical office.

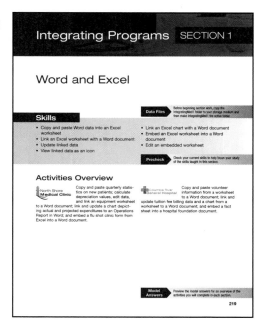

eBook Features

The student ebook provides access to the content in *Using Computers in the Medical Office* from any device (desktop, tablet, and smartphone) anywhere, through a live Internet connection. The versatile ebook platform features dynamic navigation tools including a linked table of contents and the ability to jump to specific pages, search for terms, bookmark information, highlight text, and take notes. Students can also directly link to section study tools and assessment activities provided in the *Workbook* ebook.

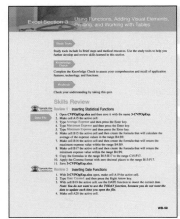

Study Tools—Study tools include In Brief steps and medical resources to help students further develop and review skills learned in this section.

Knowledge Check—is an objective completion exercise that allows students to assess their comprehension and recall of application features, technology, and functions.

Recheck—A concept quiz for each section enables students to check how their skills have improved after completing section work.

Skills Review—Completing these hands-on exercises reinforces learning of key features and skills. Instructions include some guidance, but less than is provided within the section activities.

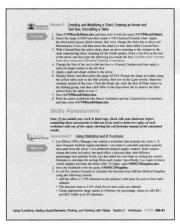

Skills Assessment—Framed within a workplace project perspective, these assessments evaluate the ability to apply section skills and concepts in solving realistic problems. They require the demonstration of program skills and decision-making, which may include additional research.

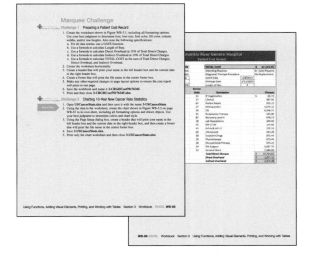

Marquee Challenge—Culminating assessments test mastery of program features and problem-solving abilities.

Instructor eResources

All instructor resources are available digitally through a web-based ebook on the Paradigm Bookshelf. The instructor materials include:

- Assessment resources, including live and PDF model answers for section work and workbook activities, section-based exam banks, and instructional teaching articles.

- Planning resources, such as course objectives, teaching suggestions, and sample course syllabi.

Information Technology Essentials

Precheck Check your current skills to help focus your study of the skills taught in this section.

The Information Processing Cycle

Computers process information in the same way that humans make decisions. We use our eyes and ears to input facts and data into our brains. We use our brains to process that data and organize it into information. The resulting output is a thought or decision that we can display or present by drawing it, writing it, or making a video or audio recording of it. If we decide to keep the results for future use, we can store the paper or recording in a file cabinet.

As shown in Figure 1, the information processing cycle can be divided into four segments: input, processing, output, and storage. It relies on computer hardware to mimic the human thought process. The term hardware refers to the devices you can physically see and touch in and on the computer.

Input

Input involves getting data into the computer so that it can be processed. Some commonly used input devices are described in the following sections.

Keyboard Designed based on the layout of keys on a typewriter, the keyboard is primarily used for typing text. Although numbers are found in a row above the letters, most PC keyboards also include a calculator-style number pad for the convenience of bookkeepers, accountants, and others who frequently work with numbers.

Twelve keys labeled F1 through F12, as well as several other named keys, can be programmed to perform special functions in software applications. For example, the F1 key usually displays a help window where you might type a request for instructions on how to print what has just been typed. The Home key might move the cursor to the left side of a line in one program, but to the upper left corner of the page in another. (The cursor, also known as the insertion point, is the flashing bar, dash, or other symbol that indicates where the next character you type will appear on the screen.)

Figure 1 The Information Processing Cycle

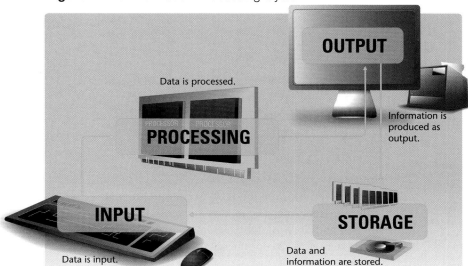

Data is processed.

PROCESSING

OUTPUT

Information is produced as output.

INPUT

Data is input.

STORAGE

Data and information are stored.

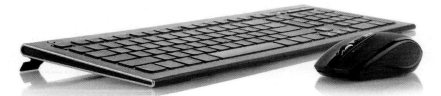

A keyboard and mouse are examples of common input devices.

Mouse A mouse is a pointing device used for issuing commands and selecting text or files for processing. Moving the mouse on the desktop causes a pointer to move on the screen. If you point to the File tab in the top left corner of the Microsoft Word screen, for example, and then click the left mouse button, the backstage area will appear, allowing you to click the *Open* option if you want to access a file you have previously saved.

If you want to delete several words or lines of text in a file, you can point to the beginning of the first word, hold down the left mouse button, drag the mouse to highlight the text, and then press the Delete key to remove the text from the document.

Touchpad Most laptop computers provide a touchpad instead of a mouse as a pointing device. To use a touchpad, move your index finger across the pad to position the cursor and then use your thumb to press the buttons at the bottom of the pad.

Touchscreen A touchscreen allows you to select items and input commands by physically touching a specific area of the monitor. Most smartphones and tablets utilize touchscreen technology. Touchscreens are also used at information kiosks to provide an easy way to select items of interest, without the necessity of a keyboard. Servers at restaurants use touchscreens to place orders since they are much easier to clean than keyboards and can be used with only one hand.

Scanner A scanner works like a photocopier to transfer pictures or text into a computer. If you don't have a digital camera, you can scan hard copies of your photos into a PC and then organize or enhance them with photo-editing software.

Digitizing Pen and Drawing Tablet Although a mouse can be used for drawing designs and pictures, it is very clumsy. Better detail can be achieved with a digitizing pen and drawing tablet. Some tablets and laptop computers now accept "handwritten" input with a digitizing pen called a stylus.

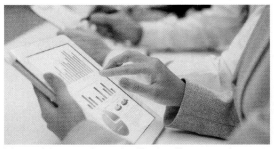

Most tablets, such as the iPad, utilize a touchscreen as the main mode of user input. Touchscreens have advanced and allow multiple fingers or thumbs to be used simultaneously on the screen.

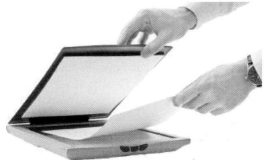

A scanner is a tool to input either pictures or text.

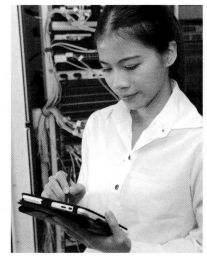

Tablet PCs are useful for writing notes by hand when in a meeting or on the road.

Engineers, architects, and designers often use a sophisticated type of graphics tablet to make precise drawings such as those used in building construction and the manufacture of circuit boards for computers. Such graphics tablets are made up of hundreds of tiny intersecting wires that form an electronic matrix embedded in the tablet surface. A stylus or crosshair cursor activates these intersection points, which collectively represent the image.

Joystick A joystick (named after the control stick used to fly fighter jets) is an input device consisting of a small box with a vertical stick that, when pushed in a certain direction, moves the cursor on the screen. Most often used to control fast-moving images in computer games, joysticks can also be used by people who have difficulty using a mouse.

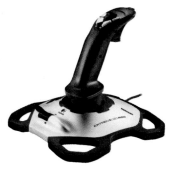

A joystick is an input device used to move objects on a computer screen and is a common input device for computer gaming.

Digital Camera Digital cameras can be used to transfer pictures and videos onto a computer. A webcam is a popular example of a video camera that can be used in combination with headphones and a microphone to communicate with people all over the world. Many computers, including all smartphones, now come with built-in cameras and microphones to make this type of communication easier.

Microphone With a microphone you can add a "sound bite" to a computerized slide presentation or speak to a friend over the Internet. Microphones can stand on a desk or be worn as part of a headset.

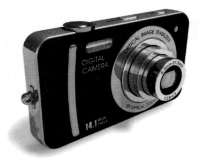

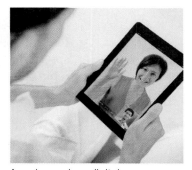

Bar Code Reader Bar code readers are used for entering the Universal Product Code (UPC) found on items in grocery and retail stores. They also are used to track medication administration in hospitals.

A digital camera captures images in a digital format and often contains an output device for viewing those images.

A webcam is a digital camera that can be controlled remotely over the Internet.

Dual Purpose Devices Although usually thought of as storage devices, compact discs (CDs), digital video discs (DVDs), flash drives, and hard drives all allow you to enter data into a computer quickly and easily.

Processing

A computer's central function is to process data. Processing can involve calculating numbers, editing text, modifying pictures, and other information management tasks. The central processing unit (CPU) is the brain of the computer that handles those tasks. The rate at which the CPU can process data is known as the clock speed.

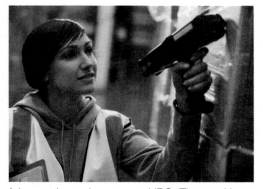

A bar code reader scans a UPC. The resulting input can be used to check a patient's identity and medication requirements.

Processors Most IBM-compatible PCs use a central processing unit made by Intel or AMD. These CPUs process data at clock speeds from 2.0 to 4.0 gigahertz (GHz). (One gigahertz equals one billion cycles per second.) The first Apple Macintosh computers ran on Motorola 68000 processors, but Macs now use Intel processors and can run IBM-compatible PC operating systems.

Many CPUs include multiple processors on a single chip. These dual-core or quad-core processors can process multiple instructions simultaneously for better performance. Some CPUs have six processors in one. Single-core processors use a technique called multitasking, in which one processor switches between programs so quickly that the user doesn't perceive any interruption, but both programs are actually running more slowly than they would with two separate processors or with one dual-core processor.

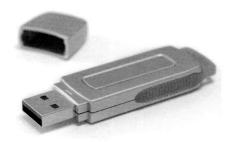

Flash drives are small, easy-to-handle, portable storage devices that many people use to carry important data with them wherever they go.

Memory Chips Memory chips are the hardware that provides the workspace for the data and instructions the computer is processing. The user workspace is called random access memory (RAM) because the CPU has quick and easy access to it. Having a large amount of RAM is like having a large work table where you can spread out books, papers, pencils, a calculator, and other tools you need to do your work. RAM is considered volatile or temporary storage because it disappears completely when the power to the computer is shut off.

The amount of RAM a personal computer needs depends on the operating system it runs. A Windows 10 or Windows 8.1 system requires at least 1 gigabyte (GB). A gigabyte equals about one billion bytes.

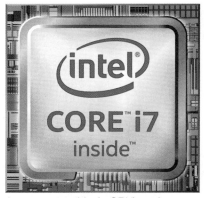

A processor chip (a CPU) performs the calculations in a computer.

Read only memory (ROM) is sometimes confused with RAM due to the similarity of their names, but ROM is nonvolatile and contains the getting-started instructions that the PC needs when the power is first turned on. As its name implies, ROM can only be used as programmed by the PC manufacturer. You can't make any changes to it; you can only cause its contents to be "read" into the computer.

The motherboard is a container for the computer's CPU and RAM, and contains slots for adding expansion cards. Figure 2 shows a typical motherboard layout.

Figure 2 Motherboard Layout

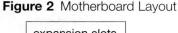

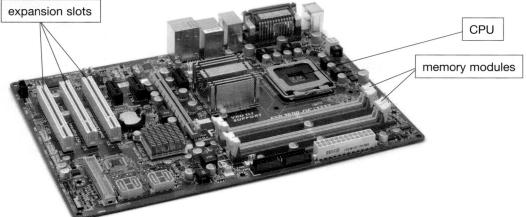

expansion slots

CPU

memory modules

Output

Output is processed data that can be used immediately or stored for later use. Output may be produced in either hard copy or soft copy, or in both forms. Hard copy is a permanent version of output, such as a letter printed on paper using a printer. Soft copy is a temporary version of output and includes any output that cannot be physically handled. Soft copy output devices include monitors and speakers.

Monitor A monitor is a screen used for displaying graphics and text. Although older cathode ray tube (CRT) monitors are still in use, new PCs are sold with flat screen, liquid crystal display (LCD) or light-emitting diode (LED) monitors. In an LCD monitor, liquid crystals are sandwiched between two sheets of material. Electric current passing through the crystals causes them to twist. This twisting effect blocks some light waves and allows other light waves to pass through, creating images on the screen. In an LED monitor, the LCD method of light transmission is enhanced by positioning red, green, and blue LEDs behind the liquid crystals. An LED monitor provides a more vibrant, colorful display than an LCD monitor.

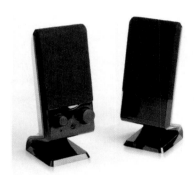

Flat screen, LCD monitors are the most commonly used output devices.

Printer Printers provide hard copy printouts on paper. Several printing technologies are available, including ink-jet, which squirts liquid ink onto the paper, and laser, which fuses powdered toner to the paper.

Speakers and Headphones Speakers and headphones provide audio output in stereo or surround sound for movies, radio programs, streaming video, online learning courses, and telephone calls.

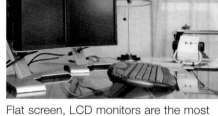

Computer speakers provide sound output.

Storage

The storage portion of the information processing cycle involves recording output so that it will be available after the computer has been shut off and RAM has been erased.

Output can be stored for future use on hard drives, CDs, DVDs, and flash drives. A drive is a PC device that can read and write data onto the surface of a round platter (disk) as it spins. Hard disk platters are made of metal; compact and digital video discs are made of plastic. Flash drives and solid-state hard drives store data in nonvolatile RAM; they have no moving parts, but they provide the same function as conventional drives.

Hard drives contain a stack of metal platters (disks), a drive motor, and read/write heads that are positioned to access the top and bottom of each platter. Hard drive capacities vary; an average desktop PC might have a hard drive that holds 500 GB.

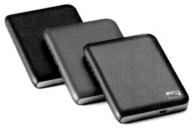

Portable external hard drives are available in a variety of sizes, styles, and colors.

Data CDs are made of the same material that is used for music CDs. In fact, you can play your favorite music CDs using the CD drive of your PC. CDs can hold about 700 MB of data. DVDs can hold from 4 GB to 8 GB,

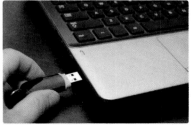

This flash drive storage device has a USB connector that fits into a standard USB port.

depending on whether they can record on one or two layers. Blu-ray discs are used both for high-definition video and for data; a Blu-ray disc can hold 25 GB to 50 GB.

The flash drives on the market today can hold from 128 megabytes to 256 gigabytes of data on a printed circuit board inside a protective plastic case. They are the size and shape of a person's thumb. Some drives even provide fingerprint authorization. Flash drives connect directly to a USB port and thus do not require the installation of any device driver programs to support them.

System Unit Ports

Ports are the sockets that the input, output, and storage devices plug into (see Figure 3). In the early days of personal computing, serial, parallel, and printer cables and ports were found on all PCs. Today, most external, or peripheral, devices use Universal Serial Bus (USB) cables and ports. USB cables and connector plugs are smaller, thinner, and more durable. They transmit data at up to 5 gigabits per second (Gbps) for a USB 3.0 port. As many as 127 devices can be connected to a computer host at once through a daisy-chain-style connection setup.

USB hubs provide extra connection options for computers with only one or two USB ports. You can even make backup copies of your data to an external hard drive connected to your computer via the USB port on your keyboard.

Exploring Technology   1

Identify the processor, clock speed, and amount of random access memory (RAM) in a computer you often use. *Hint: On a computer running Windows 10 or 8.1, right-click the Start button and then click* System *at the pop-up menu. In either operating system, if the Control Panel is displayed using Classic view, double-click the System icon.*

Exploring Technology   2

Identify the hardware you have on your computer and categorize each piece as input, output, or both.

Figure 3 System Unit Ports

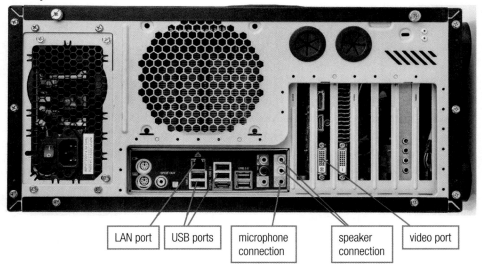

LAN port   USB ports   microphone connection   speaker connection   video port

Computer Software

Software refers to the operating instructions and applications that allow computers to process the numbers, pictures, sounds, and text we enter into them. We can touch the disc that contains the software, but not the lines of programming code that make up the software.

Personal Computer Operating Systems

The original personal computer operating system, MS-DOS (Disk Operating System), used a command-line interface, which meant that commands were typed into a text prompt and the computer returned text output to the monitor. Today, most operating systems use Graphical User Interfaces (GUIs), in which a mouse is used to manipulate graphic objects such as icons and windows on-screen.

If a PC has an older CPU with a clock speed that is too slow, or if it does not have enough RAM, the PC will run slowly or it won't be able to run the operating system at all. Windows 10 and Windows 8.1 require, at a minimum, a CPU that runs at 1 GHz and has 1 GB of RAM.

The operating system for Apple Macintosh computers is Mac OS. The tenth version of the Mac operating system is called Mac OS X. Since its initial introduction in 2001, several updates to this operating system have been released, each one with a different code name. El Capitan (version 10.11) was released in September 2015. Previous versions included Yosemite, Mavericks, Mountain Lion, Lion, and Snow Leopard.

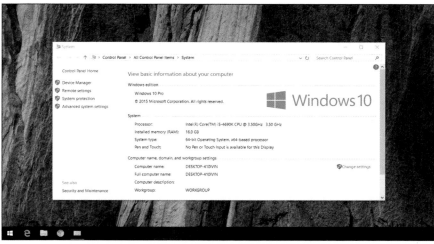

The Windows 10 operating system requires a CPU that runs at 1 GHz.

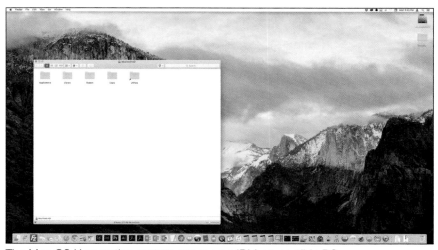

The Mac OS X operating system can run on IBM-compatible PCs.

Applications

Applications allow someone with no technical knowledge of how a PC works to use a computer to balance his or her checkbook or to insert a photograph into a personalized greeting card, print it out, and send it to a friend. Thousands of software applications are available to empower users to perform these and other tasks, ranging from mundane to amazing. This section presents the most common types of computer applications on the market today.

Word Processing Word processing software was originally designed as a replacement for the typewriter. Now a word processing program such as Microsoft Word can support photos and drawings; mathematical calculations; text in table format; text of varying sizes, shapes, and colors; and even sound bites.

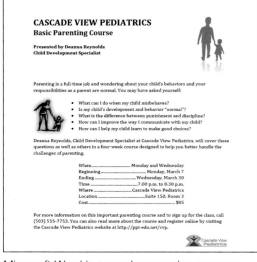

Microsoft Word is a word processing program with several formatting features that can be applied to words, lines, paragraphs, pages, or entire documents.

Spreadsheet Spreadsheet software such as Microsoft Excel can be used for both simple and complex calculations. Current versions can also support graphics and perform some database tasks, such as sorting. A series of keystrokes or clicks used to perform a task can be saved as a macro and programmed to run at the press of a key.

Because formulas are used to create calculations, you can ask, "If I spend only $2 per day on coffee instead of $5, how much money will I save per month?" When you replace one value with another, the program will automatically recalculate your budget.

Database Database software such as Microsoft Access is designed to keep track of information. It allows you to arrange data alphabetically, numerically, or chronologically, or you can filter the data to display only those items that match your criteria, such as the names of customers who spent more than $500 at your online music store last year. Database software can easily do simple calculations, such as showing monthly subtotals and an annual total for each of your customers, but complex math is usually best left to spreadsheet software.

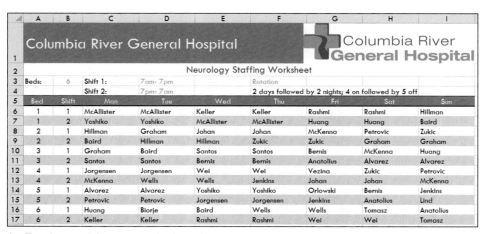

An Excel spreadsheet can calculate elements of a sales report, such as quarterly total sales, and display them in a chart.

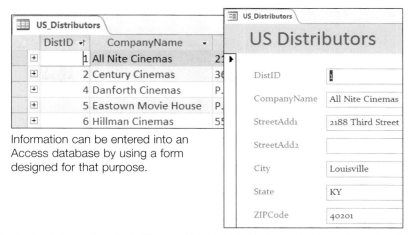

US_Distributors		
DistID	CompanyName	
1	All Nite Cinemas	2:
2	Century Cinemas	3(
4	Danforth Cinemas	P.
5	Eastown Movie House	P.
6	Hillman Cinemas	55

US Distributors

DistID	1
CompanyName	All Nite Cinemas
StreetAdd1	2188 Third Street
StreetAdd2	
City	Louisville
State	KY
ZIPCode	40201

Information can be entered into an Access database by using a form designed for that purpose.

Movies

MovieID	MovieTitle	Rating	Length	ReleaseDate	Genre
1	Ring of Roses	G	129	2/10/2014	Adventure
2	The Codebreakers of World War II	G	183	12/30/2015	History
3	The Life of Winston Churchill	G	125	1/15/2016	Biography
4	Two by Two	G	95	3/15/2017	Action
5	Going Global	G	164	9/1/2018	Documentary

An Access database report is a selection of data in a database. The user chooses which types of information should be included in the report, and the database automatically finds and organizes the corresponding data.

Presentation Presentation software such as Microsoft PowerPoint allows users to create slide shows that can be viewed on a computer monitor or projected onto a large screen. Slide shows can include clip art, graphs and charts, photos, drawings, video clips, sound, and text. Features such as arrows and boxes that "fly" into the screen and slide transition effects can add interest and emphasis to the content of a presentation.

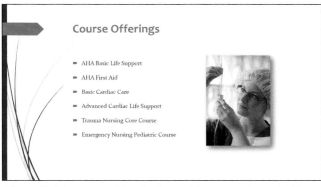

PowerPoint can combine text, graphics, sounds, and videos.

Audio, Video, and Photo Editing Photo-editing software is used for organizing, retouching, and editing photographs and videos. Programs such as PaintShop Pro and Photo Elements allow you to edit photographs by cropping, removing the red-eye effect, or by making more advanced changes such as putting one person's head on another person's body. You can also create your own slide shows with background audio and then email the results to friends and family or copy them to the cloud and display them on your TV.

Video-editing software such as Adobe Premiere can be used to edit video clips to remove the shots you took of your feet when you forgot to stop recording, or to add music, or to rearrange the scenes to create a more logical flow—or a more creative one. You can also edit the audio tracks. With some relatively inexpensive products, you can fine-tune the sound and achieve a professional level of quality.

The Internet provides many options for uploading and sharing videos, music, and photos. YouTube is a popular website that allows users to watch and post videos. Many emerging new musicians use the website SoundCloud to upload their latest tracks and share them with the community. Websites such as Imgur and Photobucket are useful for uploading and sharing images.

Graphics and Drawing Applications such as Adobe Photoshop, Adobe Illustrator, Microsoft Paint, and Corel PaintShop Pro are popular software packages that provide the tools to design graphical images that can be used for web pages, posters, marketing brochures, and greeting cards. Visio is a graphics application that focuses more on technical and business drawings, flow charts, and organizational charts to illustrate complex processes. Visio is vector graphics–based, meaning that it uses points, lines, curves, and geometric shapes to create images. Raster-based graphics programs use groups of pixels (picture elements) to make an image.

A digitized pen and tablet may seem to be a requirement for using drawing applications, but you can do amazing things with a mouse by, for example, picking a circle from a group of shapes and then making it larger or smaller or turning it into an oval. Free graphics and drawing software applications include Inkscape, Skencil, and GIMP.

Suites Software applications are often bundled into packages called suites. Widely used versions of the Microsoft Office suite contain the word processing application, Word; the spreadsheet application, Excel; the database application, Access; and the presentation application, PowerPoint.

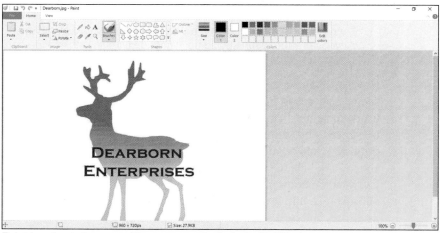
Paint is a basic image-editing program included with Windows.

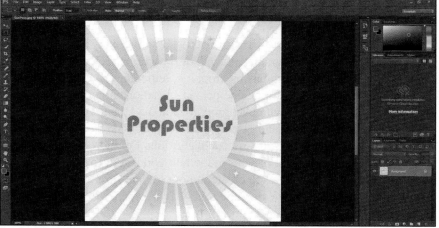
Adobe Photoshop is a high-end image-editing program used by graphics professionals.

Money management software enables users to manage their money by helping them pay bills, balance checkbooks, keep track of income and expenses, maintain investment records, and more.

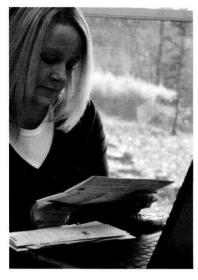

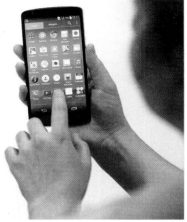

Smartphones include PIM software that tracks appointments and stores contact information.

Money Management Quicken and Microsoft Money are two software applications with an interface that resembles a checkbook. Users can not only write and print checks, but also track their spending habits, create a budget, generate cash flow reports, download their credit card charges, and keep track of their savings and investments.

TurboTax and TaxCut are income-tax preparation programs that prompt you to enter your tax information and then print duplicates of the state and federal forms with your data on the appropriate lines. They also let you file your tax returns electronically and direct your refund to your bank account.

Personal Information Management Microsoft Outlook and Lotus Organizer are examples of personal information management (PIM) programs that keep track of your to-do list, address book, and personal calendar. Many PIMs also contain a scheduler with an alarm to alert you of a meeting, whether it occurs daily, weekly, or only once. Smartphones and tablets can synchronize with your computer's PIM program so you can carry your information everywhere you go.

Collaboration Businesses often need several people to collaborate on a project. Collaborative software or groupware, such as IBM Notes, Adobe Connect, and Microsoft Office SharePoint, provides a way to keep track of who has made or suggested changes to documents or plans and to distribute everything electronically. A calendar feature allows

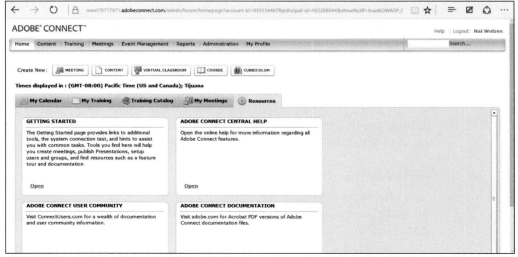

Collaboration software (groupware) can help team members stay connected.

users to schedule meetings at times when others are free. Both email and instant messaging (IM) functions are used, providing real-time communication among team members wherever they are in the world. SharePoint allows direct editing of documents through Word, Excel, or PowerPoint and also provides controlled access to shared documents via the web.

Gaming Computer games have come a long way since the Solitaire program included in the first versions of Windows. Today's games contain high-quality 3D animations, sound, and action that are very realistic. Role playing, action, sports, and fantasy games are just a small part of a fast-growing industry. You can even play games over the Internet with people in other cities and countries.

Some games, especially those that include realistic simulations, require a lot of computing power. You will need a fast CPU, plenty of RAM, and a dedicated video card for the best performance.

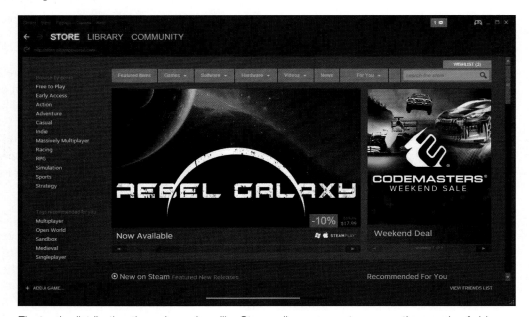

Electronic distribution through services like Steam allow gamers to access thousands of video games that can be downloaded and installed on their computers.

Open Source Open source software is the general term for applications that are provided completely free of charge, with no license fees or restrictions and no copyrights to worry about. You can download the software, copy it, and give it to your friends. The programming source code is also provided without charge and anyone is allowed to modify and improve it. Linux is a popular open source operating system. For further details about open source software, go to www.opensource.org.

OpenOffice is a suite of applications that is considered open source and includes a word processor, a spreadsheet program, a presentation application, a drawing application, and a database manager. These applications can save and open data files from Microsoft Office, and they provide many of the same capabilities as the equivalent retail products. OpenOffice can be downloaded for free from www.openoffice.org.

Networks

Computer networks are created when people want to share something such as a printer, an Internet connection, specific information within the confines of their business, or the wide and abundant variety of information found on the web. Networks allow computers to communicate and to share these resources.

Local Area Networks

The Local Area Network (LAN) illustrated in Figure 4 consists of several computers that are physically connected to one another via a central hub called a switch. The network also includes a server (a computer that manages the network) and a shared printer. Most LANs are not stand-alone systems; they connect to the Internet as well, so users can take advantage of online resources such as the web and email.

Wide Area Networks

A company might have several LANs, each in a different location or branch office, and these LANs can be connected to one another to form Wide Area Networks (WANs), as shown in Figure 5. The key difference between a LAN and a WAN is that in a WAN, the company does not own all the pathways between the computers. The data has to go out in "public" to reach its destination, whether that is via a leased optic line or the Internet. Leaving the protected local area carries security risks but also provides connectivity benefits.

Figure 4 Local Area Network

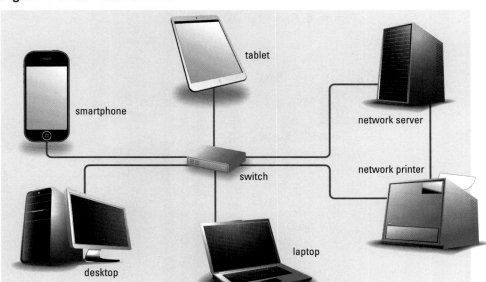

Figure 5 Wide Area Network

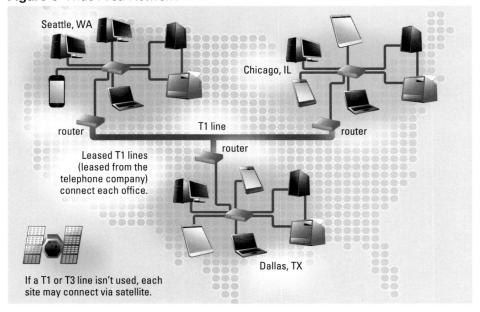

Large companies lease dedicated telephone lines (T1 or T3 lines) or satellite connections to connect their LANs. Many smaller companies find it more affordable to connect their branch offices via the existing Internet infrastructure.

Network Components

Computer networks require specialized hardware and software designed to share information and for other collaborative functions. The various components are explained in this section.

Clients Clients are the computer workstations where end users run the various applications necessary for them to do their jobs. In a client-server network, clients request information from the servers. Figure 6 shows an example of a client-server architecture. In this type of network structure, the networking paths allow a client computer to send information to a server, which can then relay the information back to that client computer or to another client on the same network. In this network, devices such as network hard drives and printers can be shared resources, available through their respective servers. In addition, the file server can provide access to a shared hard disk.

Figure 6 Client-Server Architecture

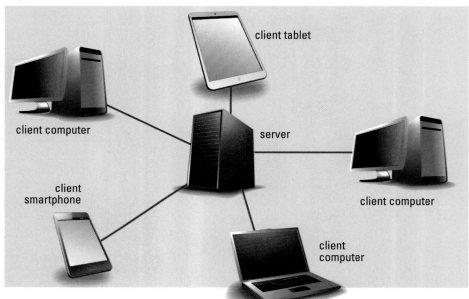

Servers Servers are data providers that are often larger and more powerful computers than clients. They house the network operating system software that organizes data sharing among the end users' PCs. They can hold large databases of information that users access to compile the reports that keep their organizations running smoothly. Servers might also be used as the storage location for everything every user creates, so that everyone else has easy access to it.

For small networks, the same computer can function as both client and server in a peer-to-peer network where all computers are equal and each one is both data requester and data provider (see Figure 7).

Figure 7 Peer-to-Peer Architecture

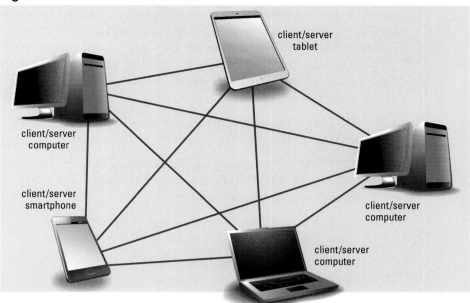

Switches and Routers Within a LAN, all the computers and other network-enabled devices (such as printers) must have a way of communicating with one another. Switches and routers serve as central hubs for that communication.

A switch is a box into which each computer connects via a cable. A switch that connects devices via radio frequency (RF) rather than via cables is called a wireless access point. A router is a more sophisticated version of a switch. A router can pass data from one LAN to another and throughout the Internet. Routers can be wired, wireless, or both.

Connectivity The PCs that make up a network have to be connected to each other in some way. The original method of connecting PCs used physical cables containing several strands of wire. The latest method is wireless and uses radio frequencies to carry data over short distances from a PC to a switch or router. All the devices are often located in the same room, but the signals are strong enough to penetrate the walls in homes and offices.

The most commonly used type of network cable is unshielded twisted pair cable (UTP). UTP cable is rated by category, and higher categories are needed for faster networks. Standard home networks use Cat 5 or Cat 5e cables; for business use, Cat 6 cable is the norm. Cat 7 and Cat 7a are the newest cable standards that provide up to 10 gigabits per second.

Wireless connections are used where cables are difficult to install or where the users are mobile or not close to a switch or router. Commonly called Wi-Fi, these connections are known by their technical 802.11 protocol specifications.

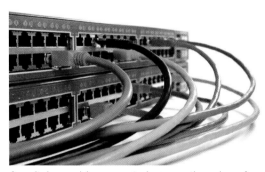

A switch provides a central connection place for cables from multiple computers.

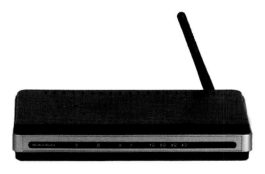

A router enables you to join two or more networks, or to join your LAN to the Internet.

Protocols A protocol is a generally accepted agreement on how to behave in a certain situation. For example, in many countries it is considered proper protocol to stand during the playing of the national anthem. Computer protocols are international agreements on how to manufacture hardware and software, and how to send data from one computer to another.

Now that wireless connectivity is becoming more common in the home computer market, more people are becoming aware of its associated technical labels. The following is a list of common protocols:

- 802.11ac is the current Wi-Fi standard. It has a maximum data rate of 1,300 Mbps and a range of about 70 meters indoors or 250 meters outdoors.

- 802.11n is the most common Wi-Fi standard; many 802.11n devices are still in use today. It has a maximum data rate of 450 Mbps and a range of about 70 meters indoors or 250 meters outdoors.

- 802.11g is an earlier Wi-Fi standard. It has a maximum data rate of 54 Mbps and a range of 38 meters indoors or 140 meters outdoors.

- 802.11b and 802.11a are now obsolete Wi-Fi standards, with maximum data rates of 54 Mbps and 11 Mbps, respectively.

- TCP/IP (Transmission Control Protocol/Internet Protocol) defines the rules for sending and receiving data between network devices. Each device has a unique IP address, which is a series of four numbers between 0 and 255, separated by periods, like this: 192.168.0.1.

- HTTP (HyperText Transfer Protocol) defines the rules for sending and receiving web pages (hypertext) on the Internet. For example, you might see http:// ParadigmCollege/myschool.edu on the uniform resource locator (URL) or Address line of your Internet browser. Figure 8 shows how data travels across the Internet.

Figure 8 Internet Infrastructure
Data moves across the Internet by traveling through a collection of physical devices.

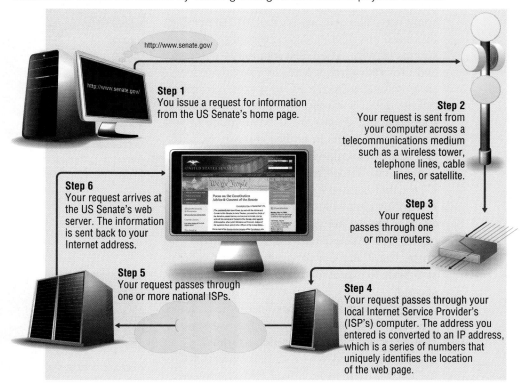

http://www.senate.gov/

Step 1
You issue a request for information from the US Senate's home page.

Step 2
Your request is sent from your computer across a telecommunications medium such as a wireless tower, telephone lines, cable lines, or satellite.

Step 3
Your request passes through one or more routers.

Step 4
Your request passes through your local Internet Service Provider's (ISP's) computer. The address you entered is converted to an IP address, which is a series of numbers that uniquely identifies the location of the web page.

Step 5
Your request passes through one or more national ISPs.

Step 6
Your request arrives at the US Senate's web server. The information is sent back to your Internet address.

- HTTPS (HyperText Transfer Protocol Secure Sockets) encrypts data before sending it over the web. You can see the letters *https* on the URL line when you reach a web page asking for your credit card number or when you are paying your bills online, such as https://emcp/mybank.com/myaccount.

- POP3 is the current version of Post Office Protocol for receiving email. POP is a store-and-forward system in which your email waits on the mail server until you pick it up via an email application such as Outlook; then it forwards it to that application.

- SMTP (Simple Mail Transfer Protocol) enables you to send email. The message is transferred to the recipient's mail server on the Internet, where it waits for the user to pick it up via his or her email application.

- FTP (File Transfer Protocol) provides an efficient, fast way to transfer files between computers. It is commonly used for files that are too large for email attachments and for large repositories of files.

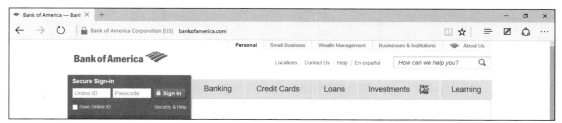

HTTPS is a protocol that protects your personal data. Note the padlock at the left side of the Address bar and the website name in green at the top of the screen.

Connectors and Ports Wired network connections commonly use RJ-45 connectors. These are similar to telephone connectors (which are RJ-11 or RJ-14) but they use eight wires instead of the usual 2 or 4. An RJ-45 connector is slightly wider than its telephone counterpart.

Exploring Technology 5

If you have Windows 10, display the Start menu, type **network**, and then click *View network connections* in the list that appears. A list of the computers and other devices in your LAN appears. Open the Network and Sharing Center and explore the icons and links there to learn more about your network. What protocols are installed? What is your connection speed?

Exploring Technology 6

Ask your instructor if your school has wireless connectivity. If yes, find out where wireless is active and then go to that area to see if you can locate the wireless access point(s) (antennas) that are installed. For example, if the school cafeteria has wireless connectivity, you may be able to see the hardware that provides the access to the Internet mounted on the ceiling or walls.

The Internet

The Internet is a global network of computers that allows data of all types and formats to be passed freely from one computer to another (see Figure 9). The web, email, and FTP are different parts of the Internet.

Figure 9 The Internet Network

Communications systems include computer hardware and communications software that allow computer users to exchange data around the house or around the world.

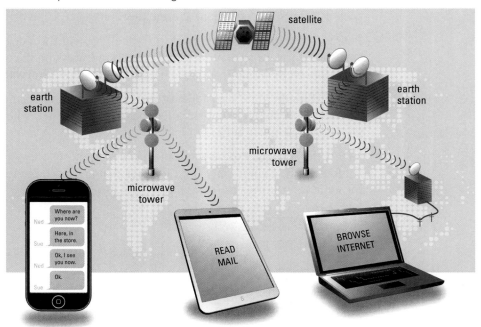

World Wide Web

The World Wide Web is a collection of hypertext files containing graphics, audio, and video that can be accessed on the Internet. The web is only a part of the Internet, albeit a very large part.

Electronic Mail

Electronic mail (email) uses its own protocols (such as SMTP and POP3) to route a message between computers on the Internet and hold it at a destination mail server until the recipient picks it up.

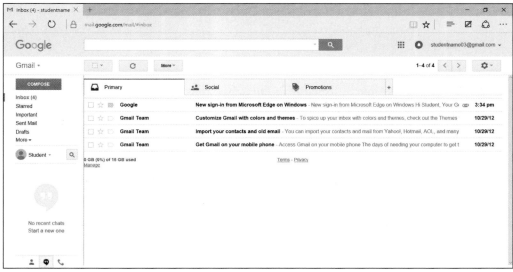

Google's Gmail is a popular web-based email application.

File Transfer Protocol

Like email and the web, File Transfer Protocol (FTP) is an information workspace on the Internet. It was originally used for exchanging data between incompatible mainframe systems, such as those made by IBM and those made by UNIVAC, but is now used to transfer files. A FTP server can be accessed through a web browser or a dedicated FTP application such as FileZilla.

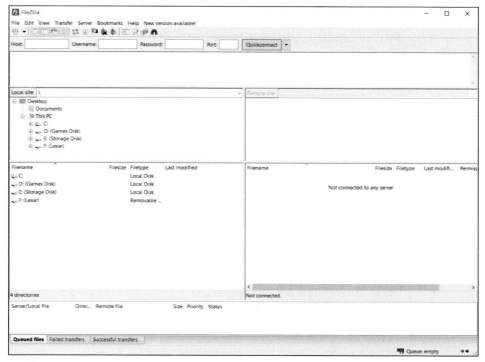

FileZilla is a commonly used application for transferring files through an FTP site.

Web 2.0

When the World Wide Web became popular in the mid 90's, content hosted on websites was relatively static and created by publishers. Users didn't have much of a chance to interact and be active members in creating and managing the content. Websites were only updated when the content creators felt the need to do so.

As the infrastruture of the Internet grew and became more capable of delivering users more bandwidth and speed, the way users interacted with the World Wide Web changed. Websites began allowing users to interact more and add content to websites. For example, the video-sharing website YouTube relies entirely upon users uploading videos and providing feedback in the form of comments. A service such as YouTube would have not been viable in the past because of the bandwidth requirements for watching a video on the Internet. A few key elements of Web 2.0 are mass user participation, user created and shared content, social connectivity, and web-integrated applications.

Social Networking With the advent of Web 2.0, social networking websites became very popular. Facebook and MySpace were the pioneers of social networking, which consists of users creating and maintaining a profile with which other users can view and interact. When Facebook and MySpace were first introduced, they had very limited features that expanded over time. MySpace's popularity waned as Facebook became an

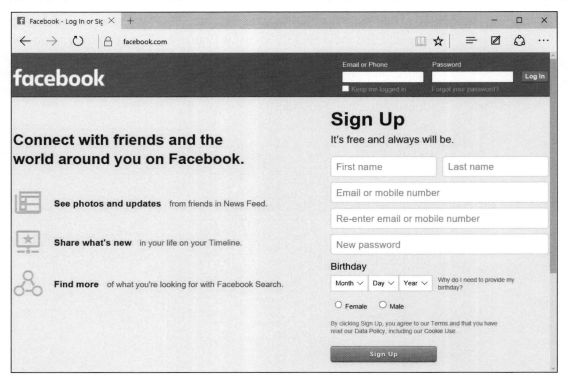

Facebook is currently the most commonly used social networking website.

easier-to-use, more streamlined platform. Facebook allows users to interact with their friends and families by sharing pictures, videos, stories, hyperlinks, event information and so on.

Currently, the most widely used social networking sites are Facebook, Twitter, and LinkedIn. Other social networking sites tend to be based on certain interests. For example, Pinterest is a social networking website that allows users to share ideas through media, primarily pictures. Users can go on Pinterest and find an activity or craft another user has "pinned" on his or her profile.

Media Sharing Increased bandwidth and user interaction led to websites being designed to provide users a place to share media such as pictures, music, and videos. These websites generate money by providing users a platform to share their media and then placing advertisements on the website. Imgur, Tumblr, SoundCloud, and YouTube are all examples of media-sharing websites. While these websites allow you to upload media, you must be the rightful owner of the media in order to share it online. Websites like YouTube will take down any content that contains copyrighted materials.

Since so much user-created media is available on the Internet, finding specific content can be difficult. Fortunately, there are websites dedicated to providing you with links and information to find content. For example, the website Reddit allows users to post links to pictures, videos, music, articles, and so on in an online bulletin board system. Once a link to content has been posted on Reddit, every user can either "up vote" or "down vote" the post. This voting system allows users to control the content that other users may or may not see.

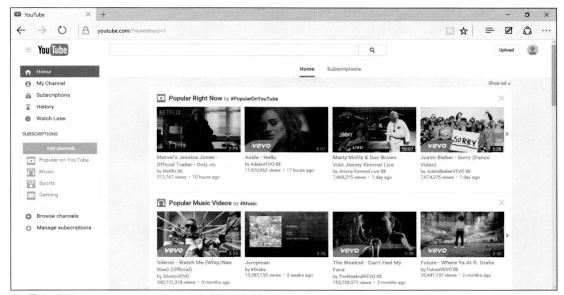

YouTube is the most commonly used video-sharing website.

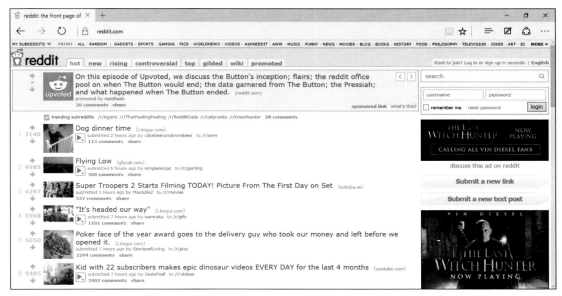

Reddit is a website where users post links to content and other users can vote on it.

Security Issues

Malware is a term describing computer programs that have malicious intent. Viruses, spyware, ransomware, worms, and adware programs all fall into this category.

Viruses

A computer virus is a string of code written to hurt others by damaging or destroying their computer files or making their computer experience difficult. Viruses are stored in executable (program) files; when the program runs, the virus code executes, causing damage and copying the virus into the computer's memory, where it infects other programs (see Figure 10). A virus is typically spread via an email attachment. Some viruses send themselves out via automatically generated emails to everyone in your address book.

Figure 10 How a Virus Attacks
When you forward an email with an attachment such as a picture, you may be spreading a damaging virus.

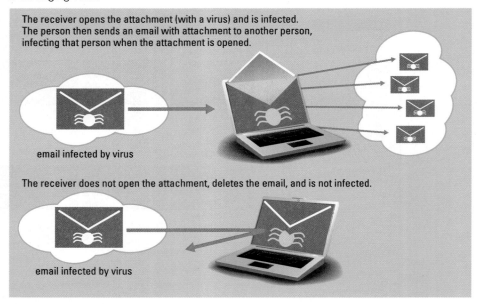

The receiver opens the attachment (with a virus) and is infected. The person then sends an email with attachment to another person, infecting that person when the attachment is opened.

email infected by virus

The receiver does not open the attachment, deletes the email, and is not infected.

email infected by virus

Spyware

Spyware tracks your activity as you surf the Internet and reports it to companies that want to sell you their products—or steal your identity. Spyware takes advantage of cookies, the small files that websites put on your computer to remember who you are on your next visit.

Ransomware

Ransomware is malicious code that takes control of either your computer or files on your computer and restricts access to them until a ransom is paid to the attacker.

Worms

A worm is a self-replicating computer program that distributes itself via a network, as shown in Figure 11. Unlike a virus, it does not necessarily attach itself to another file. Worms are usually designed to damage a network, in many cases by simply clogging up the network's bandwidth and slowing its performance.

Figure 11 How a Worm Attacks
A worm reproduces itself and attacks all the computers on a network.

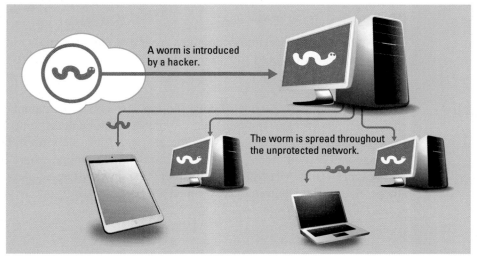

A worm is introduced by a hacker.

The worm is spread throughout the unprotected network.

Figure 12 How a Trojan Attacks
A Trojan pretends to be a useful program but instead opens your system to hackers.

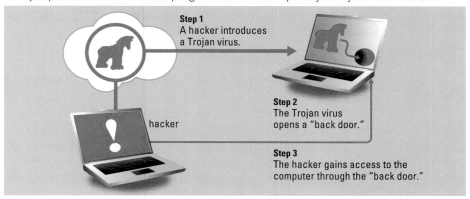

Trojan

Named after the infamous Trojan horse of the Greek legend, a Trojan is malware that masquerades as a useful program. When you run the program, you let the Trojan into your system (see Figure 12). Trojans open a "back door" to your system for malicious hackers.

Adware

Adware looks at files on your computer and then sends pop-up advertisements that try to sell you products and services. Although annoying, adware is not usually destructive, but it can slow down your processor and Internet speed significantly.

Privacy Threats and Information Theft

Spyware programs can steal your personal information and tell it or sell it to other people who might be able to impersonate you and take money from your bank account or charge large purchases to your credit card.

Phishing is a method of convincing people to reveal their passwords, credit card numbers, social security numbers, and other private or confidential information. Phishers pretend to

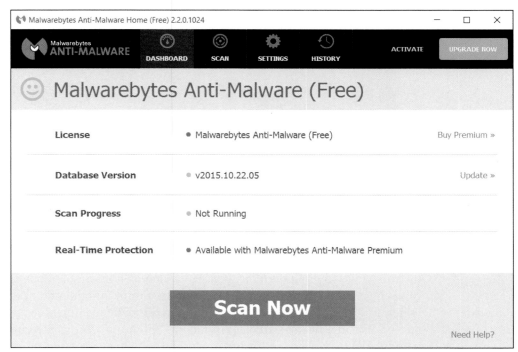

Products such as Malwarebytes scan your computer for malware and help prevent it from downloading in the first place.

be representatives of the victim's bank or a government agency by sending official-looking emails with obscure links back to websites that look exactly like the real website. The information they gather is then used in schemes involving identity theft that allow them to gain access to the victim's bank account, which they empty of its funds.

Protection Software

Several computer programs are available to protect against virus attacks and the installation of spyware or adware on your computer. Some examples of anti-virus applications are McAfee VirusScan and BitDefender AntiVirus. Spybot Search & Destroy, SpySweeper, AdAware, and Spyware Detector are used for spyware and adware. Windows 10 and Windows 8.1 include an anti-spyware program called Windows Defender.

To minimize infection, always update your computer with the latest security patches as they become available. Keep your protection software up to date by downloading the latest "signature" files of known viruses.

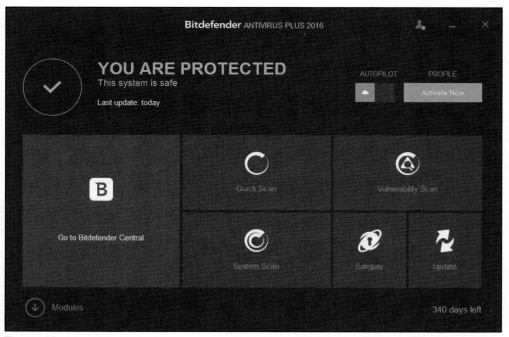

The installation of an antivirus software program such as Bitdefender AntiVirus Plus is essential for computers connected to the Internet. Keeping these virus definitions up to date will significantly help in the fight against viruses.

Email Etiquette and Computer Ethics

Two types of rules govern and guide behavior: etiquette and ethics. Etiquette refers to the rules that govern courteous behavior, such as holding the door open for someone, or saying "please" and "thank you." We often think of etiquette in terms of knowing which fork to use in a fancy restaurant, but etiquette also involves the rules for language appropriate in a businesslike environment. "Fighting words" are embarrassing to some people, and they can also lead to anger and violence. Showing proper etiquette is a way of showing a person respect. If you show disrespect to someone, that is not proper etiquette.

When applied to computer communication, improper etiquette can result in serious misunderstandings or ill will among coworkers. It can even lead to the loss of a lucrative business contract or even a job.

Ethics are the moral principles that govern behavior. In the news, we often see reports about corporate executives who have been charged or convicted of funneling company money into their own personal bank accounts. Politicians are accused of taking bribes from lobbyists in return for a favorable vote on a piece of legislation that will be profitable for the lobbyist's organization. Taxpayers claim tax deductions they are not entitled to. Students submit reports that were written by someone else. People offer to copy the latest music CD or software program they just purchased and give it to their friends. Where do you stand on these ethical issues?

Both etiquette and ethics have direct application to computers, especially in relation to email and copyright issues.

Email Etiquette

Everyone—friends, relatives, schoolmates, coworkers, employers, teachers, businesses, government officials, and sales and marketing departments—is sending email these days. Speedy communication with other people all over the world can be fun, exciting, and productive. However, it can also cause problems. What you write in an email message can hurt someone's feelings, be misinterpreted, or be accidentally sent to the wrong person. You can cause yourself embarrassment or even get yourself fired.

Here are 10 rules of email etiquette. You might want to add a few of your own.

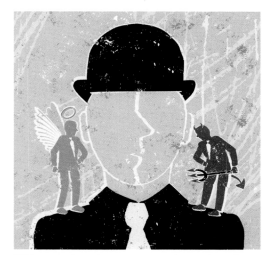

Ethics are the rules we use to determine what is right and wrong, and these rules help guide our choices and actions, both in our personal and business lives.

1. Be brief and to the point. Emails are supposed to be a fast way to communicate. Don't slow down the process.
2. Don't use ALL CAPITAL letters. It looks and feels like you're shouting or angry.
3. Remember to attach the attachment. Mentioning what you are "attaching" in any type of email is a good idea. Get in the habit of stopping as soon as you type the phrase "I am attaching…" and immediately clicking the button for attaching the file.
4. Use spell check (even if you're a great speller). Using the spelling check feature only takes a few seconds and it shows that you care about quality. But watch out! It is easy to click "Change" instead of "Ignore" and change a person's name to a common word and that, whether humorous or not, is an embarrassing mistake.
5. Reread what you wrote from the perspective of the receiver. Ask yourself how the recipient is likely to interpret your words. Did you leave out or misspell a word that completely changes the meaning?
6. Double-check the address in the *To* box. Confirm that you clicked the correct name in your address list. Once you click the Send button, there is *no* way to stop the message or undo an address mistake.
7. Watch your language. Profanity can come back to haunt you.
8. Assume your email will be read by *lots* of other people. Emails are often forwarded so others can take action or to inform a supervisor. Avoid cute or friendly asides and comments that you only want a close friend to see.

9. Always put something in the *Subject* line. A well-written subject will help the receiver decide where to file your message and whether to read it now or wait until later.

10. Privacy does not exist in emails, especially those in a corporate environment. The email administrator can potentially see the contents of any email. Company policy may allow checking emails to ensure that no company secrets are exposed, or to stop harassing or abusive email.

Software Piracy and Copyright Infringement

When you install a software application, you must accept the license agreement that describes the legal contract between the user (you) and the software developer. If you do not accept the agreement, the installation process will stop. By accepting the agreement, you agree to everything it says. The contract often covers the number of people who may use the program at the same time. That would usually be one person, but organizations can purchase agreements that cover a specific number of users.

Most software is copyrighted, with the exception of open source software, mentioned earlier. Copyright laws in the United States and most (but not all) other countries state that authors, music composers, TV show and movie creators, artists, and publishers own the works they create and distribute and that no one is allowed to use or copy their work without specific permission. Software license agreements might specify that you can make one backup copy, but you cannot give that copy to a friend. The same rules apply to all copyrighted material including music CDs, DVDs, and songs available on the web. Infringing on a copyright is illegal, and this law is enforced.

Warning: This computer program is protected by copyright law and international treaties. Unauthorized reproduction or distribution of this program, or any portion of it, may result in severe civil and criminal penalties, and will be prosecuted to the maximum extent possible under the law.

OK

Software manufacturers usually obtain a copyright that prohibits the illegal copying and distribution of software. Warnings such as this one are designed to remind users of the copyright law.

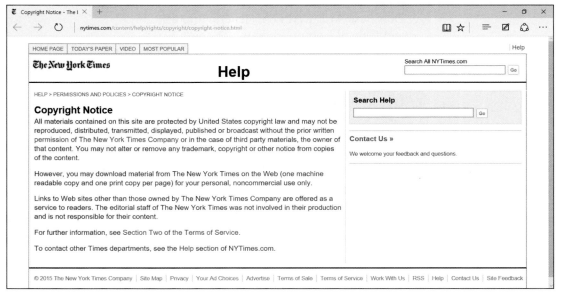

The copyright notice on *The New York Times* web page reminds visitors that the content of the site is copyrighted.

Formerly known as the Software Publishers Association, the Software & Information Industry Association (SIIA, www.siia.net) encourages people who witness software piracy to inform them so that they can investigate the situation. Once they gather enough evidence, they will contact the organization's executives, ask them to prove they have enough licenses, and encourage them to purchase the software legally. In most cases the pressure works, but if necessary, the SIIA may take legal action.

Software piracy is a felony, but even if it were not, other compelling reasons exist for why you should not copy programs, music, or DVDs. For one, doing so hurts the people who spend a lot of time and money creating products for your enjoyment. They do research. They buy computers, musical instruments, or video cameras. They pay money for studio time to record their songs, and then more money to advertise them and ship them to music stores. They may sell their creations to publishing companies who agree to pay them royalties based on sales. Will you send money to your favorite band every time you give a friend a copy of their latest CD? If graphic artists and musicians can't pay their expenses and cover the cost of making the songs, movies, computer games, and other software you enjoy, how can an individual artist, or even a large company, continue to create more?

Exploring Technology 8

Check to see who is the registered user of each of the applications on your computer by running it and watching for the name on the startup screen. If it isn't registered to your organization, your department, or yourself, ask a supervisor why not. Your action could actually help save your organization from costly litigation and potential fines.

Exploring Technology 9

Navigate to www.riaa.com and click the Report Piracy tab. Read about what you can do to help stop software piracy.

Exploring Technology 10

Use your word processor to write the explanation you will use when you decline to give or receive an unauthorized copy of a music CD, software program, DVD, or any other copyrighted material.

Glossary

802.11 protocol a protocol for wireless LAN technology that specifies an over-the-air interface between the wireless client device and a server, or between two wireless devices, approved by the IEEE in 1997; also called *Wi-Fi*

802.11ac protocol approved in January 2014, this protocol for wireless LAN technology is built on 802.11n but has approximately three times the transfer rate

802.11g protocol approved in June 2003, this protocol for wireless LAN technology operates in the same frequency range as 802.11b but with transfer rates similar to 802.11a

802.11n protocol this protocol for wireless LAN technology provides for speeds of up to 150 Mbps at a range of up to 250 meters (820 feet)

adware software that tracks the websites that a user visits to collect information for marketing or advertising

bar code reader an electronic device that uses photo technology to read the lines in a bar code; the lines and spaces contain symbols that the computer translates into information

cathode ray tube (CRT) monitor a large, sealed glass tube housed in a plastic case; used with older desktop computers

central processing unit (CPU) the part of a computer that interprets and carries out instructions that operate the computer and manage the computer's devices and resources; consists of components, each of which performs specific functions; also called the *microprocessor* or *processor*

client a smaller computer, terminal, or workstation capable of sending data to and from a larger computer (host computer) in a network

client-server architecture a type of network architecture in which a personal computer, workstation, or terminal (called a *client*) is used to send information or a request to another computer (called a *server*) that then relays the information back to the user's client computer or to another computer (another client)

collaboration software programs that enable people at separate computer workstations to collaborate on a single document or project; also called *groupware*

compact disc (CD) a plastic disc 4.75 inches in diameter and about 1/20th of an inch thick; uses laser technologies to store information and data

connectivity refers to the ability to link with other programs and devices

copyright the legal protection of an individual's or business's original work, such as software applications, music, and books, that prohibits others from duplicating or illegally using such work or products; an artist or author whose work is copyrighted has the right to charge others for its use

database a computer application in which data is organized and stored in a way that allows for specific data to be accessed, retrieved, and used

digital camera a type of camera that records and stores images, including people, scenery, documents, and products, in a digitized form that can be entered into and stored by a computer

digital versatile disc (DVD) an extremely high-capacity optical disc; also called a *digital video disc (DVD)*

digitizing the process of converting analog information to digital information; sometimes referred to as "going digital"

digitizing pen an electronic pen device, resembling a standard writing pen, used with a drawing tablet to simulate drawing on paper

drawing tablet a tablet with wires under the surface that, when used with a digitizing pen, allows the user to create and capture drawings that can be entered and stored on a computer

dual-core processor a central processing unit (CPU) chip that contains two complete processors along with their cache memory

electronic mail (email) a text, voice, or video message sent or received remotely or over a computer network, or the system by which such a message is sent

ethics rules used to determine the right and wrong things to do

etiquette rules governing courteous behavior

File Transfer Protocol (FTP) a transmission standard that enables a user to send and receive large files, such as reports, over the Internet

flash drive storage device with a USB connector

gigabyte unit of memory equal to 1,073,741,824 bytes

graphical user interface (GUI) a computer interface that enables a user to control the computer and launch commands by pointing and clicking at graphical objects such as windows, icons, and menu items

graphics computer-generated pictures produced on a computer screen, paper, or film, ranging from a simple line or bar chart to a detailed, colorful image or picture; also called *graphical images*

graphics tablet a flat tablet used with a pen-like stylus or a crosshair cursor to capture an image; the user grasps a stylus or crosshair cursor and traces an image or drawing placed on the tablet surface

hard copy a permanent, tangible version of output, such as a letter printed on paper

hard drive a device for reading and writing to the magnetic storage medium known as a hard disk; consists of one or more rigid metal platters (disks) mounted on a metal shaft in a container that contains an access mechanism

Hypertext Transfer Protocol (HTTP) the communications standard used to transfer documents on the World Wide Web

information processing cycle a cycle during which a computer enters, processes, outputs, and/or stores information

ink-jet printer a nonimpact printer that forms images by spraying thousands of tiny droplets of electrically charged ink onto a page; the printed images are in dot-matrix format, but of a higher quality than images printed by dot-matrix printers

input data that is entered into a computer or other device, or the act of capturing such data

input device any hardware component that enables a computer user to enter data and programs into a computer system; keyboards, point-and-click devices, and scanners are among the more popular input devices, and a desktop or laptop computer system may include one or more input devices

Internet a worldwide network of computers linked together via communications software and media for the purpose of sharing information; the largest and best-known network in the world; also called *the Net*

Internet service provider (ISP) an organization that has a permanent connection to the Internet and provides temporary access to individuals and others for free or for a fee

joystick an input device (named after the control lever used to fly fighter planes) consisting of a small box with a vertical lever that, when pushed in a certain direction, moves the cursor correspondingly on the screen; often used for computer games

keyboard an electronically controlled hardware component used to enter alphanumeric data (letters, numbers, and special characters)

laser printer a nonimpact printer that produces output of exceptional quality using a technology similar to that of photocopy machines

light emitting diode (LED) a small light that is used in an LCD to improve color and image appearance

liquid crystal display (LCD) a display device in which liquid crystals are sandwiched between two sheets of material

local area network (LAN) a computer network physically confined to a relatively small geographical area, such as a single building or a college campus

malware malicious software

megabyte a unit of memory that stores approximately 1 million bytes

memory a chip-based data storage system in which each bit of data is represented by a binary on/off state; a series of 1s and 0s

monitor the screen, or display device, on which computer output appears

motherboard the main circuit board inside a personal computer to which other circuit boards can be connected; contains electrical pathways, called *traces*, etched onto it that allow data to move from one component to another

mouse an input device that, when moved about on a flat surface, causes a pointer on the screen to move in the same direction

multitasking the ability of an operating system to run more than one software program at a time; the use of different areas in Windows RAM makes this possible

network a group of two or more computers, software, and other devices that is connected by one or more communications media

nonvolatile storage that retains its data even when there is no power being supplied to it; a hard disk and a flash drive are both nonvolatile

open-source software software whose programming code is owned by the original developer but made available for free to the general public, who is encouraged to experiment with the software, make improvements, and share the improvements with the user community

operating system (OS) a type of software that creates a user interface and supports the workings of computer devices and software programs that perform specific jobs

output information that is written or displayed as a result of computer processing; also the act of writing or displaying such data

peer-to-peer architecture a network design in which each computer or workstation comprising the network has equivalent capabilities and responsibilities

personal information manager (PIM) software software that helps users organize contact information, appointments, tasks, and notes

phishing an activity characterized by attempts to fraudulently acquire another person's sensitive information, such as a credit card number

Photo-editing software an application that allows users to create and modify images and output them in one of the various image file formats.

port a plug-in slot on a computer to which you can connect a device, such as a printer or, in the case of accessing the Internet, a telephone line; also called an *interface*

Post Office Protocol (POP) server a special type of server that holds email messages until they are accessed and read by their recipients

presentation software an application that allows a user to create a presentation of slides

printer the most common type of hard-copy output device that produces output in a permanent form

processing the manipulation of data by the computer's electrical circuits

processor the part of a computer that interprets and carries out instructions that operate the computer and manages the computer's devices and resources; consists of components, each of which performs specific functions; also called the *central processing unit (CPU)*

protocol a set of rules and procedures for exchanging information between network devices and computers

quad-core processor a CPU that contains four complete processors in a single chip

random access memory (RAM) a computer chip or group of chips containing the temporary, or volatile, memory in which programs and data are stored while being used by a computer

read-only memory (ROM) a computer chip on the motherboard of a computer containing permanent, or nonvolatile, memory that stores instructions

router a hardware device that connects two or more networks

scanner a light-sensing electronic device that can read and capture printed text and images, such as photographs and drawings, and convert them into a digital form a computer can understand; once scanned, the text or image can be displayed on the screen, edited, printed, stored on a disk, inserted into another document, or sent as an attachment to an email message; also called an *optical scanner*

server a computer and its associated storage devices that users access remotely over a network

Simple Mail Transfer Protocol (SMTP) a communications protocol installed on the ISP's or online service's mail server that determines how each message is to be routed through the Internet and then sends the message

soft copy a temporary version of output, typically the display of data on a computer screen

software programs containing instructions that direct the operation of the computer system and the written documentation that explains how to use the programs; types include system software and application software

software piracy the act of copying or using a piece of software without the legal right to do so

software suite a combination of application programs (usually integrated) bundled as a single package; may contain applications such as word processing, spreadsheet, database, and other programs

spreadsheet software a productivity program that provides a user with a means of organizing, calculating, and presenting financial, statistical, and other numeric information; used to manipulate numbers electronically instead of using a pencil and paper

spyware software that tracks the activity of Internet users for the benefit of a third party

stylus a sharp, pointed instrument used for writing or marking on a graphics tablet or other device

switch a small hardware device that joins multiple computers together within one local area network (LAN)

T1 line a high-speed telephone line that allows for both voice and data transmission and can carry data at a speed of 1.544 megabits per second

touchpad an input device that enables a user to enter data and make selections by moving a finger across the pad; also called a *track pad*

touchscreen an input device that allows the user to choose options by pressing a finger (or fingers) on the appropriate part of the screen

Transmission Control Protocol/Internet Protocol (TCP/IP) protocol that governs how packets are constructed and sent over the Internet to their destination

Universal Product Code (UPC) a type of code printed on products and packages consisting of lines and spaces that a computer translates into a number; the computer then uses this number to find information about the product or package, such as its name and price, in a computerized database

Universal Serial Bus (USB) port a type of port that is widely used for connecting high-speed modems, scanners, and digital cameras to a computer; a single USB port can accommodate several peripheral devices connected together in sequence

video-editing software software that allows users to edit sound and video and output it in various digital formats

virus a program that is designed to harm computer systems and/or any users, typically sent via email

volatile storage that loses its data when power is lost; the RAM on a motherboard is volatile, for example

webcam a digital video camera that captures real-time video for transmission to others via a web server or an instant messaging tool

wide area network (WAN) a network that spans a large geographical area

Windows a Microsoft-developed GUI operating system for personal computers

word processing software a type of computer application that allows the user to create, edit, manipulate, format, store, and print a variety of documents, including letters, memos, announcements, and brochures

World Wide Web (www) a global system of linked computer networks that allows users to jump from one site to another by way of programmed links on web pages; also called *the web*

worm a program that actively transmits copies of itself over the Internet, using up resources and causing other problems; also called a *software worm*

Workbook

The *Workbook* ebook includes study tools and an assessment activity. These resources are designed to help you further develop and demonstrate mastery of the concepts learned in this section.

Getting Started

Adjusting Monitor Settings, Copying Data Files, and Changing View Options

Skills

- Set monitor resolution
- Modify DPI settings
- Copy files from OneDrive
- Copy files from a network location
- Change view options
- Display file extensions

The Microsoft Office product line has evolved over time, becoming available on Apple computers, tablets, phones, and through the Internet. This textbook and the accompanying ebook were written using a typical personal computer (tower/box, monitor, keyboard and mouse) or laptop. While you may be able to perform some of the activities in this textbook on a different operating system or tablet, not all of the steps will work as written and may jeopardize any work you may be required to turn in to your instructor. If you do not have access to a compatible computer, explore what options you have at your institution such as where and when you can use a computer lab.

One of the evolutions of the Microsoft Office product is that it is now offered in a subscription-based plan called Microsoft Office 365. An advantage of having a Microsoft Office 365 subscription is that it includes and incorporates new features or versions as they are released, as long as your subscription is active. For example, when Microsoft released Office 2016, any Office 365 users with the Office 2013 version were automatically upgraded. This new direction Microsoft is taking may impact section activities and assessments. For example, new features and tweaks may alter how some of the steps are completed. The ebook will contain the most up-to-date material and will be updated as new features become available.

In Activity 1 you will customize your monitor settings so that what you see on the screen matches the images in this textbook. In Activity 2 you will obtain the data files you will be using throughout this textbook from OneDrive. Activity 3 includes instructions on how to change the view settings so that your view of files in a File Explorer window matches the images in this textbook.

Before beginning projects in this textbook, you may need to customize your monitor's settings and turn on the display of file extensions. Projects in the sections in this textbook assume that the monitor display is set at 1920 × 1080 pixels, the DPI is set at 125%, and that the display of file extensions is turned on. Adjusting a monitor's display settings is important because the ribbon in the Microsoft Office applications adjusts to the screen resolution setting of your computer monitor. A monitor set at a high resolution will have the ability to show more buttons in the ribbon than a monitor set to a low resolution. The illustrations in this textbook were created with a screen resolution display set at 1920 × 1080 pixels. In Figure GS1 at the bottom of the page, the Word ribbon is shown two ways: at a lower screen resolution (1600 × 900 pixels) and at the screen resolution featured throughout this textbook. Note the variances in the ribbon in both examples.

What You Will Do   Adjust the monitor settings for your machine to match the settings used to create the images in the textbook. If using a lab computer, check with your instructor before attempting this activity.

1 Right-click a blank area of the desktop and then click the *Display settings* option at the shortcut menu.

2 At the Settings window with the *Display* option selected, scroll down and click the <u>Advanced display settings</u> hyperlink.

3 Scroll down and look at the current setting displayed in the *Resolution* option box. For example, your screen may be currently set at 1600 × 900. If your screen is already set to 1920 × 1080, skip ahead to Step 7.

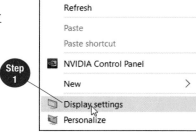

> Screen resolution is set in pixels. Pixel is the abbreviation of picture element and refers to a single dot or point on the display monitor. Changing the screen resolution to a higher number of pixels means that more information can be seen on the screen as items are scaled to a smaller size.

Figure GS1 Word Ribbon with Two Screen Resolutions

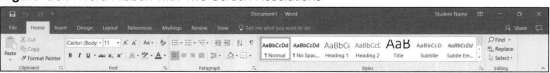
1600 x 900 Screen Resolution

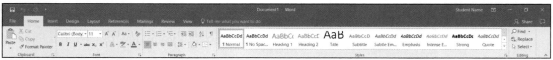
1920 x 1080 Screen Resolution

4 Click the *Resolution* option box and then click the 1920 × 1080 option. If necessary, check with your instructor for alternate instructions. ***Note: Depending on the privileges you are given on a school machine, you may not be able to complete these steps.***

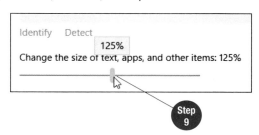

Resolution

1920 × 1080 (Recommended)
1680 × 1050
1600 × 900
1440 × 900
1280 × 1024
1280 × 960
1280 × 800
1280 × 768
1280 × 720

Step 4

> If the machine you are using has more than one monitor, make sure the proper monitor is selected. (The active monitor displays as a blue rectangle.)

5 Click the Apply button.

6 Click the Keep changes button at the message box asking if you want to keep the display settings.

> Some monitor settings will render the computer unusable because objects on the desktop or in a window will become inaccessible and hidden. In this case, Windows will automatically revert the settings to the previous configuration after 30 seconds.

7 Click the Back button.

8 At the Settings window with the *Display* option active, look at the percentage in which the size of text, apps, and other items currently display (also known as the DPI setting). For example, items on your screen may display at 100%. If the percentage is 125%, skip to Step 12.

> As the resolution on monitors has increased, text, application windows, buttons, options, and so on start to appear smaller and smaller on the screen. To counter this, Windows allows you to increase the size of these objects by changing the DPI setting. The computers used to create the images in this textbook uses the 125% DPI setting, which slightly increases the size of text, applications, buttons, and options.

9 Click and hold down the left mouse button on the button on the slider bar below the text *Change the size of text, apps, and other items*, drag the slider button until *125%* displays, and then release the mouse button.

Identify   Detect
125%
Change the size of text, apps, and other items: 125%

Step 9

10 Click the Apply button.

11 At the message indicating that you must sign out of your computer, click the Sign out later button.

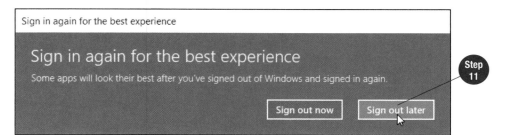

Sign in again for the best experience

Sign in again for the best experience
Some apps will look their best after you've signed out of Windows and signed in again.

Sign out now   Sign out later

Step 11

12 Click the Close button.

While working through the activities in this book, you will often be using data files as starting points. These files need to be obtained from OneDrive or other locations such as your school's network drive. All of the files required to complete the bookwork are provided through OneDrive, which you can access through links in the textbook's ebook. Make sure you have Internet access before trying to retrieve the data files from OneDrive. Ask your instructor if alternate locations are available for retrieving the files, such as a network drive or online resource such as D2L, BlackBoard, or Canvas. Retrieving data files from an alternate location will require different steps, so check with your instructor for additional steps or tasks to complete.

What You Will Do   In order to complete the activities in this textbook, you will need to obtain the data files from OneDrive. Make sure you have access to OneDrive or an alternate location containing the files.

1 Insert your USB flash drive into an available USB port.

2 Navigate to this textbook's ebook. To access this textbook's ebook, launch your browser, go to http://paradigm.bookshelf.emcp.com, log in, click the textbook ebook thumbnail, and then click the Open Book to Last Page Viewed button. *Note: The steps in this activity assume you are using the Microsoft Edge browser. If you are using a different browser, the following steps may vary.*

3 Navigate to the ebook page that corresponds to this textbook page.

4 Click the Ancillary Links button in the Toolbar at the bottom of the window.

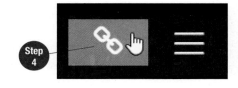

Data Files

5 At the Ancillary Links dialog box that appears, click the Data Files: All Files hyperlink.

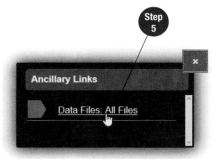

6 Click the Download hyperlink at the top of the window.

A zip file containing the student data files will automatically begin downloading from the OneDrive website.

7 Click the Open button in the message box saying that the DataFiles.zip has finished downloading.

8 Right-click the *ExcelMedS2* folder in the Content pane.

9 Click the *Copy* option at the shortcut menu.

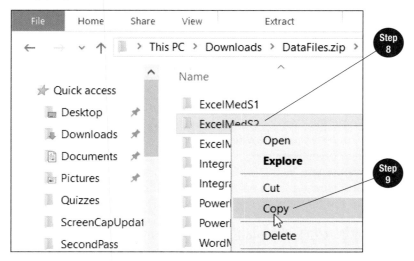

10 Click your USB flash drive that displays in the Navigation pane at the left side of the File Explorer window.

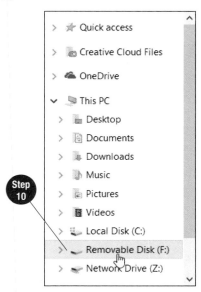

11 Click the Home tab and then click the Paste button in the Clipboard group.

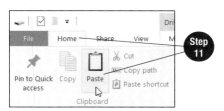

12 Close the File Explorer window by clicking the Close button in the upper right corner of the window.

Activity 3 Changing View Options

You can change the view of the File Explorer window to show the contents of your current location (drive or folder) in various formats, including icons, tiles, or a list, among others. With the Content pane in Details view, you can click the column headings to change how the contents are sorted and whether they are sorted in ascending or descending order. You can customize a window's environment by using buttons and options on the File Explorer View tab. You can also change how panes are displayed, how content is arranged in the Content pane, how content is sorted, and which features are hidden.

What You Will Do Before getting started with the textbook material, you need to adjust the view settings so that items in the File Explorer window appear the same as the images in the textbook.

1 Click the File Explorer button on the taskbar.

> By default, a File Explorer window opens at the Quick access location, which contains frequently-used folders such as Desktop, Documents, Downloads, Pictures and so on. It also displays recently used files at the bottom of the Content pane.

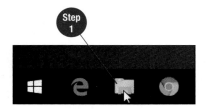

2 Click the drive letter representing your storage medium in the Navigation pane.

3 Double-click the *ExcelMedS2* folder in the Content pane.

4 Click the View tab below the Title bar.

5 Click the *Large icons* option in the Layout group.

> After you click an option on the View tab, the View tab collapses to provide more space in the File Explorer window.

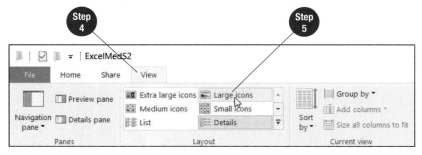

6 Click the View tab.

7 Click the *Details* option in the Layout group.

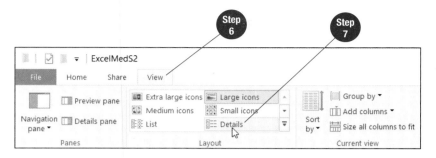

8 With files now displayed in Details view, click the *Name* column heading to sort the list in descending order by name.

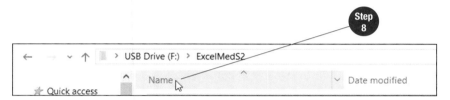

9 Click the *Name* column heading again to restore the list to ascending order by name.

10 Click the View tab and then click the *File name extensions* check box in the Show/hide group to insert a check mark. ***Note: If the check box appears with a check mark in it, then file extensions are already turned on—skip this step.***

> Inserting a check mark in a check box makes the option active. The files in the File Explorer window will now display any files with a file extension.

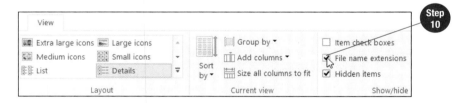

11 Close the File Explorer window by clicking the Close button in the upper right corner of the window.

In Addition

Changing the Default View for All Folders

You can set a view to display by default for all folders of a similar type (such as all disk drive folders or all documents folders). To do this, change the current view to the desired view for the type of folder that you want to set. Next, click the Options button on the View tab and then click the View tab at the Folder Options dialog box. Click the Apply to Folders button in the Folder views section and then click OK. Click Yes at the Folder Views message asking if you want all folders of this type to match this folder's view settings.

Using Word in the Medical Office

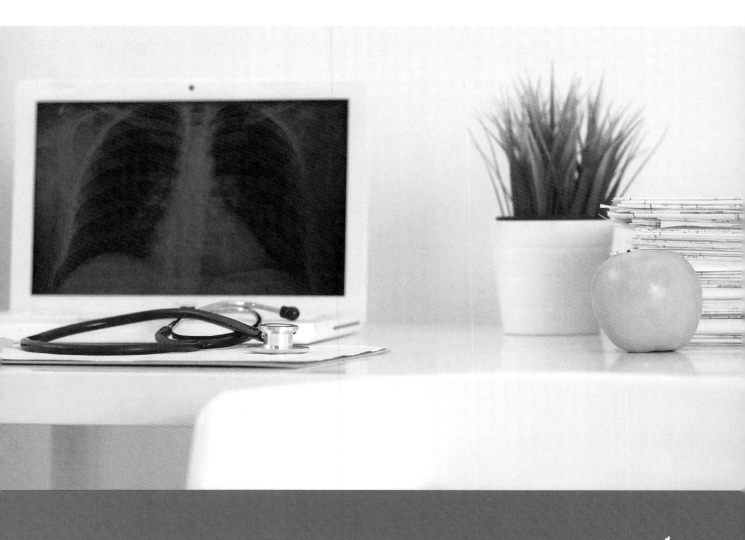

Introducing
Word 2016

Microsoft Word 2016 is a word processing program used to create documents such as memos, letters, medical reports, medical research papers, brochures, announcements, newsletters, envelopes, labels, and much more. Word provides a wide variety of editing and formatting features as well as sophisticated visual elements.

This unit on Microsoft Word 2016 in the medical office contains four sections that guide you in learning and applying the features of Word 2016. In Section 1, you will create and edit medical documents by inserting, replacing, and deleting text; checking the spelling and grammar in documents; using the AutoCorrect feature and Thesaurus; changing document views; creating documents using a template; and managing documents. Section 2 focuses on formatting characters and paragraphs and includes applying fonts, aligning text in paragraphs, indenting text, changing line and paragraph spacing, inserting bullets and numbers, inserting symbols, setting tabs, adding borders and shading, inserting quick parts, and applying styles and style sets. In Section 3, you will learn how to format and enhance documents by finding and replacing text; cutting, copying, and pasting text; using the Clipboard task pane; inserting page breaks and page numbers; changing margins and page orientation; inserting headers and footers, images, WordArt, and shapes in a document; and preparing envelopes and labels. In Section 4, you will learn how to merge main documents with data sources, sort and filter records, create and modify tables, and prepare and edit forms.

In each of the four Word sections, you will prepare medical documents for two clinics and a hospital as described below.

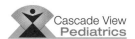

Cascade View Pediatrics is a full-service pediatric clinic that provides comprehensive primary pediatric care to infants, children, and adolescents.

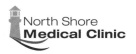

North Shore Medical Clinic is an internal medicine clinic dedicated to providing exceptional care to all patients. The physicians in the clinic specialize in a number of fields including internal medicine, family practice, cardiology, and dermatology.

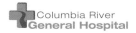

Columbia River General Hospital is an independent, not-for-profit hospital with the mission of providing high-quality, comprehensive care to patients and improving the health of the community.

Word

Creating and Editing a Document

Data Files Before beginning section work, copy the WordMedS1 folder to your storage medium and then make WordMedS1 the active folder.

Skills

- Create, save, and print a document
- Close a document and close Word
- Move the insertion point
- Insert and delete text
- Scroll in a document
- Select, replace, and delete text
- Use Undo and Redo
- Check the spelling and grammar in a document
- Use AutoCorrect
- Use the Thesaurus

- Change document views
- Hide and show white space
- Change the display percentage
- Navigate and find text using the Navigation pane
- Use the Tell Me and Help features
- Preview and print a document
- Create a document using a template
- Create, rename, and delete a folder
- Save a document in a different format

Precheck Check your current skills to help focus your study of the skills taught in this section.

Activities Overview

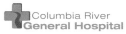

Edit and format a history and physical examination document, manage files, and edit and format a consultation report document.

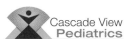

Prepare a memo regarding well-child checkups and edit and format a document containing information on scheduling appointments.

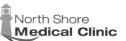

Prepare an x-ray report document, prepare a letter requesting interpreting services, edit and format a notice to employees regarding a diabetes presentation, research a medical spelling dictionary, prepare a letter to a doctor, and prepare a chart note.

Model Answers Preview the model answers for an overview of the activities you will complete in each section.

Creating, Saving, and Printing a Document

Microsoft Word is a word processing program you can use to create, save, edit, and print documents. To create a document in Word, open the Word program and then click the *Blank document* template. This opens a blank document with the insertion point positioned at the beginning of the document. The document screen contains a variety of features for working with a document, such as the Title bar, Quick Access Toolbar, ribbon, and Status bar. Type text in a document and press the Enter key, and the insertion point moves down to the next line with extra spacing above the line. If you want to create a new line without including the extra spacing, use the New Line command: Shift + Enter. When entering text, Word includes an AutoCorrect feature that will automatically correct certain words that are entered incorrectly. After creating a document, save the document so it is available for future use. Save a document at the Save As dialog box.

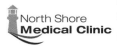

What You Will Do   As the medical office assistant for North Shore Medical Clinic, you are responsible for preparing and updating medical records. You need to type the results of a portable chest x-ray for a patient at the clinic.

Tutorial
Opening a Blank
Document

Tutorial
Exploring the Word
Screen

Tutorial
Entering Text

Tutorial
Undoing an
AutoCorrect Correction

Tutorial
Saving with a New
Name

Tutorial
Printing a Document

1 At the Windows 10 desktop, click the Start button and then click the Word 2016 tile.

   Depending on your system configuration, these steps may vary.

2 At the Word 2016 opening screen, click the *Blank document* template.

3 At the blank Word document, identify the various features by comparing your screen with the one shown in Figure W1.1.

   Refer to Table W1.1 for a description of the screen features.

Figure W1.1 Word Document Screen

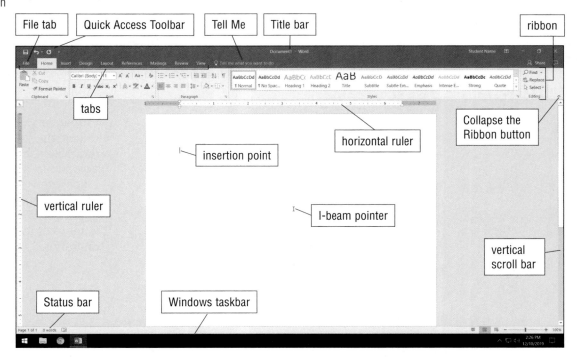

Table W1.1 Word Screen Features and Descriptions

Feature	Description
Collapse the Ribbon button	when clicked, removes the ribbon from the screen (redisplay the ribbon by clicking a tab [except the File tab] and then clicking the Pin the ribbon button [previously the Collapse the Ribbon button])
File tab	when clicked, displays the backstage area that contains options for working with and managing documents
horizontal ruler	used to set margins, indents, and tabs
I-beam pointer	used to move the insertion point or to select text
insertion point	indicates location of next character entered at the keyboard
Quick Access Toolbar	contains buttons for commonly used commands
ribbon	area containing tabs with options and buttons divided into groups
Status bar	displays number of pages and words, view buttons, and Zoom slider bar
tabs	contain commands and buttons organized into groups
Tell Me	used to look up a feature and provide options for using the feature
Title bar	displays document name followed by program name
vertical ruler	used to set top and bottom margins
vertical scroll bar	used to view parts of the document beyond the screen
Windows taskbar	divided into three sections—the Start button, the task buttons area, and the Notification area

4 Type Name: Joseph Ingram as shown in Figure W1.2. When you have finished typing, hold down the Shift key, press the Enter key, and then release the Shift key.

Shift + Enter is the New Line command. Use this command to keep lines of text within the same paragraph, which creates less space between one line and the next.

5 Type Procedure: Portable chest x-ray and then press Shift + Enter.

6 Type Date of Procedure: 05/16/2019 and then press the Enter key.

Pressing the Enter key begins a new paragraph in the document.

7 Type the remainder of the text shown in Figure W1.2.

Type the text as shown. When you type *teh* and then press the spacebar, the AutoCorrect feature will automatically change it to *the*. When you type *adn* and then press the spacebar, AutoCorrect changes it to *and*. Do not press the Enter key to end a line of text within a paragraph. Word will automatically wrap text to the next line.

Figure W1.2 Steps 4–7

Name: Joseph Ingram
Procedure: Portable chest x-ray
Date of Procedure: 05/16/2019

Comparison: A single portable view of teh chest is provided and comparison is made with earlier study of the same date.

Findings: Endotracheal tube adn right chest tubes are in place. Heart appears to be generous in size and right border is somewhat indistinct of perihilar vascular structure. No sign of pneumothorax was observed.

8 Click the File tab to display the backstage area.

The File tab is in the upper left corner of the screen at the left side of the Home tab.

9 Click the *Save As* option.

10 At the Save As backstage area, click the *Browse* option.

If you are saving to your OneDrive, click the *OneDrive - Personal* option. Click the desired folder in the right panel, click in the *File name* text box at the Save As dialog box, type the desired document name, and then press the Enter key.

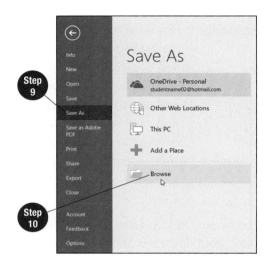

11 At the Save As dialog box, click the drive in the Navigation pane that contains your storage medium.

Press the F12 function key to display the Save As dialog box without displaying the Save As backstage area.

12 Double-click the *WordMedS1* folder in the Content pane.

13 Click in the *File name* text box, type 1-Results, and then press the Enter key (or click the Save button).

Word automatically adds the file extension *.docx* to the end of a document name.

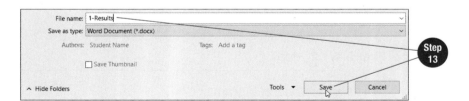

14 Print the document by clicking the File tab, clicking the *Print* option, and then clicking the Print button at the backstage area.

When you click the File tab, the backstage area displays with options for working with and managing documents. Refer to Table W1.2 for descriptions of the options and information you will find at each option's backstage area.

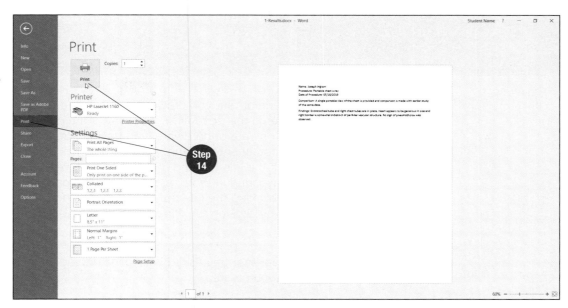

In Brief

Save Document to Removable Disk
1. Press F12.
2. At Save As dialog box, click removable disk drive in Navigation pane.
3. Double-click folder in Content pane.
4. Click in *File name* text box.
5. Type document name.
6. Click Save or press Enter.

Print Document
1. Click File tab.
2. Click *Print*.
3. Click Print button.

Table W1.2 Backstage Area Options

Tab	Options and Information
Info	permissions, possible issues with sharing the document, document versions, properties (number of pages, number of words), date created, date last modified, date last printed, author
New	available templates, such as Blank document, as well as templates from Office.com
Open	options for opening documents and list of recently opened documents
Save	saves previously saved document or displays Save As backstage area with options for saving a document, current folder, and recent folders
Save As	options for saving a document, current folder, and recent folders
Print	number of copies, printer, settings (one-sided pages, letter size, normal margins, one page per sheet)
Share	share document with specific people, share document using email, present document online, and share as a blog post
Export	export document as PDF or XPS document; change file type
Close	close currently open document
Account	user information, connected services, product information
Feedback	opens window with options for providing feedback to Microsoft on Microsoft products
Options	opens Word Options dialog box with options for customizing Word

Check Your Work — Compare your work with the model answer to ensure that you have completed the activity correctly.

In Addition

Understanding Default Document Formatting

A Word document is based on a template that applies default formatting. Default formatting refers to formatting automatically applied by Word. Some of the default settings include 11-point Calibri font, line spacing of 1.08, and 8 points of spacing after each paragraph (added when you press the Enter key). You will learn more about fonts and paragraph spacing in Section 2.

Correcting Errors

Word contains a spelling feature that inserts wavy red lines below words it cannot find in the spelling dictionary. You can edit these words or leave them as written. The wavy red lines do not print. You will learn more about checking for and correcting spelling errors in Activity 1.5.

As you are working in a document that you previously saved and named, consider saving any new information you enter in the document. This way, if the power is disrupted or some other issue occurs with the software or hardware, you have the most recent version of your document saved. To save a document with the same name, click the Save button on the Quick Access Toolbar or click the File tab and then click the *Save* option at the backstage area. When you are finished working in Word, close any open documents and then close Word. Close a document by clicking the File tab and then clicking the *Close* option at the backstage area. Close Word by clicking the Close button in the upper right corner of the screen.

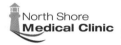
North Shore
Medical Clinic

Tutorial
Saving with the Same
Name

Tutorial
Closing a Document
and Closing Word

What You Will Do   Your supervisor has asked you to include additional information in the procedure results document you created.

1   With **1-Results.docx** open, make sure the insertion point is positioned at the end of the paragraph and then press the Enter key.

2   Type Option: Satisfactory post median sternotomy chest.

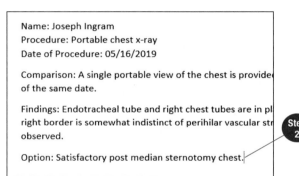

Name: Joseph Ingram
Procedure: Portable chest x-ray
Date of Procedure: 05/16/2019

Comparison: A single portable view of the chest is provide
of the same date.

Findings: Endotracheal tube and right chest tubes are in pl
right border is somewhat indistinct of perihilar vascular str
observed.

Option: Satisfactory post median sternotomy chest.

Step 2

3   Save the document with the added text by clicking the Save button 🖫 on the Quick Access Toolbar.

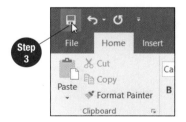

Step 3

4   Add additional text to the document by pressing the Enter key and then typing Prepared by Terrence Decker.

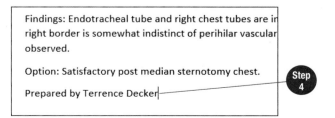

Findings: Endotracheal tube and right chest tubes are ir
right border is somewhat indistinct of perihilar vascular
observed.

Option: Satisfactory post median sternotomy chest.

Prepared by Terrence Decker

Step 4

In Brief

Save Document with Same Name
Click Save button on Quick Access Toolbar.
OR
1. Click File tab.
2. Click *Save*.

Close Document
1. Click File tab.
2. Click *Close*.

Close Word
Click Close button.

5 Save the document with the added text by clicking the File tab and then clicking the *Save* option at the backstage area.

> If you are working in a document that has not been saved, clicking the Save button on the Quick Access Toolbar or clicking the File tab and then clicking the *Save* option will cause the Save As backstage area to display.

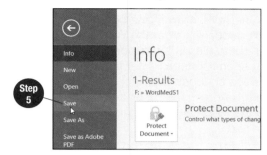

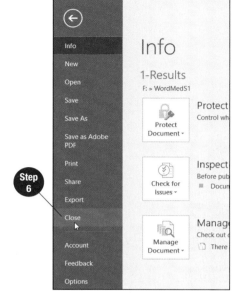

6 Close the document by clicking the File tab and then clicking the *Close* option at the backstage area.

7 Close Word by clicking the Close button in the upper right corner of the screen.

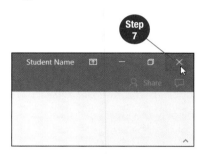

Check Your Work | Compare your work with the model answer to ensure that you have completed the activity correctly.

In Addition

Naming a Document

Document names created in Word and other applications in the Office suite can be up to 255 characters in length, including the drive letter, folder names, server name, and spaces. File names cannot include any of the symbols in the table at the right.

Symbol Name	Symbol
forward slash	/
backslash	\
greater-than symbol	>
less-than symbol	<
asterisk	*
question mark	?
quotation mark	"
colon	:
pipe symbol	|

Activity 1.3 — Opening and Editing a Document; Moving the Insertion Point

An existing document can be opened from the *Recent* option list at the Open backstage area, from a folder in OneDrive, or from the computer's hard drive or removable disk. In this activity, you will open a document from the WordMedS1 folder on your USB flash drive. (If you saved your student data files in a location or folder other than a USB flash drive, check with your instructor for specific steps.) After you create a document, you will often want to make changes to it. These changes may include adding text, called inserting, or removing text, called deleting. Before inserting or deleting text, position the insertion point at the desired location using the keyboard or the mouse. Use the Backspace key or Delete key on the keyboard to delete text.

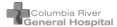
Columbia River
General Hospital

What You Will Do   As a medical office assistant for Columbia River General Hospital, you are responsible for typing history and physical examination documents for patients admitted to the hospital.

Tutorial
Opening a Document
from a Removable
Disk

Tutorial
Moving the Insertion
Point and Inserting
and Deleting Text

1 Open Word and then click the <u>Open Other Documents</u> hyperlink in the bottom left corner of the opening screen.

> If Word is already open and a blank Word screen displays, click the File tab to display the Open backstage area. If an existing document that contains text or objects is open, click the File tab and then click the *Open* option to display the Open backstage area.

2 At the Open backstage area, click the *Browse* option.

3 At the Open dialog box, click the drive in the Navigation pane where your USB flash drive is located (such as *Removable Disk (F:)*).

> Press Ctrl + F12 to display the Open dialog box without displaying the Open backstage area.

4 Double-click the *WordMedS1* folder in the Content pane.

5 Double-click ***CRGHh&p.docx*** in the Content pane.

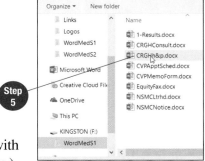
Step 5

6 With the document open, click the File tab and then click the *Save As* option.

7 At the Save As backstage area, click the *Browse* option. (This should display the Save As dialog box with the WordMedS1 folder active on your storage medium.)

> To open the Save As dialog box without displaying the Save As backstage area, press F12.

8 At the Save As dialog box, press the Home key to move the insertion point to the beginning of the file name in the *File name* text box, type 1-, and then press the Enter key. (The file name in the *File name* text box should display as **1-CRGHh&p.docx**.)

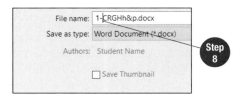
Step 8

> Pressing the Home key saves you from having to type the entire document name.

9 Position the mouse pointer at the beginning of the *HISTORY OF PRESENT ILLNESS* paragraph and then click the left mouse button.

> This moves the insertion point to the location of the mouse pointer.

In Brief

Open Document from Removable Disk
1. Press Ctrl + F12.
2. In Navigation pane, click drive containing removable disk.
3. Double-click folder in Content pane.
4. Double-click document.

10 Press the Up Arrow, Down Arrow, Left Arrow, and Right Arrow keys at the right of the regular keys on the keyboard.

> Pressing the arrow keys is one way to move the insertion point in a document. Use the information shown in Table W1.3 to practice using other methods for moving the insertion point.

11 Move the insertion point to the beginning of the name *Shawn Lipinski, MD* near the beginning of the document and then type Physician:. Press the spacebar after typing the colon.

> By default, text you type in a document is inserted in the document and existing text is moved to the right.

12 Click immediately to the right of the last number in the ID# *10572* and then press the Backspace key until all of the numbers are deleted.

> Press the Backspace key to delete any character immediately to the left of the insertion point.

Steps 12-13

Step 11

Name: Arlo Lorenzo
ID#: 11345|
Room: 3307
Physician: Shawn Lipinski, MD
Admitted: 02/25/2019
Date of Birth: 10/19/1972

HISTORY OF PRESENT ILLNESS

13 Type 11345.

14 Click any character in the last sentence in the *HISTORY OF PRESENT ILLNESS* section (the sentence that begins *He notes that he usually*).

15 Press the Backspace key until the insertion point is positioned immediately to the right of the period that ends the previous sentence. Press the Delete key until you have deleted the remainder of the sentence.

> Press the Delete key to delete any character immediately to the right of the insertion point.

16 Click the Save button on the Quick Access Toolbar.

> Clicking the Save button saves the document with the same name (**1-CRGHh&p.docx**).

Table W1.3 Insertion Point Movement Keys

Press	To move insertion point
End	to end of line
Home	to beginning of line
Page Up	up one screen
Page Down	down one screen
Ctrl + Home	to beginning of document
Ctrl + End	to end of document

Check Your Work Compare your work with the model answer to ensure that you have completed the activity correctly.

In Addition

Adding Buttons to the Quick Access Toolbar

You can add buttons to the Quick Access Toolbar that represent commonly used features. For example, you might want to add the Open button to save steps when opening a document or the Quick Print button to save steps when printing a document. To add a button to the Quick Access Toolbar, click the Customize Quick Access Toolbar button ▾ at the right side of the toolbar and then click the desired button name at the drop-down list or click *More Commands* to access more button options.

Scrolling; Selecting, Replacing, and Deleting Text; Using Undo and Redo

In addition to moving the insertion point to a specific location, you can use the mouse to move the display of text in the document screen. Use the mouse with the vertical scroll bar to scroll through text in a document. The vertical scroll bar displays toward the right side of the screen. Scrolling in a document changes the text displayed but does not move the insertion point. Previously, you learned to delete text by pressing the Backspace key or the Delete key. You can also select the text and then delete it, replace it with other text, or apply formatting to it. If you make a change to text, such as deleting it, and then change your mind, use the Undo and/or Redo buttons on the Quick Access Toolbar.

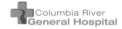
Columbia River
General Hospital

What You Will Do   To minimize the need for additional editing, you have decided to review carefully the History and Physical Examination document you have open on your screen.

Tutorial
Scrolling

Tutorial
Selecting, Replacing, and Deleting Text

Tutorial
Using Undo and Redo

1 With **1-CRGHh&p.docx** open, press Ctrl + Home to move the insertion point to the beginning of the document.

2 Position the mouse pointer on the down scroll arrow on the vertical scroll bar and then click the left mouse button several times.

> This scrolls down the lines of text in the document. Scrolling changes the display of text but does not move the insertion point.

3 Position the mouse pointer on the vertical scroll bar below the scroll box and then click the left mouse button two times.

> The scroll box on the vertical scroll bar indicates the location of the text in the document screen in relation to the remainder of the document. Clicking below the scroll box on the vertical scroll bar scrolls down one screen of text at a time.

4 Position the mouse pointer on the scroll box on the vertical scroll bar, click and hold down the left mouse button, drag the scroll box to the top of the vertical scroll bar, and then release the mouse button.

5 Position the mouse pointer on the word *leg* (the last word in the first sentence in the *HISTORY OF PRESENT ILLNESS* section) and then double-click the left mouse button. (This selects the word *leg*.)

> Selected text displays with a gray background. You can also click and drag through text with the mouse to select the text. When you select text, the Mini toolbar displays. You will learn more about the Mini toolbar in Activity 2.1.

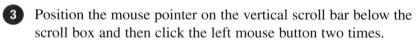

6 Type extremity.

> When you type *extremity*, it replaces *leg*.

7 Move the insertion point immediately to the left of the comma after the word *healthy* (located in the third sentence in the *HISTORY OF PRESENT ILLNESS* section) and then press the F8 function key on the keyboard. Press the Right Arrow key until the words *never been hospitalized* and the comma that follows *hospitalized* are selected.

> Pressing the F8 function key turns on Extend mode. Use the insertion point movement keys to select text in Extend mode.

8 Press the Delete key.

9 Hold down the Ctrl key, click anywhere in the second sentence in the *HISTORY OF PRESENT ILLNESS* section (begins *He was brought to the hospital*), and then release the Ctrl key.

> Holding down the Ctrl key while clicking the mouse button selects the entire sentence.

10 Press the Delete key to delete the selected sentence.

11 Click the Undo button 	on the Quick Access Toolbar.

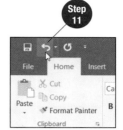

> When you click the Undo button, the deleted sentence reappears. Clicking the Undo button reverses the last command or deletes the last entry you typed. Click the arrow at the right side of the Undo button and a drop-down list displays the changes made to the document since it was opened. Click an action to undo it and any actions listed above it in the drop-down list.

12 Click the Redo button 	on the Quick Access Toolbar.

> Clicking the Redo button deletes the selected sentence. If you click the Undo button and then decide you do not want to reverse the original action, click the Redo button.

13 Position the mouse pointer between the left edge of the page and the heading *CONSULTATION* until the pointer turns into an arrow pointing up and to the right (instead of the left) and then click the left mouse button.

> The space between the left edge of the page and the text is referred to as the selection bar. Use the selection bar to select specific amounts of text. Refer to Table W1.4 for more information on selecting text.

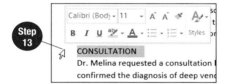

14 Deselect the text by clicking in the document.

> Deselecting cancels the selection of text.

15 Save the document by clicking the Save button on the Quick Access Toolbar.

Table W1.4 Selecting Text with the Mouse

To select	Complete these steps using the mouse
a word	Double-click the word.
a line of text	Click in the selection bar to the left of the line.
multiple lines of text	Drag in the selection bar to the left of the lines.
a sentence	Hold down the Ctrl key and then click anywhere in the sentence.
a paragraph	Double-click in the selection bar next to the paragraph or triple-click anywhere in the paragraph.
multiple paragraphs	Drag in the selection bar.
an entire document	Triple-click in the selection bar.

Check Your Work Compare your work with the model answer to ensure that you have completed the activity correctly.

In Addition

Resuming Reading or Editing in a Document

When you work in a multiple-page document and then close the document, Word remembers where the insertion point was last positioned. When you reopen the document, Word displays a Welcome Back message at the right side of the screen near the vertical scroll bar.

The message tells you that you can pick up where you left off and identifies the page where your insertion point was last located. Click the message and the insertion point is positioned at the top of that page.

Activity 1.5   Checking Spelling and Grammar

Use Word's spelling checker to find and correct misspelled words and find and delete duplicated words (such as *and and*). The spelling checker compares words in your document with words in its dictionary. If a match is found, the word is passed over. If no match is found for the word, the spelling checker stops, selects the word, and offers replacements. The grammar checker will search a document for grammar, punctuation, and word usage errors. The spelling checker and the grammar checker can help you create a well-written document, but these features do not replace the need for proofreading.

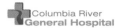
Columbia River
General Hospital

What You Will Do   Continuing with the editing process, you are ready to check the spelling and grammar in the History and Physical Examination document.

Tutorial
Checking Spelling and Grammar

1 With **1-CRGHh&p.docx** open, press Ctrl + Home to move the insertion point to the beginning of the document.

2 Click the Review tab and then click the Spelling & Grammar button ☑ in the Proofing group.

> When you click the Spelling & Grammar button, Word selects the first misspelled word and displays the Spelling task pane at the right side of the screen with options for correcting the error, ignoring the error, or adding the word to the spelling dictionary. It also contains a brief definition of the selected word in the list box. If a grammar error is selected, the Grammar task pane displays.

3 When the word *traetment* is selected in the document and *treatment* is selected in the list box in the Spelling task pane, click the Change button in the task pane.

> Refer to Table W1.5 for an explanation of the buttons in the Spelling task pane and Grammar task pane.

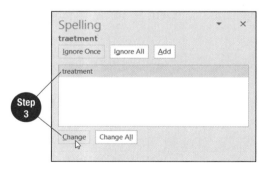

4 When the word *swolen* is selected in the document and *swollen* is selected in the list box in the Spelling task pane, click the Change button.

5 When the word *juandice* is selected in the document and *jaundice* is selected in the list box in the Spelling task pane, click the Change button.

6 When the word *Their* is selected in the document and *There* is selected in the list box in the Grammar task pane, click the Change button.

7 If the word *thyromegaly* is selected in the document, click the Ignore All button in the Spelling task pane.

This medical term is spelled correctly.

8 When the word *were* is selected (this word occurs twice), click the Delete button in the Spelling task pane.

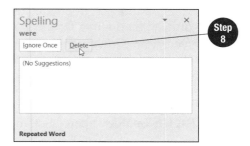

9 If the text *SL:SN* is selected in the document, click the Ignore Once button in the Spelling task pane.

10 Click OK at the message box telling you the spelling and grammar check is complete.

11 Click the Save button on the Quick Access Toolbar to save the changes made to the document.

Table W1.5 Spelling Task Pane and Grammar Task Pane Buttons

Button	Function
Ignore Once	during spell checking, skips that occurrence of the word; in grammar checking, leaves currently selected text as written
Ignore All	during spell checking, skips that occurrence and all other occurrences of the word in the document
Add	adds selected word to the main spelling dictionary
Delete	deletes currently selected word(s)
Change	replaces selected word in sentence with selected word in list box
Change All	replaces selected word in sentence, and all other occurrences of the word, with selected word in list box

Check Your Work Compare your work with the model answer to ensure that you have completed the activity correctly.

In Addition

Changing Spelling Options

Control spelling and grammar checking options at the Word Options dialog box with the *Proofing* option selected. Display this dialog box by clicking the File tab and then clicking *Options*. At the Word Options dialog box, click *Proofing* in the left panel. Using options at the dialog box, you can tell the spelling checker to ignore certain types of text, create custom dictionaries, show readability statistics, and hide spelling and/or grammar errors in the document.

Editing While Checking Spelling and Grammar

When checking a document, you can temporarily leave the Spelling task pane or Grammar task pane by clicking in the document. To resume the spelling and grammar check, click the Resume button in the Spelling task pane or Grammar task pane.

Activity 1.6   Using AutoCorrect and the Thesaurus

The AutoCorrect feature automatically detects and corrects some typographical errors, misspelled words, and incorrect capitalization. In addition to correcting errors, you can use the AutoCorrect feature to insert frequently used text. Use the Thesaurus to find synonyms, antonyms, and other related terms for a particular word.

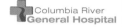
Columbia River
General Hospital

What You Will Do   You need to insert additional text in the History and Physical Examination document. To speed up the process, you will create a new AutoCorrect entry. You will also use the Thesaurus to find synonyms for specific words in the document.

Tutorial ▶
Adding and Deleting
an AutoCorrect Entry

Tutorial ▶
Using the Thesaurus

1 With **1-CRGHh&p.docx** open, click the File tab and then click *Options*.

2 At the Word Options dialog box, click *Proofing* in the left panel and then click the AutoCorrect Options button in the *AutoCorrect options* section.

3 At the AutoCorrect dialog box with the AutoCorrect tab selected, type tc in the *Replace* text box and then press the Tab key.

4 Type tachycardia in the *With* text box and then click the Add button.

5 With the *tc* selected in the *Replace* text box, type pl and then press the Tab key.

6 With *tachycardia* selected in the *With* text box, type pulmonary, click the Add button, and then click OK to close the AutoCorrect dialog box.

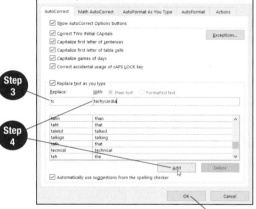

7 Click OK to close the Word Options dialog box.

8 Press Ctrl + End to move the insertion point to the end of the document. Move the insertion point so it is positioned immediately to the right of the period after the sentence *Neurologic assessment was normal* (below the *NEUROLOGIC* heading) and then press the Enter key.

9 Type DIAGNOSIS and then press Shift + Enter.

10 Type the remaining text shown in Figure W1.3. *Note: Type the text exactly as shown. AutoCorrect will change* **tc** *to* **tachycardia** *and* **pl** *to* **pulmonary.** *Do not press the Enter key at the end of each line in the figure. Word will automatically wrap text to the next line.*

Figure W1.3 Steps 9–10

DIAGNOSIS
Patient is diagnosed with deep vein thrombophlebitis in the lower left extremity and tc. This patient will be admitted. A pl ventilation perfusion scan is mandated by the presence of tc. A baseline study needs to be done to exclude the presence of plembolization. He will be treated with bed rest and anticoagulation. Further notation will be made as the case progresses. Appropriate studies for coagulopathy were performed.

Add AutoCorrect Entry
1. Click File tab.
2. Click *Options*.
3. Click *Proofing*.
4. Click AutoCorrect Options button.
5. Type text in *Replace* text box.
6. Type text in *With* text box.
7. Click Add button.
8. Click OK.
9. Click OK.

Use Thesaurus
1. Click in a word.
2. Click Review tab.
3. Click Thesaurus button.
4. Right-click word in Thesaurus task pane list box.
5. Click *Insert*.

⑪ Click anywhere in the word *done* (located in the fourth sentence of the paragraph you just typed), click the Review tab, and then click the Thesaurus button 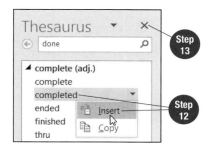 in the Proofing group.

⑫ At the Thesaurus task pane, right-click the word *completed* in the list box and then click *Insert* at the drop-down list.

⑬ Close the Thesaurus task pane by clicking the Close button ☒ in the upper right corner.

⑭ Position the mouse pointer on the word *exclude* (located in the fourth sentence of the paragraph you just typed) and then click the right mouse button.

⑮ At the shortcut menu that displays, point to *Synonyms* and then click *eliminate* at the side menu.

⑯ Click the Save button to save the document with the same name.

⑰ Click the File tab and then click *Options*. Click *Proofing* in the left panel of the dialog box and then click the AutoCorrect Options button.

⑱ At the AutoCorrect dialog box, type pl in the *Replace* text box.

> This selects the *pulmonary* entry in the list box.

⑲ Click the Delete button.

⑳ Type tc in the *Replace* text box and then click the Delete button.

㉑ Click OK to close the AutoCorrect dialog box and then click OK to close the Word Options dialog box.

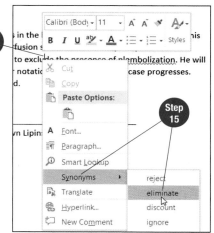

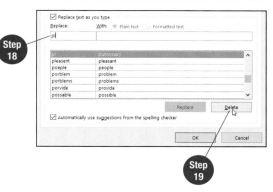

Check Your Work — Compare your work with the model answer to ensure that you have completed the activity correctly.

In Addition

Using the Thesaurus Task Pane

Depending on the word you are looking up, the words in the Thesaurus task pane list box may display followed by (n.) for *noun*, (v.) for *verb*, (adj.) for *adjective*, or (adv.) for *adverb*. Click a word in the list box and a definition of the word displays below the list box. You may need to install a dictionary before you can see a definition. To install a dictionary, click the <u>Get a Dictionary</u> hyperlink. At the Dictionaries pane, click the desired dictionary and then click the Download button.

By default, a document displays in Print Layout view. This view displays the document on the screen as it will appear when printed. Other views are available, such as Read Mode, Web Layout, Outline, and Draft. Change views with buttons in the view area on the Status bar or with options in the Views group on the View tab. Change to Draft view and the document displays in a format for efficient editing and formatting. Read Mode displays a document in a format for easy viewing and reading. Change to Web Layout view to display a document as it would appear as a web page. In Print Layout view, a page displays as it will appear when printed, including the white space at the top and bottom of the page representing the document's margins. To save space on the screen, the white space can be removed using the Hide White Space icon. Redisplay white space using the Show White Space icon.

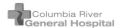

What You Will Do   Your supervisor, as well as Dr. Lipinski, will be reviewing the History and Physical Examination document electronically, so you decide to experiment with various views to determine the best one to use for on-screen reviewing.

Tutorial
Changing Document
Views

Tutorial
Hiding and Showing
White Space

1 With **1-CRGHh&p.docx** open, press Ctrl + Home to move the insertion point to the beginning of the document.

2 Change to Draft view by clicking the View tab and then clicking the Draft button ▦ in the Views group.

Change to Draft view to display the document in a format designed for efficient editing and formatting. In Draft view, margins and other features such as headers and footers do not display.

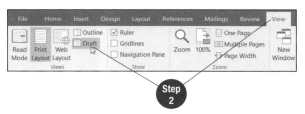

3 Change to Web Layout view by clicking the Web Layout button in the view area on the Status bar (see Figure W1.4).

Change to Web Layout view to display the document as it would appear as a web page.

4 Change to Read Mode by clicking the Read Mode button ▣ in the Views group.

Read Mode displays a document for easy viewing and reading. You can also display a document in Read Mode by clicking the Read Mode button in the view area on the Status bar.

5 Display the next two pages on the screen by clicking the Next button (right-pointing arrow in a circle) that displays at the right side of the screen.

Figure W1.4 View Buttons in View Area on Status Bar

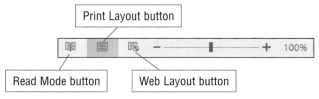

6 Display previous pages by clicking the Previous button (left-pointing arrow in a circle) that displays at the left side of the screen.

7 Continue navigating in Read Mode using the keyboard commands shown in Table W1.6.

8 Return to Print Layout view by pressing the Esc key.

Pressing the Esc key displays the document in Print Layout view. You can also return to Print Layout view by clicking the View tab and then clicking *Edit Document* at the drop-down list.

9 To save space on the screen, remove the white space that displays at the top and bottom of each page as well as the gray space between pages. To do this, position the mouse pointer on the gray space above the page until the pointer turns into the hide white space icon and then double-click the left mouse button.

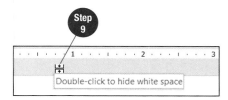

10 Scroll through the document and then redisplay the white and gray space at the top and bottom of each page. To do this, position the mouse pointer on the gray line at the top of the page until the pointer turns into the show white space icon and then double-click the left mouse button.

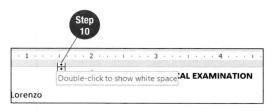

Table W1.6 Navigating in Read Mode

Press this key	To complete this action
Page Down or spacebar	Move to next page or section.
Page Up or Backspace key	Move to previous page or section.
Right Arrow	Move to next page.
Left Arrow	Move to previous page.
Home	Move to first page in document.
End	Move to last page in document.
Esc	Return to previous view.

In Addition

Zooming In on an Object in Read Mode

If your document contains an object such as an image, shape, SmartArt, or table, you can zoom in on the object in Read Mode by double-clicking the object. The object appears larger on the screen and a button con-taining a diagonally pointing arrow displays just outside the upper right corner of it. Click this button to zoom in even more on the object. Click once outside the object to return it to its original size.

By default, a document displays at 100%. This display percentage can be changed with the Zoom slider bar at the right side of the Status bar and with options in the Zoom group on the View tab. To change display percentage with the Zoom slider bar, drag the button on the bar to increase or decrease the percentage, or click the Zoom Out button to decrease the display percentage or the Zoom In button to increase the percentage. Use buttons in the Zoom group on the View tab to return to the 100% display percentage, display one page or multiple pages, expand the document across the screen, and display the Zoom dialog box.

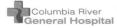
Columbia River General Hospital

What You Will Do   Several people will be reviewing the History and Physical Examination document on the screen, so you decide to experiment with various views and zoom percentages to determine the best view for on-screen reviewing.

Tutorial
Changing the Display Percentage

1 With **1-CRGHh&p.docx** open, press Ctrl + Home to move the insertion point to the beginning of the document.

2 Click the Zoom Out button — at the left side of the Zoom slider bar to decrease the display percentage to 90%.

> Figure W1.5 identifies the Zoom slider bar along with the Zoom Out and Zoom In buttons.

3 Click the Zoom In button + at the right side of the Zoom slider bar to increase the display percentage to 100%.

4 Position the mouse pointer on the Zoom slider button on the Zoom slider bar, click and hold down the left mouse button, drag to the right to increase the display percentage, and then release the mouse button.

5 Click the View tab.

6 Click the 100% button in the Zoom group to return to the default display percentage of 100%.

7 Click the One Page button in the Zoom group to display just the first page on the screen.

8 Click the Multiple Pages button in the Zoom group to display all of the pages on the screen.

9 Click the Zoom button in the Zoom group to display the Zoom dialog box.

> You can also display the Zoom dialog box by clicking the Zoom level button (the percentage that displays at the right side of the Zoom slider bar).

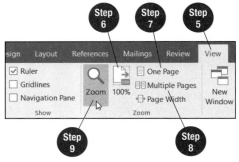

⑩ Click the *75%* option in the *Zoom to* section of the dialog box.

⑪ Click OK to close the Zoom dialog box.

The document displays at 75%.

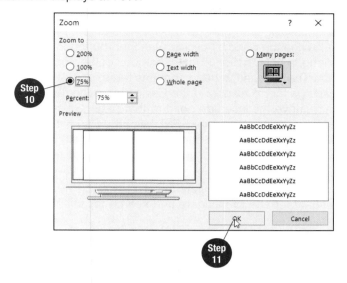

⑫ Click the 100% button in the Zoom group to return to the default display percentage.

Figure W1.5 View Buttons in View Area on Status Bar

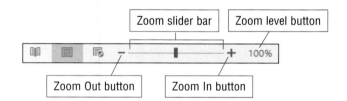

In Addition

Working with Windows

The Windows group on the View tab contains a number of buttons for working with windows. Click the New Window button to open a new window containing the same document. This is useful if you want to view a portion of the document while editing in another location. If more than one document is open, the documents can be arranged so that a portion of each is visible. To do this, click the Arrange All button in the Window group. Click the Split button in the Window group to split the open document in two with a split bar and another horizontal ruler. Splitting a window is useful if you want to view different parts of a document at one time. Compare the contents of two documents by opening both documents and then clicking the View Side by Side button in the Window group. Both documents display on the screen arranged side by side. By default, synchronous scrolling is active, which means that scrolling in one document results in the same scrolling in the other document. Turn off synchronous scrolling by clicking the Synchronous Scrolling button.

Use the Navigation pane to browse in a document or search for specific text or items. Display the Navigation pane by clicking the Find button in the Editing group on the Home tab or by clicking the *Navigation Pane* check box in the Show group on the View tab to insert a check mark. The Navigation pane contains three tabs—Headings, Pages, and Results. Click the Headings tab to display in the Navigation pane thumbnails of each page. Click a page thumbnail to move the insertion point to that page. Search for text by clicking in the search text box and then typing the desired text. With the Pages tab active, each occurrence of the search text is highlighted in the pages. Click the Results tab to display each occurrence of the search text along with the text that displays before and after each occurrence.

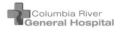

What You Will Do Review the History and Physical Examination document by using the Navigation pane to navigate and search for specific text in the document.

Tutorial
Navigating Using the
Navigation Pane

Tutorial
Finding Text

1 With **1-CRGHh&p.docx** open, display the Navigation pane by clicking the View tab and then clicking the *Navigation Pane* check box to insert a check mark.

> You can also display the Navigation pane by clicking the Find button in the Editing group on the Home tab.

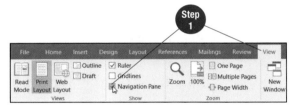

2 Click the Pages tab in the Navigation pane.

> Clicking the Pages tab displays thumbnails of each page in the Navigation pane.

3 Click the page 2 thumbnail in the Navigation pane.

> Clicking the page 2 thumbnail moves the insertion point to the beginning of page 2.

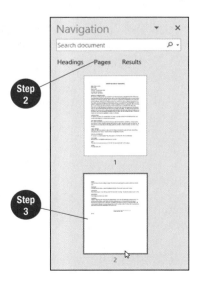

In Brief

Display Navigation Pane
1. Click View tab.
2. Click *Navigation Pane* check box.
OR
1. Click Home tab.
2. Click Find button.

4 Click the page 1 thumbnail in the Navigation pane.

5 Click in the search text box in the Navigation pane (contains the text *Search document*) and then type LUNGS.

> After you type *LUNGS*, each occurrence of the text is highlighted in the document.

6 Click the Next Search Result button (displays as a down arrow) in the Navigation pane to select the next occurrence of *LUNGS* (note that both lowercase and uppercase versions appear in the results of the search). Click the button again to select the next occurrence.

> You can click the Previous Search Result button (displays as an up arrow) to display the previous occurrence of the search text.

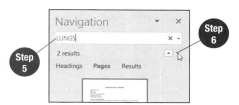

7 Click the Results tab to display in the Navigation pane each occurrence of the search text *LUNGS* along with the text that displays before and after each occurrence.

8 Select the first occurrence of *LUNGS* in the document by clicking the first item in the Navigation pane.

9 Click the X at the right side of the search text box.

> Clicking this button ends the current search, removes the search text in the Navigation pane, and selects the current search result in the document.

10 Close the Navigation pane by clicking the Close button in the upper right corner of the pane.

> You can also close the Navigation pane by clicking the *Navigation Pane* check box in the Show group on the View tab to remove the check mark.

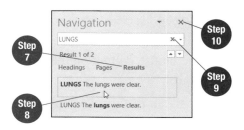

In Addition

Displaying Ribbon Options

Control how much of the ribbon displays on screen with the Ribbon Display Options button in the upper right corner of the screen. Click this button to display a drop-down list with options for hiding the ribbon, showing only the tabs, or showing tabs and commands. You can also hide the ribbon by clicking the Collapse the Ribbon button above the vertical scroll bar or with the keyboard shortcut Ctrl + F1. Redisplay the ribbon by double-clicking any tab or by pressing Ctrl + F1.

Activity 1.10 — Using the Tell Me and Help Features; Previewing and Printing

Word includes the Tell Me feature, which provides information and guidance on how to complete a function. To use Tell Me, click in the *Tell Me* text box on the ribbon to the right of the View tab and then type the function for which you want help. As you type, a drop-down list displays with options that are refined as you continue typing, a feature referred to as word-wheeling. The drop-down list displays options for completing the function, displaying the top three help links most related to the search, or displaying the Help task pane. The Help task pane can be opened through the Tell Me feature or by pressing the F1 function key on the keyboard. You can also display the Help task pane by hovering the mouse pointer over certain buttons on the ribbon and then clicking the *Tell me more* hyperlink in the ScreenTip that displays. The Help task pane displays with information about the button feature. The Print backstage area provides options for previewing the document before printing, indicating the number of copies, specifying the pages for printing, and customizing the document.

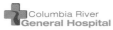
Columbia River
General Hospital

What You Will Do   To enhance the appearance of the History and Physical Examination document, you decide to use the Tell Me feature to change the font color of the heading *HISTORY AND PHYSICAL EXAMINATION*. You are also ready to print the History and Physical Examination document, but first you want to learn more about printing a document. You decide to experiment with the Help feature to learn about printing.

Tutorial
Using the Tell Me
Feature

Tutorial
Using the Help Feature

Tutorial
Previewing and
Printing

1 With **1-CRGHh&p.docx** open, select the heading *HISTORY AND PHYSICAL EXAMINATION* by positioning the mouse pointer in the heading and then triple-clicking the left mouse button.

2 Click in the *Tell Me* text box.

The *Tell Me* text box is on the ribbon to the right of the View tab and contains the text *Tell me what you want to do*. When you click in the text box, the last five functions entered display in a drop-down list.

3 Type font color in the *Tell Me* text box.

A drop-down list displays with options such as *Font Color, Font Size, Border Color, Text Highlighter Color,* and *Font*.

4 Position the mouse pointer on the arrow at the right of the *Font Color* option in the drop-down list.

5 At the side menu that displays, click the *Blue* color option in the *Standard Colors* section.

The Blue font color is applied to the selected heading. The Tell Me feature guided you through the process of applying font color without you having to learn how to apply font color using a button on the ribbon or an option at a dialog box.

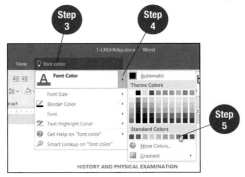

6 Press Ctrl + Home to move the insertion point to the beginning of the document and then press the F1 function key.

> Pressing the F1 function key displays the Help task pane.

7 At the Help task pane, click in the search text box, type print, and then press the Enter key.

8 At the Help task pane, click the <u>Print a document in Word</u> hyperlink.

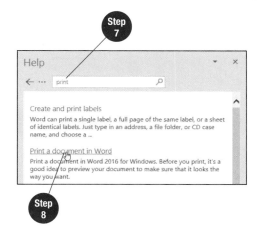

9 Read the information and then close the Help task pane by clicking the Close button in the upper right corner of the task pane.

10 Display the Help task pane with information on the Format Painter feature by hovering the mouse pointer over the Format Painter button in the Clipboard group on the Home tab and then clicking the <u>Tell me more</u> hyperlink at the bottom of the ScreenTip that displays.

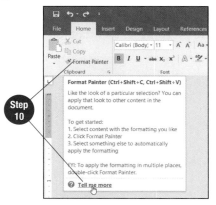

11 Read the information and then close the Help task pane.

12 Click the File tab and then click the *Print* option to display the Print backstage area.

> At the Print backstage area, your document displays at the right side of the screen and looks as it will when printed. The left side of the Print backstage area displays three categories—*Print*, *Printer*, and *Settings*. Click the Print button in the *Print* category to send the document to the printer. Specify the number of copies you want printed with the *Copies* option in the *Print* category. Use the gallery in the *Printer* category to specify the desired printer. The *Settings* category contains a number of galleries, each with options for specifying how you want your document printed, such as whether or not you want the pages collated when printed; the orientation, page size, and margins of your document; and how many pages of your document you want to print on each sheet of paper.

13 Click two times on the Zoom In button (contains a plus symbol) that displays at the right side of the Zoom slider bar.

Click the Zoom In button to increase the size of the page or click the Zoom Out button (contains a minus symbol) to decrease the size of the page.

14 Click the Zoom to Page button at the right side of the Zoom slider bar.

Click the Zoom to Page button to increase or decrease the page size so an entire page displays in the preview area.

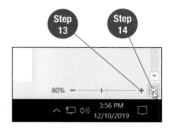

15 Click the Next Page button below and to the left of the preview page to display the next page in the document.

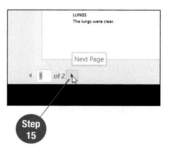

16 Print only page 2 of the document by clicking in the *Pages* text box in the *Settings* category, typing 2, and then clicking the Print button.

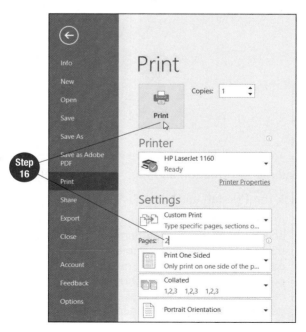

17 Position the insertion point anywhere in page 1, click the File tab, and then click the *Print* option.

18 Click the top gallery in the *Settings* category and then click *Print Current Page* at the drop-down list.

19 Click the Print button.

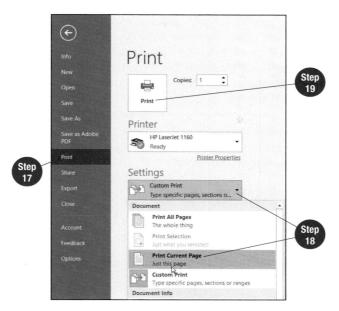

20 Save and then close **1-CRGHh&p.docx**.

Check Your Work Compare your work with the model answer to ensure that you have completed the activity correctly.

In Addition

Printing a Range of Pages

Identify a specific page, multiple pages, and/or a range of pages for printing at the Print backstage area. To print specific pages, click in the *Pages* text box and then type the page numbers of the pages you want to print. If you want to print multiple pages, use a comma to indicate *and* and a hyphen to indicate *through*. For example, to print pages 2 and 5, you would type *2,5* in the *Pages* text box. To print pages 6 through 10, you would type *6-10*. You can enter both commas and hyphens when specifying page numbers.

Getting Help in a Dialog Box and Backstage Area

Display a dialog box and then click the Help button in the upper right corner and the Microsoft online help files related to the dialog box display in a web browser. You can also display a backstage area and then click the Help button in the upper right corner of the screen to display the Microsoft online help files related to the backstage area in a web browser.

Activity 1.11 Creating a Document Using a Template

Word includes a number of template documents formatted for specific uses. Each Word document is based on a template document, with the Normal template as the default. With Word templates (and Microsoft online templates), you can easily create a variety of documents with specialized formatting, such as letters, reports, and awards. Display available templates by clicking the File tab and then clicking the *New* option. At the New backstage area, click in the search text box, type a category, and then press the Enter key. Word displays templates matching the category. Click the desired template and then click the Create button. You must be connected to the Internet to download online templates.

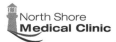
North Shore
Medical Clinic

What You Will Do Your supervisor at North Shore Medical Clinic has asked you to send a letter requesting information on interpreting services. You decide to use a letter template to help you format the letter.

Tutorial
Creating a Document
Using a Template

1 Click the File tab and then click the *New* option.

2 At the New backstage area, click in the search text box (contains the text *Search for online templates*), type business letter equity theme, and then press the Enter key.

3 Click the first *Letter (Equity theme)* template in the backstage area.

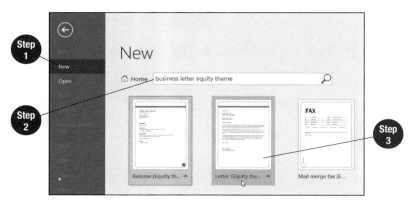

4 Click the Create button.

5 At the letter document, click the placeholder text *[Pick the date]* and then type the current date. (Your date will automatically change to numbers when you click outside the placeholder.)

6 If necessary, select the name that displays below the date and then type your first and last names.

7 Click the placeholder text *[Type the sender company name]* and then type North Shore Medical Clinic.

8 Click the placeholder text *[Type the sender company address]*, type 7450 Meridian Street, Suite 150, press the Enter key, and then type Portland, OR 97202.

9 Click the placeholder text *[Type the recipient name]* and then type Community Interpreting Services.

10 Click the placeholder text *[Type the recipient address]*, type 4525 Lawrence Street, press the Enter key, and then type Portland, OR 97216.

In Brief

Create Document Using Template
1. Click File tab.
2. Click *New*.
3. Click template.
4. Click Create button.

11 Click the placeholder text *[Type the salutation]* and then type Ladies and Gentlemen:.

12 Click any character in the three paragraphs of text in the body of the letter and then type the text shown in Figure W1.6.

13 Click the placeholder text *[Type the closing]* and then type Sincerely,.

14 Make sure your name displays below *Sincerely,*. If not, select the name that displays and then type your first and last names.

15 Click the placeholder text *[Type the sender title]* and then type Medical Office Assistant.

16 Click the Save button on the Quick Access Toolbar.

17 At the Save As backstage area, navigate to the *WordMedS1* folder on your storage medium.

18 At the Save As dialog box, with the WordMedS1 folder active, type 1-RequestLtr in the *File name* text box and then press the Enter key (or click the Save button).

> If a dialog box displays telling you that your document will be upgraded to the newest file format, click OK.

19 Print the letter by clicking the File tab, clicking the *Print* option, and then clicking the Print button.

20 Close the document by clicking the File tab and then clicking the *Close* option.

Figure W1.6 Step 12

At North Shore Medical Clinic, our goal is to provide the best possible medical care for our patients. Since some of our patients are non-English speakers, we occasionally need interpreting services. Up to this point, we have been hiring interpreters from various agencies. We recently determined that we would like to contract with one agency to provide all interpreting services at our clinic.

We are interested in learning about all interpreting services available at your agency and would like a representative to contact us to schedule a face-to-face meeting. Please call our clinic at (503) 555-2330 and ask for the clinic director. We look forward to working with your agency.

Check Your Work Compare your work with the model answer to ensure that you have completed the activity correctly.

In Addition

Specifying a Category

When you search for online templates at the New backstage area, a *Category* list box displays at the right side of the screen. The list box displays the category name and the number of templates that fit within the category. Click the desired category in the list box, and only templates matching that category will display in the New backstage area.

Managing Folders and Documents; Saving in a Different Format

As you continue working with documents, consider document management tasks such as creating a folder and copying, moving, and deleting documents. You can complete many document management tasks related to one or more documents at the Open dialog box or Save As dialog box. By default, Word saves a file as a Word document and adds the extension *.docx* to the name. With the *Save as type* option at the Save As dialog box, you can save a document in a different format, such as an earlier version of Word, rich text format, a web page, or a plain text file.

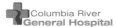
Columbia River
General Hospital

What You Will Do   To begin managing your documents, you decide to create a folder named H&P in which you will save all history and physical examination documents. You will also save a document in an older version of Word.

Tutorial
Managing Folders

Tutorial
Managing Documents

Tutorial
Saving in a Different Format

1. At the blank Word screen, click the File tab.

2. At the Open backstage area, click the *Browse* option.

3. At the Open dialog box, navigate to the *WordMedS1* folder on your storage medium.

4. Click the New folder button.

5. Type H&P and then press the Enter key.

6. In the Content pane of the Open dialog box, click **CRGHh&p.docx**, hold down the Ctrl key, click **1-CRGHh&p.docx**, click **1-Results.docx**, and then release the Ctrl key.

   Use the Ctrl key to select nonadjacent documents. Use the Shift key to select adjacent documents.

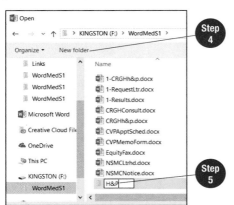

7. Right-click one of the selected documents and then click *Copy* at the shortcut menu.

8. Double-click the *H&P* folder.

   In the Open dialog box Content pane, folders display before documents. Folders display preceded by a folder icon and documents display preceded by a document icon.

9. Right-click in a white portion of the Open dialog box Content pane and then click *Paste* at the shortcut menu.

   The copied documents are inserted in the H&P folder.

10. You need to send **1-CRGHh&p.docx** to a colleague who uses Word 2003, so you need to save the document in that format. At the Open dialog box with the H&P folder active, double-click **1-CRGHh&p.docx**.

11. Click the File tab and then click the *Save As* option.

12. At the Save As backstage area, click the *Browse* option.

13 At the Save As dialog box, make WordMedS1 the active folder and then type 1-CRGHh&pW2003 in the *File name* text box.

14 Click the *Save as type* option box and then click *Word 97-2003 Document (*.doc)* at the drop-down list.

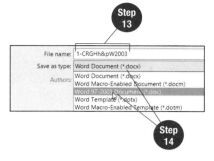

Step 13

Step 14

15 Click the Save button in the lower right corner of the dialog box.

> If a compatibility checker message displays, click the Continue button.

16 Close the document.

17 Press Ctrl + F12 to display the Open dialog box. If the WordMedS1 folder on your storage medium is not already the active folder, navigate to the WordMedS1 folder.

18 At the Open dialog box, rename the H&P folder by right-clicking the folder name and then clicking *Rename* at the shortcut menu.

19 Type H&PEDocs and then press the Enter key.

> The new folder name replaces the original folder name. You can also rename a folder by selecting the folder, clicking the Organize button, clicking *Rename* at the drop-down list, and then typing the new folder name.

20 Delete the H&PEDocs folder by first making sure the folder is selected. If necessary, click the folder to select it.

21 Click the Organize button and then click *Delete* at the drop-down list.

22 At the message asking if you are sure you want to delete the folder and all of its contents, click the Yes button.

> You can also delete a folder by clicking the folder and then pressing the Delete key or by right-clicking the folder and then clicking *Delete* at the shortcut menu.

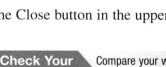

Step 21

23 Close the Open dialog box.

24 Close Word by clicking the Close button in the upper right corner of the screen.

Check Your Work Compare your work with the model answer to ensure that you have completed the activity correctly.

In Addition

Editing a PDF File in Word

PDF stands for Portable Document Format and is a common format for sharing files. A PDF file can be opened and edited in Word. When you open a PDF file, Word converts it to a .docx file, and the data in the file may not display in the exact format as in the PDF file. Converting a PDF file to a Word document works best with text-based documents.

Features Summary

Feature	Ribbon Tab, Group	Button	Quick Access Toolbar	File Tab Option	Keyboard Shortcut
AutoCorrect dialog box				*Options, Proofing, AutoCorrect Options*	
close document				*Close*	Ctrl + F4
close Word		×			Alt + F4
Draft view	View, Views				
Extend mode					F8
Help					F1
hide white space					
Move insertion point to end of document					Ctrl + End
Move insertion point to beginning of document					Ctrl + Home
Navigation pane	View, Show				Ctrl + F
New backstage area				*New*	
New Line command					Shift + Enter
Open backstage area				*Open*	Ctrl + O
Open dialog box					Ctrl + F12
Print backstage area				*Print*	Ctrl + P
Print Layout view	View, Views				
Read Mode	View, Views				
redo (repeat) an action			⤷		Ctrl + Y
Save As backstage area				*Save* OR *Save As*	
Save As dialog box					F12
save document			💾		Ctrl + S
show white space					
Spelling & Grammar	Review, Proofing	ABC ✓			F7
Tell Me feature	*Tell Me* text box				Alt + Q
Thesaurus	Review, Proofing				Shift + F7
undo an action			↩		Ctrl + Z
Word Options dialog box				*Options*	

> **Workbook** ▷ Section study tools and assessment activities are available in the Workbook pages of the ebook. These resources are designed to help you further develop and demonstrate mastery of the skills learned in this section.

Word

Formatting Characters and Paragraphs

Skills

- Apply fonts and font effects
- Apply formatting with Format Painter
- Repeat a command
- Align text in paragraphs
- Indent text
- Change line spacing
- Change paragraph spacing
- Create bulleted and numbered lists
- Insert symbols

- Insert special characters
- Set tabs and tabs with leaders
- Add borders and shading to text
- Apply a page border
- Apply styles and style sets
- Apply themes
- Insert the date and time
- Insert quick parts

Data Files Before beginning section work, copy the WordMedS2 folder to your storage medium and then make WordMedS2 the active folder.

Precheck Check your current skills to help focus your study of the skills taught in this section.

Activities Overview

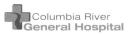

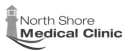

Edit and format an informational document on heart disease and format legal documents on records storage and maintenance.

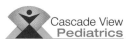

Edit and format a document on well-child checkup appointment recommendations and suggestions and prepare a document containing information on clinic hours.

Edit and format a document on diabetes, format a document on cystic fibrosis, edit and format a document on how to request medical records, prepare a letter to the local community college indicating the availability of an internship, prepare a memo describing Word features, prepare a memo describing aspects of the medical assisting field, prepare a job announcement, and prepare a flyer advertising a free diabetes presentation.

Model Answers Preview the model answers for an overview of the activities you will complete in each section.

Applying Formatting with the Font Group and the Mini Toolbar

Apply character formatting to text with buttons in the Font group on the Home tab. Formatting a document changes how the document displays and prints. The top row of the Font group contains options and buttons for changing the font and font size of text as well as changing text case and clearing formatting. The bottom row contains buttons for applying formatting to text such as bold, italics, underlining, strikethrough, subscript, superscript, text effects, highlighting, and font color. Microsoft Word has taken some commonly used commands and placed them on the Mini toolbar. When you select text, the Mini toolbar displays above the selected text. The Mini toolbar disappears when you move the mouse pointer away from it.

Columbia River General Hospital

What You Will Do Your supervisor at Columbia River General Hospital has asked you to format and edit an informational document on heart disease. You decide to improve the appearance of the document by applying different types of fonts and effects to the text.

Tutorial
Applying Font Formatting Using the Font Group

Tutorial
Applying Font Formatting Using the Mini Toolbar

Tutorial
Highlighting Text

1 Open **CRGHHeartDisease.docx** and then save it with the name **2-CRGHHeartDisease**.

2 Select the text *Heart Disease* and then click the Bold button B in the Font group on the Home tab.

3 With *Heart Disease* still selected, click the Change Case button Aa ▼ in the Font group and then click *UPPERCASE* at the drop-down list.

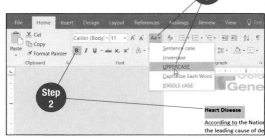

4 With *Heart Disease* still selected, click the Text Effects and Typography button A ▼ and then click the blue outline option in the fourth column, first row of the drop-down gallery.

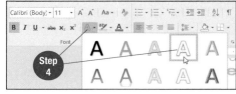

5 Select *Aortic disease* and then click the Underline button U ▼ in the Font group.

6 Select and then underline the remaining headings: *Arrhythmia (abnormal heart rhythm)*, *Cardiomyopathy (heart muscle disease)*, *Congenital heart disease*, *Coronary artery disease*, *Heart failure*, *Heart valve disease*, *Pericardial disease*, and *Vascular disease*.

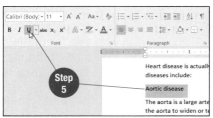

7 Select the words *abnormal heart rhythm* in the parentheses after the word *Arrhythmia* in the second underlined heading and then click the Italic button I on the Mini toolbar that displays above the selected text.

The Mini toolbar disappears when you move the mouse pointer away from it.

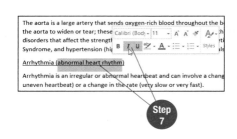

8 Select the words *heart muscle disease* in the parentheses after the word *Cardiomyopathy* and then click the Italic button on the Mini toolbar.

9 Select the heading *HEART DISEASE* and then click the Clear All Formatting button in the Font group.

10 Select the entire document by clicking the Select button in the Editing group on the Home tab and then clicking *Select All* at the drop-down list.

11 Click the *Font* option box arrow in the Font group. Hover the mouse pointer over various typefaces at the drop-down gallery and notice how the text in the document reflects the selected font.

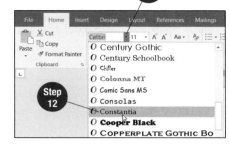

> This feature is referred to as live preview. It provides you with an opportunity to see how the document will appear with formatting before you make a final choice.

12 Scroll down the gallery and then click *Constantia*.

13 Click the *Font Size* option box arrow and then click *12* at the drop-down gallery.

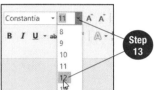

14 Click the Font Color button arrow and then click the *Dark Blue* option at the drop-down gallery (second color from the right in the *Standard Colors* row).

15 Deselect the text by clicking anywhere in the document.

16 You decide to highlight specific text to identify it for review by colleagues. To do this, click the Text Highlight Color button in the Font group and then select the first sentence under the heading *Aortic disease* (the sentence that begins *The aorta is a large artery that*).

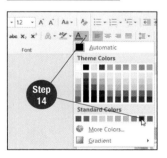

> When you click the Text Highlight Color button, the mouse pointer displays with a highlighter pen attached. To turn off highlighting, click the Text Highlight Color button again.

17 Select the sentence under the *Arrhythmia* heading to highlight it and then click the Text Highlight Color button to turn off highlighting.

18 Remove the text highlighting by pressing Ctrl + A, clicking the Text Highlight Color button arrow, and then clicking *No Color* at the drop-down list.

19 Save and then print **2-CRGHHeartDisease.docx**.

Check Your Work Compare your work with the model answer to ensure that you have completed the activity correctly.

In Addition

Using Typefaces

A **typeface** is a set of characters with a common design and shape. It can be decorative or plain and either monospaced or proportional. Word refers to typefaces as fonts. A monospaced typeface allots the same amount of horizontal space for each character, while a proportional typeface allots a varying amount of space for each character. Proportional typefaces are divided into two main categories: serif and sans serif. A serif is a small line at the end of a character stroke. Consider using a serif typeface for text-intensive documents because the serifs help move the reader's eyes across the page. Use a sans serif typeface for headings, headlines, and advertisements.

In addition to buttons in the Font group, you can apply font formatting with options at the Font dialog box. Display the Font dialog box by clicking the Font group dialog box launcher. With options at this dialog box, you can change the font, font size, and font style; change the font color; choose an underline style; and apply formatting effects. Once you apply formatting to text, you can copy that formatting to different locations in the document using the Format Painter. If you apply formatting to text in a document and then want to repeat the formatting for other text, use the Repeat command. Apply the Repeat command by pressing the F4 function key or Ctrl + Y.

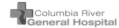
Columbia River
General Hospital

What You Will Do   The changes you made to the heart disease document have enhanced the readability and appearance of the text. Now you will turn your attention to the headings.

Tutorial
Applying Font Formatting Using the Font Dialog Box

Tutorial
Formatting with Format Painter

Tutorial
Repeating the Last Command

1 With **2-CRGHHeartDisease.docx** open, press Ctrl + Home to move the insertion point to the beginning of the page and then press Ctrl + A to select the entire document.

2 Click the Font group dialog box launcher.

The dialog box launcher displays as a small button containing a diagonal arrow.

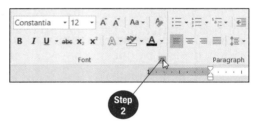

Step
2

3 At the Font dialog box, click *Cambria* in the *Font* list box (you will need to scroll up the list box to display this option) and then click *11* in the *Size* list box.

4 Click the *Font color* option box arrow and then click the *Black, Text 1* option (second column, first row in the *Theme Colors* section).

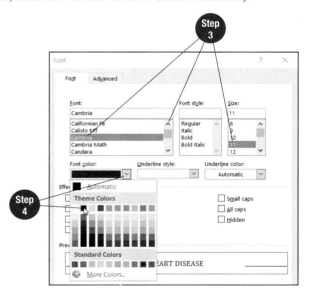

Step
3

Step
4

5 Click OK to close the Font dialog box.

6 Select the heading *HEART DISEASE* near the beginning of the document and then click the Font group dialog box launcher.

7 At the Font dialog box, click *Candara* in the *Font* list box (you will need to scroll down the list box to display this option), and then click *14* in the *Size* list box (you will need to scroll down the list box to display this option).

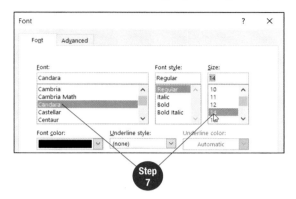

8 Click OK to close the Font dialog box.

9 With the heading still selected, click the Format Painter button in the Clipboard group on the Home tab.

When Format Painter is active, the mouse pointer displays with a paintbrush attached.

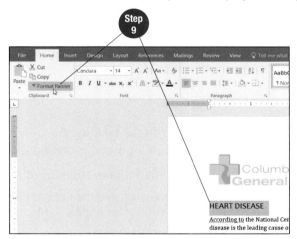

10 Scroll down the document and then select the heading *HEART DISEASE FACTS*.

Selecting the heading applies the formatting from the first heading and also turns off Format Painter.

11 Select the heading *Aortic disease* and then click the Font group dialog box launcher.

12 Click *Candara* in the *Font* list box (you will need to scroll down the list box to display this option), click *Bold* in the *Font style* list box, and then click *14* in the *Size* list box (you will need to scroll down the list box to display this option).

13 Click the *Underline style* option box arrow and then click *(none)* at the drop-down list.

14 Click OK to close the dialog box and then deselect the heading.

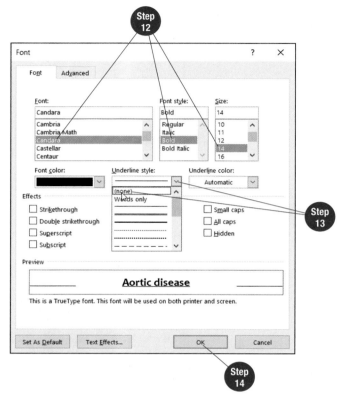

15 Click any character in the heading *Aortic disease* and then double-click the Format Painter button in the Clipboard group on the Home tab.

16 Select the heading *Arrhythmia (abnormal heart rhythm)*.

> Because you double-clicked the Format Painter button, the feature remains active even after you select the text and apply the formatting.

17 Select individually the remaining headings: *Cardiomyopathy (heart muscle disease)*, *Congenital heart disease*, *Coronary artery disease*, *Heart failure*, *Heart valve disease*, *Pericardial disease*, and *Vascular disease*.

18 Click the Format Painter button in the Clipboard group to turn off Format Painter.

19 Select the text *National Center for Chronic Disease Prevention and Health Promotion* in the first paragraph.

20 Click the Text Effects and Typography button in the Font group, point to *Shadow*, and then click the shadow option in the first column, first row in the *Outer* section.

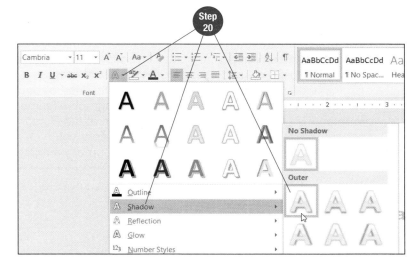

21 Select the text *American Heart Association* in the second paragraph and then press the F4 function key.

> Pressing F4 repeats the previous command and applies the shadow effect to the selected text.

22 Select the text *Marfan Syndrome* in the first paragraph in the *Aortic disease* section and then press F4.

23 Save **2-CRGHHeartDisease.docx**.

Check Your Work — Compare your work with the model answer to ensure that you have completed the activity correctly.

In Addition

Using Font Keyboard Shortcuts

Along with options and buttons in the Font group and the Font dialog box, you can apply font formatting with the keyboard shortcuts shown here.

Font Group Button	Keyboard Shortcut
Font	Ctrl + Shift + F
Font Size	Ctrl + Shift + P
Increase Font Size	Ctrl + Shift + >
Decrease Font Size	Ctrl + Shift + <
Change Case	Shift + F3
Bold	Ctrl + B
Italic	Ctrl + I
Underline	Ctrl + U
Subscript	Ctrl + =
Superscript	Ctrl + Shift + +

Activity 2.3 Aligning Text

Paragraphs of text in a document are aligned at the left margin by default. This default alignment can be changed to center (used for titles, headings, or other text you want centered), right (used for addresses, dates, times, or other text you want aligned at the right margin), and justified (used for text you want aligned at both the left and right margins, such as text in a report or an article). Change paragraph alignment with buttons in the Paragraph group on the Home tab, the *Alignment* option at the Paragraph dialog box, or with keyboard shortcuts. Text alignment can be changed before you type a paragraph, or you can change the alignment of an existing paragraph or group of paragraphs.

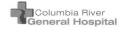

What You Will Do   You decide to improve the appearance of the heart disease document by changing the text alignment.

1   With **2-CRGHHeartDisease.docx** open, center the heading *HEART DISEASE* by clicking anywhere within the title and then clicking the Center button ≡ in the Paragraph group on the Home tab.

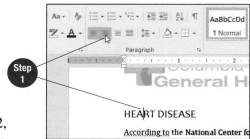

2   Click any character in the heading *HEART DISEASE FACTS* (near the middle of page 2, after the *HEART DISEASE* section) and then click the Center button.

3   Press Ctrl + Home to move the insertion point to the beginning of the document and then select from the middle of the third paragraph to the end of the document.

> The entire third paragraph does not have to be selected, only a portion.

4   Click the Justify button ≡ in the Paragraph group.

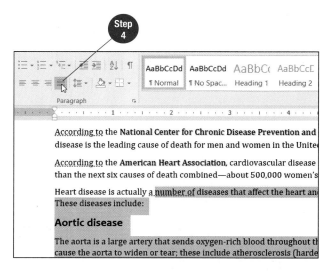

5   Move the insertion point to any character in the heading *HEART DISEASE FACTS* and then click the Center button.

> When you justified the text, *HEART DISEASE FACTS* was moved to the left.

6 Press Ctrl + End to move the insertion point to the end of the document and then press the Enter key.

7 Click the Center button in the Paragraph group.

8 Click the Bold button in the Font group to turn on bold formatting and then type your first and last names.

9 Press Shift + Enter.

10 Type Date:, press the spacebar, and then press Alt + Shift + D.

> Alt + Shift + D is the keyboard shortcut to insert the current date.

11 Press Shift + Enter, type Time:, press the spacebar, and then press Alt + Shift + T.

> Alt + Shift + T is the keyboard shortcut to insert the current time.

12 Press the Enter key.

13 Return paragraph alignment back to the default (left alignment) by pressing Ctrl + Q.

> Ctrl + Q is the keyboard shortcut to return all paragraph formatting to the default.

14 After looking at the centered text you just typed, you decide to remove the formatting and apply different formatting. To do this, first select the three lines of text you just typed.

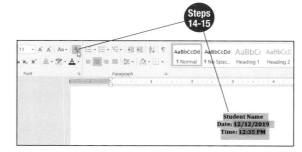

Steps
14-15

15 Click the Clear All Formatting button in the Font group on the Home tab.

> Clicking the Clear All Formatting button returns all paragraph and character formatting to the default.

16 With the three lines still selected, click the Align Right button ≡ in the Paragraph group, click the *Font* option box arrow, click *Cambria* at the drop-down gallery, click the *Font Size* option box arrow, and then click *10* at the drop-down gallery.

17 Deselect the text and then save **2-CRGHHeartDisease.docx**.

> **Check Your Work** Compare your work with the model answer to ensure that you have completed the activity correctly.

In Addition

Understanding Methods for Changing Alignment

You can change paragraph alignment with the *Alignment* option box at the Paragraph dialog box. Display the Paragraph dialog box by clicking the Paragraph group dialog box launcher. At the Paragraph dialog box, click the *Alignment* option box arrow and then click the desired alignment at the drop-down list. You can also change alignment with the keyboard shortcuts shown here.

Alignment	Keyboard Shortcut
Left	Ctrl + L
Center	Ctrl + E
Right	Ctrl + R
Justified	Ctrl + J

Activity 2.4 Indenting Text

A paragraph of text in a document can be indented. For example, you can indent the first line of text in a paragraph, all lines of text in a paragraph, or the second and subsequent lines of a paragraph (called a hanging indent). Several methods are available for indenting text, including buttons in the Paragraph group on the Home tab and the Layout tab, markers on the horizontal ruler, options at the Paragraph dialog box with the Indents and Spacing tab selected, and keyboard shortcuts.

Columbia River General Hospital

What You Will Do   You want to emphasize certain paragraphs of information in the heart disease document, and you have decided to accomplish this by indenting.

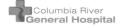
Indenting Text

1. With **2-CRGHHeartDisease.docx** open, click anywhere in the paragraph below the *Aortic disease* heading.

2. Position the mouse pointer on the Left Indent marker on the horizontal ruler, click and hold down the left mouse button, drag the marker to the 0.5-inch mark on the ruler, and then release the mouse button.

   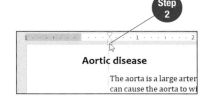
   Step 2
   Aortic disease
   The aorta is a large arter can cause the aorta to w

   If the horizontal ruler is not visible, click the View tab and then click the *Ruler* check box in the Show group to insert a check mark. The ruler indent markers are shown in Figure W2.1. To precisely position a marker on the ruler, hold down the Alt key while dragging the marker.

3. Drag the Right Indent marker to the 6-inch mark on the horizontal ruler.

   Step 3
   t the body. Certain
   le atherosclerosis
   the strength of the

4. Click anywhere in the paragraph below the *Arrhythmia (abnormal heart rhythm)* heading and then click the Increase Indent button in the Paragraph group on the Home tab.

   This indents text 0.5 inches from the left margin.

   Step 4
   Arrhythmia (abnormal heart rhythm)
   Arrhythmia is an irregular or abnormal heartbeat and uneven heartbeat) or a change in the rate (very slow

5. Drag the Right Indent marker to the 6-inch mark on the horizontal ruler.

6. Click anywhere in the paragraph below *Cardiomyopathy (heart muscle disease)* and then click the Layout tab.

7. In the *Indent* section of the Paragraph group, click in the *Left* measurement box and then type 0.5.

8. Click the *Right* measurement box up arrow until *0.5"* displays.

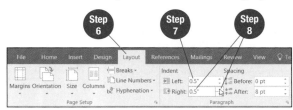
Step 6   Step 7   Step 8

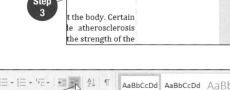
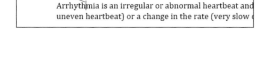

⑨ Click anywhere in the paragraph below the *Congenital heart disease* heading and then use the Paragraph dialog box to change the left and right indents. Begin by clicking the Paragraph group dialog box launcher.

⑩ At the Paragraph dialog box, click the *Left* measurement box up arrow in the *Indentation* section until *0.5″* displays in the box.

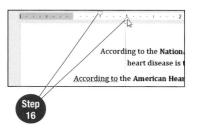

⑪ Click the *Right* measurement box up arrow in the *Indentation* section until *0.5″* displays in the box.

⑫ Click OK to close the Paragraph dialog box.

⑬ Click anywhere in the paragraph below the *Coronary artery disease* heading and then press F4.

⑭ Indent the paragraph of text below each of the headings *Heart failure, Heart valve disease, Pericardial disease,* and *Vascular disease* by clicking in each paragraph and then pressing F4.

⑮ Click anywhere in the first paragraph of text below the title *HEART DISEASE* (the paragraph that begins *According to the National Center for Chronic Disease*).

⑯ Drag the First Line Indent marker to the 0.5-inch mark on the horizontal ruler and then drag the Hanging Indent marker to the 1-inch mark on the ruler.

> This creates a hanging indent in the paragraph.

⑰ Click anywhere in the second paragraph of text below the heading *HEART DISEASE*, click the Home tab, click the Increase Indent button in the Paragraph group, and then press Ctrl + T.

> Ctrl + T is the keyboard shortcut to create a hanging indent. For additional keyboard shortcuts, refer to the In Addition at the bottom of this page.

⑱ Save **2-CRGHHeartDisease.docx**.

Figure W2.1 Ruler Indent Markers

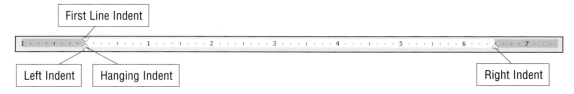

> **Check Your Work** Compare your work with the model answer to ensure that you have completed the activity correctly.

In Addition

Indenting Text Using Keyboard Shortcuts
Indent text with the keyboard shortcuts shown here.

Command	Keyboard Shortcut
Indent text from left margin	Ctrl + M
Decrease indent from left margin	Ctrl + Shift + M
Create a hanging indent	Ctrl + T
Remove hanging indent	Ctrl + Shift + T

Activity 2.5 Changing Line and Paragraph Spacing

By default, line spacing is set at 1.08. This default line spacing can be changed with the Line and Paragraph Spacing button in the Paragraph group on the Home tab, keyboard shortcuts, or with the *Line spacing* and *At* options at the Paragraph dialog box. Control spacing above and below paragraphs with options in the Line and Paragraph Spacing button drop-down gallery, the *Before* and *After* measurement boxes in the *Spacing* section of the Paragraph group on the Layout tab, or with the *Before* and *After* options in the *Spacing* section of the Paragraph dialog box with the Indents and Spacing tab selected.

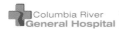
Columbia River
General Hospital

What You Will Do   Your supervisor needs the heart disease document in a few hours. You decide to make a few spacing changes in the document before printing the final version.

Tutorial
Changing Line Spacing

Tutorial
Changing Spacing
Before and After
Paragraphs

Tutorial
Keeping Text Together

1 With **2-CRGHHeartDisease.docx** open, press Ctrl + A to select the entire document.

2 Click the Line and Paragraph Spacing button in the Paragraph group on the Home tab and then click *1.5* at the drop-down gallery.

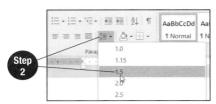

3 Deselect the text and then scroll through the document. After viewing the document, you decide to decrease the line spacing to 1.3. To begin, press Ctrl + A to select the entire document, click the Line and Paragraph Spacing button, and then click *Line Spacing Options* at the drop-down gallery.

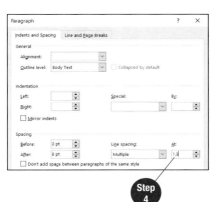

4 Type *1.3* in the *At* measurement box in the *Spacing* section of the Paragraph dialog box.

> The Paragraph dialog box also contains a *Line spacing* option box. Click the *Line spacing* option box arrow to display a drop-down list of spacing choices.

5 Click OK to close the dialog box and then deselect the text.

6 You decide to single-space the text in the *HEART DISEASE FACTS* section. To do this, select from the beginning of the heading *HEART DISEASE FACTS* to the end of the document.

7 Click the Line and Paragraph Spacing button and then click *1.0* at the drop-down gallery.

> Choosing this option changes the line spacing to single for the selected paragraphs of text. You can also change line spacing with keyboard shortcuts. Press Ctrl + 1 to change to single spacing, Ctrl + 2 to change to double spacing, and Ctrl + 5 to change to 1.5 line spacing.

8 Click anywhere in the *Aortic disease* heading and then click the Layout tab.

9 Click the *After* measurement box up arrow in the Paragraph group. (The text *12 pt* should display.) Click in the *Before* measurement box (this selects *0 pt*), type 15, and then press the Enter key. (The text *15 pt* should display.)

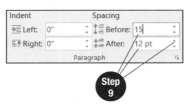

In Brief

Change Line Spacing
1. Click Line and Paragraph Spacing button.
2. Click line spacing option.
OR
1. Click Line and Paragraph Spacing button.
2. Click *Line Spacing Options*.
3. Type line spacing in *At* measurement box.
4. Click OK.

10 After looking at the extra spacing before and after the heading, you decide to remove it. To do this, make sure the insertion point is positioned in the heading *Aortic disease* and then click the Paragraph group dialog box launcher.

11 At the Paragraph dialog box, click three times on the *Before* measurement box down arrow in the *Spacing* section and then click two times on the *After* measurement box down arrow.

Both the *Before* and *After* measurement boxes should now display *0 pt*.

12 Click OK to close the Paragraph dialog box.

13 Click anywhere in the heading *Arrhythmia (abnormal heart rhythm)* and then press F4.

Pressing F4 repeats the paragraph spacing command.

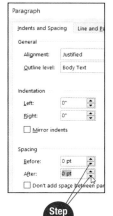

Step 11

14 Continue clicking in each of the remaining headings [*Cardiomyopathy (heart muscle disease), Congenital heart disease, Coronary artery disease, Heart failure, Heart valve disease, Pericardial disease,* and *Vascular disease*] and pressing F4.

15 You decide to change the justified paragraph to left alignment. To do this, select all the text in the *HEART DISEASE* section except the title, click the Home tab, and then click the Align Left button ☰ in the Paragraph group.

16 Select all of the text in the *HEART DISEASE FACTS* section, except the title and the right-aligned text, and then click the Align Left button in the Paragraph group.

17 You also decide to remove the hanging indents. To do this, select the two paragraphs of text below the *HEART DISEASE* title, press Ctrl + Shift + T, and then click the Decrease Indent button ☰ in the Paragraph group.

Ctrl + Shift + T is the keyboard shortcut to remove a hanging indent.

18 Scroll down the page and notice that the heading *Coronary artery disease* displays at the bottom of the first page while the paragraph that follows it displays at the top of the second page. To keep the heading with the paragraph of text, begin by clicking in the heading *Coronary artery disease* and then clicking the Paragraph group dialog box launcher.

19 At the Paragraph dialog box, click the Line and Page Breaks tab, click the *Keep with next* check box to insert a check mark, and then click OK.

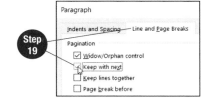

Step 19

20 Save, print, and then close **2-CRGHHeartDisease.docx**.

Check Your Work Compare your work with the model answer to ensure that you have completed the activity correctly.

In Addition

Changing Spacing Above or Below Paragraphs

Spacing above or below paragraphs is added in points. For example, to add 9 points of spacing below selected paragraphs, click the Layout tab or display the Paragraph dialog box with the Indents and Spacing tab selected. Select the current measurement in the *After* measurement box and then type *9*. You can also click the up or down arrows to increase or decrease the amount of spacing before or after paragraphs.

If you want to draw the reader's attention to a list of items, consider inserting a bullet before each item using the Bullets button in the Paragraph group on the Home tab. If the list of items is in a sequence, consider inserting numbers before each item with the Numbering button in the Paragraph group. Create multiple-level bulleted or numbered lists with options at the Multilevel List button drop-down list in the Paragraph group.

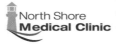
North Shore
Medical Clinic

What You Will Do   Dr. St. Claire has asked you to edit and format a document on diabetes. The medical staff will provide this informational document to patients who have been diagnosed with diabetes or are interested in learning more about diabetes. To improve the readability of the document, you decide to add numbering and bullets to specific paragraphs.

Tutorial
Creating Numbered Lists

Tutorial
Creating Bulleted Lists

1 Open **NSMCDiabetes.docx** and then save it with the name **2-NSMCDiabetes**.

2 Select the three paragraphs of text below the *Types of Diabetes* heading and then click the Numbering button in the Paragraph group on the Home tab.

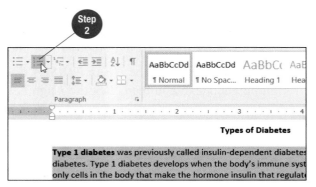

3 Position the insertion point at the end of the third numbered paragraph and then press the Enter key.

> Pressing the Enter key automatically inserts the number *4.* and indents the position of the insertion point.

4 Type the first four words, Other types of diabetes, as shown in Figure W2.2, click the Bold button in the Font group to turn off bold formatting, and then type the remaining text shown in Figure W2.2.

> Because the first words of the existing numbered paragraphs are bold, Word automatically turned on bold when you started a new numbered paragraph.

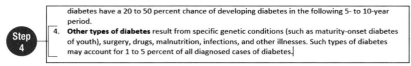

Figure W2.2 Step 4

> **Other types of diabetes** result from specific genetic conditions (such as maturity-onset diabetes of youth), surgery, drugs, malnutrition, infections, and other illnesses. Such types of diabetes may account for 1 to 5 percent of all diagnosed cases of diabetes.

In Brief

Insert Numbers
1. Select text.
2. Click Numbering button.

Insert Bullets
1. Select text.
2. Click Bullets button.

5 Select the four lines of text below the *Heart Disease and Stroke* heading and then click the Bullets button ☰▾ in the Paragraph group.

> Clicking the Bullets button in the Paragraph group inserts a round bullet before each paragraph.

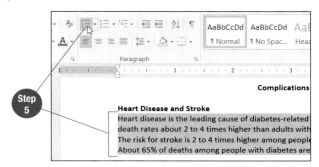

6 With the text still selected, replace the round bullets with custom bullets by clicking the Bullets button arrow and then clicking a bullet that you like in the *Bullet Library* section of the drop-down gallery.

> The choices at the Bullets button drop-down gallery vary depending on the most recent bullets selected.

7 Select the text below the *High Blood Pressure* heading and then press F4.

> Pressing F4 repeats the last command (inserting bullets).

8 Continue selecting text below each of the remaining headings (*Blindness*, *Kidney Disease*, *Nervous System Disease*, *Amputations*, *Dental Disease*, *Complications of Pregnancy*, and *Other Complications* [except for the text in parentheses]) and pressing F4 to insert bullets.

9 Save **2-NSMCDiabetes.docx**.

Check Your Work Compare your work with the model answer to ensure that you have completed the activity correctly.

In Addition

Inserting Multilevel List Numbering
Use the Multilevel List button in the Paragraph group on the Home tab to specify the type of numbering for lists that have more than one level. Apply predesigned multilevel numbering to text in a document by clicking the Multilevel List button and then clicking the desired numbering style at the drop-down list.

Creating Numbered and/or Bulleted Text
If you type *1.* and then press the spacebar, Word indents the number approximately 0.25 inch and then hang indents the text in the paragraph approximately 0.5 inch from the left margin. When you press the Enter key after typing text, *2.* is inserted 0.25 inch from the left margin at the beginning of the next paragraph. Continue typing items and Word will continue numbering them. Press the Enter key two times to turn off numbering or click the Numbering button in the Paragraph group. Bulleted lists with hanging indents are automatically created when you begin a paragraph with the symbol *, >, or -. Type one of the symbols and then press the spacebar, and the symbol bullet is inserted in the document. The type of bullet inserted depends on the type of character entered. For example, if you use the asterisk symbol (*), a round bullet is inserted.

Turning Off Automatic Numbering and/or Bulleting
If you do not want automatic numbering or bulleting in a document, turn off the features at the AutoCorrect dialog box with the AutoFormat As You Type tab selected. To display this dialog box, click the File tab and then click *Options*. At the Word Options dialog box, click the *Proofing* option and then click the AutoCorrect Options button. At the AutoCorrect dialog box, click the AutoFormat As You Type tab. Click the *Automatic numbered lists* check box and/or *Automatic bulleted lists* check box to remove the check mark(s).

Activity 2.7 — Inserting Symbols and Special Characters

Insert special symbols such as é, ö, and Å with options at the Symbol palette or the Symbol dialog box. Display the Symbol palette by clicking the Insert tab and then clicking the Symbol button in the Symbols group. Click a symbol to insert it in the document. To display additional symbols, display the Symbol dialog box by clicking the Symbol button and then clicking the *More Symbols* option. Click the desired symbol at the dialog box, click the Insert button, and then click the Close button. At the Symbols dialog box with the Symbols tab selected, you can change the font and display different symbols. Click the Special Characters tab to display a list of special characters and the keyboard shortcuts to insert them.

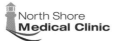
North Shore **Medical Clinic**

What You Will Do   You need to include a registered trademark symbol after the organization name *American Diabetes Association* and insert Spanish text indicating that the diabetes document is also available in Spanish. You will use the Symbol dialog box to insert the registered trademark symbol and the necessary Spanish characters.

Tutorial
Inserting Symbols

Tutorial
Inserting Special Characters

1. With **2-NSMCDiabetes.docx** open, move the insertion point to the end of the document.

2. Position the insertion point immediately after the word *Association* inside the parentheses.

3. Click the Insert tab, click the Symbol button Ω in the Symbols group, and then click *More Symbols* at the bottom of the drop-down list.

4. At the Symbol dialog box, click the Special Characters tab.

5. At the Symbol dialog box with the Special Characters tab selected, click the ® symbol in the *Character* list box.

6. Click the Insert button and then click the Close button.

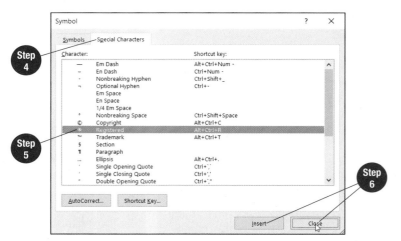

7. Press Ctrl + End to move the insertion point to the end of the document and then press the Enter key.

8. Type the text shown in Figure W2.3 up to the *é* in *También*. To insert the é symbol, begin by clicking the Symbol button and then clicking *More Symbols*.

The text in Figure W2.3 is in Spanish and translates as (*Also available in Spanish.*)

9 At the Symbol dialog box with the Symbols tab selected, click the *Font* option box arrow and then click *(normal text)* at the drop-down list. You may need to scroll up to see this option. Skip this step if *(normal text)* is already selected.

10 Scroll down the list box and then click the *é* symbol (the location of this symbol may vary).

11 Click the Insert button and then click the Close button.

12 Type the text shown in Figure W2.3 up to the *ñ* symbol, click the Symbol button, and then click *More Symbols* at the drop-down list.

13 At the Symbol dialog box, click the *ñ* symbol (the location of this symbol may vary).

14 Click the Insert button and then click the Close button.

15 Type the remaining text shown in Figure W2.3.

16 Save **2-NSMCDiabetes.docx**.

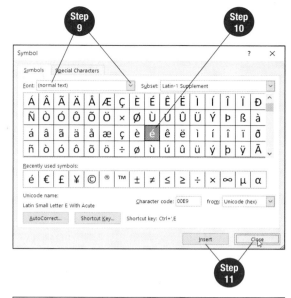

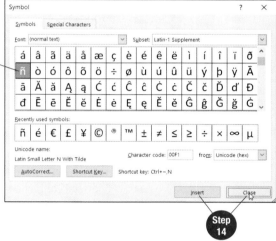

Figure W2.3 Steps 8–15

(También disponible en español.)

Check Your Work Compare your work with the model answer to ensure that you have completed the activity correctly.

In Addition

Inserting Symbols with Keyboard Shortcuts or Character Codes

Another method for inserting symbols in a document is to use keyboard shortcuts. Click a symbol at the Symbol dialog box and the keyboard shortcut displays toward the bottom of the dialog box. For example, click the ø symbol and the keyboard shortcut Ctrl + /,O displays. To insert the ø symbol in a document using the keyboard shortcut, hold down the Ctrl key and then press the / key. Release the Ctrl key and then press the O key. Not all symbols have a corresponding keyboard shortcut. Each symbol has an identifying character code. If you

know the character code of a symbol, type the code in the *Character code* text box in the Symbol dialog box. Click a symbol at the Symbol dialog box and the symbol code displays in the *Character code* text box.

Inserting Symbols Using the Palette

When you click the Symbol button in the Symbols group, a drop-down palette displays with symbol choices. The palette displays the most recently used symbols. If the palette contains the symbol you need, click the symbol to insert it in the document.

Activity 2.8 Setting Tabs

Word offers a variety of default settings, including left tabs set every 0.5 inch. You can set, move, and delete your own tabs using the horizontal ruler or the Tabs dialog box. The default tabs display as tiny vertical lines along the bottom of the horizontal ruler. With a left tab, text aligns at the left edge of the tab. The other types of tabs that can be set on the horizontal ruler are center, right, decimal, and bar. Switch between these tab types by clicking the Alignment button above the vertical ruler. To set a tab, display the desired alignment symbol on the Alignment button and then click the horizontal ruler at the desired position. You can also add leaders to every type of tab except bar tabs. Leaders are useful for directing the reader's eyes across the page and can be periods, hyphens, or underlines. Tabs with leaders are set with options at the Tabs dialog box. At the Tabs dialog box, you can choose the type of tab, the type of leader, and the tab position measurement.

North Shore Medical Clinic

What You Will Do   Dr. St. Claire has done some additional research on diabetes and has asked you to include the information in the document. You think that the information would be easiest to read if it were set in three columns and decide to set tabs to create this formatting.

Tutorial
Setting and Modifying Tabs on the Horizontal Ruler

Tutorial
Setting and Clearing Tabs at the Tabs Dialog Box

1 With **2-NSMCDiabetes.docx** open, move the insertion point to the end of the paragraph of text below the *Statistics on Diabetes* heading and then press the Enter key two times.

2 Type the first sentence shown in Figure W2.4 and then press the Enter key two times.

3 Make sure the left tab symbol ⌊ displays in the Alignment button at the left side of the horizontal ruler.

> If the horizontal ruler is not visible, click the View tab and then click the *Ruler* check box in the Show group to insert a check mark.

4 Position the arrow pointer below the 0.5-inch mark on the horizontal ruler and then click the left mouse button.

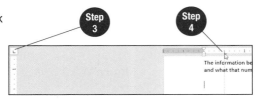

5 Click the Alignment button to display the center tab symbol ⊥, position the arrow pointer below the 3.25-inch mark on the ruler, and then click the left mouse button.

6 Click the Alignment button to display the right tab symbol ⌟, position the arrow pointer below the 6-inch mark on the ruler, and then click the left mouse button.

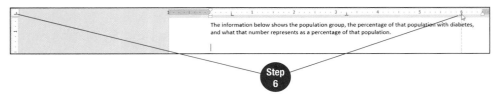

7 Type the rest of the text shown in Figure W2.4, pressing the Tab key before typing each entry, including those in the first column. Make sure to bold and underline the text as shown in the figure.

In Brief

Set Tab on Horizontal Ruler
1. Display alignment symbol in Alignment button.
2. Click position on horizontal ruler.
OR
1. Click Paragraph group dialog box launcher.
2. Click Tabs button.
3. Type tab measurement.
4. Click alignment option.
5. Click leader option.
6. Click Set.
7. Click OK.

The information below shows the population group, the percentage of that population with diabetes, and what that number represents as a percentage of that population.

Population	Number with diabetes	Percentage
Under 20	210 thousand	0.26%
20 and older	18 million	8.70%
Men 20 and older	8.7 million	8.70%
Women 20 and older	9.3 million	8.70%

8 After typing the last entry in the third column, press the Enter key and then press Ctrl + Q to remove paragraph formatting.

Pressing Ctrl + Q removes the tabs you set from the ruler.

9 You decide to add leaders to the center and right tabs. To begin, select all the text you typed at the left, center, and right tabs *except* the headings (***Population***, ***Number with diabetes***, and ***Percentage***).

10 Click the Paragraph group dialog box launcher.

11 At the Paragraph dialog box, click the Tabs button in the lower left corner.

12 At the Tabs dialog box, click *3.25″* in the *Tab stop position* section, click *2....* in the *Leader* section, and then click the Set button.

13 Click *6″* in the *Tab stop position* section, click *2....* in the *Leader* section, and then click the Set button.

14 Click OK to close the dialog box.

15 Position the insertion point immediately to the right of the last *8.70%* in the ***Percentage*** column and then press the Enter key.

16 Press the Tab key, type 60 and older, press the Tab key, type 8.6 million, press the Tab key, and then type 18.30%.

17 Save **2-NSMCDiabetes.docx**.

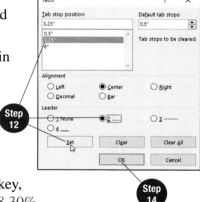

Check Your Work Compare your work with the model answer to ensure that you have completed the activity correctly.

In Addition

Moving a Tab

Move a tab on the horizontal ruler by positioning the mouse pointer on the tab symbol on the horizontal ruler, clicking and holding down the left mouse button, dragging the tab symbol to the new location on the ruler, and then releasing the mouse button.

Setting a Decimal Tab

Set a decimal tab for column entries you want aligned at the decimal point. To set a decimal tab, click the Alignment button above the vertical ruler until the decimal tab symbol ⌐ displays and then click the desired position on the horizontal ruler.

Deleting a Tab

Delete a tab from the horizontal ruler by positioning the arrow pointer on the tab symbol, clicking and holding down the left mouse button, dragging the tab symbol down into the document screen, and then releasing the mouse button.

Clearing Tabs at the Tabs Dialog Box

At the Tabs dialog box, you can clear an individual tab or all tabs. To clear all tabs, click the Clear All button. To clear an individual tab, specify the tab position and then click the Clear button.

Activity 2.9 Adding Borders and Shading

Insert a border around text and/or apply shading to text in a paragraph or selected text with the Borders button and the Shading button in the Paragraph group on the Home tab or at the Borders and Shading dialog box. At the Borders and Shading dialog box with the Borders tab selected, specify the border type, style, color, and width. Click the Shading tab and the dialog box displays options for choosing a fill color and pattern style. Click the Page Border tab and the dialog box displays options for applying a page border. You can also display the Borders and Shading dialog box with the Page Border tab selected by clicking the Design tab and then clicking the Page Borders button in the Page Background group.

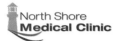
North Shore
Medical Clinic

What You Will Do   To highlight certain information in the diabetes document, you will add borders to specific text, apply shading behind the title, apply shading and a border to the information in tabbed columns, and apply a page border to the entire document.

Tutorial
Applying Borders

Tutorial
Applying Shading

Tutorial
Inserting a Page
Border

1 With **2-NSMCDiabetes.docx** open, select the numbered paragraphs of text below the heading *Types of Diabetes*.

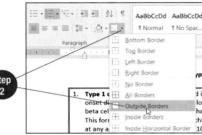

2 Click the Borders button arrow in the Paragraph group on the Home tab and then click *Outside Borders* at the drop-down gallery.

> The button image changes depending on the most recently selected option at the drop-down gallery.

3 Select the title, *UNDERSTANDING DIABETES*; change the font size to 16 points; and then apply bold formatting.

4 Click anywhere in the title, click the Shading button arrow, and then click *More Colors* at the drop-down gallery.

5 At the Colors dialog box with the Standard tab selected, click the light purple color as shown at the right.

6 Click OK to close the Colors dialog box.

7 Select the text from the sentence that begins *The information below shows the population group* through the line of text containing the column entries *60 and older*, *8.6 million*, and *18.30%*.

8 Click the Borders button arrow and then click *Borders and Shading* at the bottom of the drop-down list.

9 At the Borders and Shading dialog box with the Borders tab selected, scroll down at the right side of the *Style* list box until the first double-line option displays and then click the double-line option.

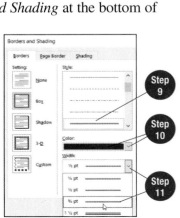

10 Click the *Color* option box arrow and then click the *Dark Blue* option (second option from the right in the *Standard Colors* section).

11 Click the *Width* option box arrow and then click *¾ pt* at the drop-down list.

12 Click the Shading tab.

13 Click the *Fill* option box arrow and then click *More Colors* at the drop-down list.

14 At the Colors dialog box, click the same light purple color you selected in Step 5.

15 Click OK to close the Colors dialog box.

16 With the Borders and Shading dialog box displayed, insert a page border around all pages in the document. Begin by clicking the Page Border tab.

> You can also display the Borders and Shading dialog box with the Page Border tab selected by clicking the Design tab and then clicking the Page Borders button in the Page Background group.

17 Click the *Shadow* option in the *Setting* section.

18 Click the *Color* option box arrow and then click the *Dark Blue* option in the *Standard Colors* section (second option from the right).

19 Click the *Width* option box arrow and then click *2 ¼ pt* at the drop-down list.

20 Click OK to close the Borders and Shading dialog box.

21 Select the entire document and then change the font to Georgia.

22 Click in the heading *Dental Disease*, display the Paragraph dialog box with the Line and Page Breaks tab selected, click the *Keep with next* check box to insert a check mark, and then click OK.

23 Save, print, and then close **2-NSMCDiabetes.docx**.

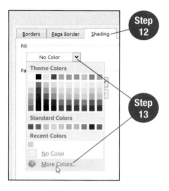

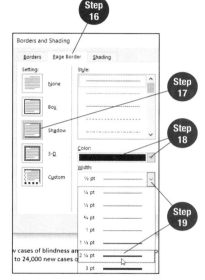

Check Your Work Compare your work with the model answer to ensure that you have completed the activity correctly.

In Addition

Applying Borders

The Borders and Shading dialog box, with the Borders tab or the Page Borders tab selected, contains a *Preview* section you can use to insert borders at specific locations. A diagram displays in the *Preview* section and you can click the sides, top, or bottom of the diagram to insert or remove a border line. Buttons display around the diagram that you can also use to insert or remove borders.

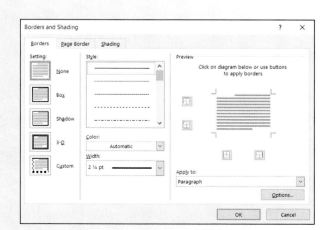

Activity 2.10   Applying Styles, Style Sets, and Themes

A Word document is based on a template that applies default formatting such as 11-point Calibri font, 1.08 line spacing, and 8 points of spacing after each paragraph. You can change these default formats with buttons and options on the ribbon and also with styles. A style is a set of formatting instructions you can apply to text. To apply a predesigned style, click the desired style in the styles gallery in the Styles group on the Home tab. Click the More Styles button at the right side of the styles gallery to display a drop-down gallery of additional styles. Word groups styles that apply similar formatting into style sets. Style sets are available in the Document Formatting group on the Design tab. If you choose a different style set, the styles in the Styles group on the Home tab change to reflect the currently selected style set. A style set changes the formatting applied by styles. In addition to a style set, you can also apply formatting to a document with a theme. A theme is a set of formatting choices that includes a color theme (a set of colors), a font theme (a set of heading and body text fonts), and an effects theme (a set of lines and fill effects). Apply a theme with the Themes button in the Document Formatting group on the Design tab. Customize a theme (or style set) with the Colors, Fonts, and Effects buttons.

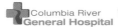
Columbia River General Hospital

What You Will Do   You have been asked by Douglas Brown, legal counsel, to format a document that explains records storage and maintenance at the hospital. You decide to apply styles and a theme to enhance the appearance of the document.

Tutorial
Applying Styles and Style Sets

Tutorial
Applying and Modifying a Theme

1 Open **CRGHRecords.docx** and then save it with the name **2-CRGHRecords**.

2 Apply a heading style to the title by clicking anywhere in the title *Maintaining Medical Records* and then clicking the *Heading 1* option in the Styles group on the Home tab.

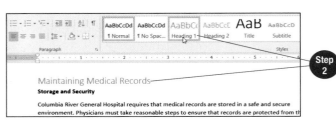

3 Click anywhere in the heading *Storage and Security* and then click the *Heading 2* option.

> The Heading 1 and Heading 2 styles apply both paragraph and character formatting. Some styles apply only paragraph formatting and others apply only character formatting.

4 Apply the Heading 2 style to the headings *Creating a Patient Profile* and *Creating Progress Notes*.

5 Apply a different style set by clicking the Design tab, clicking the More Style Sets button ⬇ at the right of the style set thumbnails in the Document Formatting group, and then clicking the *Lines (Stylish)* option.

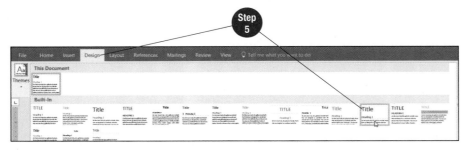

6 Change the paragraph spacing by clicking the Paragraph Spacing button in the Document Formatting group and then clicking *Relaxed* at the drop-down gallery.

7 Apply a theme by clicking the Themes button in the Document Formatting group and then clicking the *Organic* option at the drop-down gallery.

8 Change the theme colors by clicking the Colors button in the Document Formatting group and then clicking the *Blue II* option at the drop-down gallery.

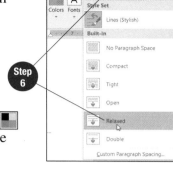

Step 6

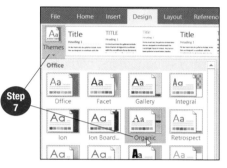

Step 7

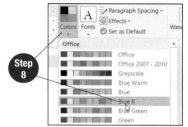

Step 8

9 Change the theme fonts by clicking the Fonts button in the Document Formatting group and then clicking the *Corbel* option at the drop-down gallery.

10 Save, print, and then close **2-CRGHRecords.docx**.

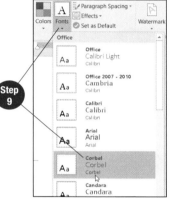

Step 9

Check Your Work — Compare your work with the model answer to ensure that you have completed the activity correctly.

In Addition

Applying the No Spacing Style

By default, a blank document contains line spacing of 1.08 and 8 points of spacing after paragraphs. The increase in line spacing and spacing after paragraphs creates more space between lines and is designed to make text easier to read on a computer screen. You can change the line spacing to 1.0 and remove the spacing after paragraphs by clicking the *No Spacing* style in the Styles group on the Home tab.

Collapsing and Expanding Headings

When you apply heading styles to text in a document, you can collapse text below the headings. By collapsing text, you can view the headings in your document and use them to easily navigate to specific locations. Collapse text in a document by clicking the gray triangle that displays when you hover the mouse pointer over

text with a heading style applied. Expand collapsed text by clicking the white triangle before a heading with a style applied.

Applying Styles at the Styles Window

The Styles window provides additional styles. Display this window by clicking the Styles group dialog box launcher. The styles in the currently selected style set display in the window followed by a paragraph symbol (¶), indicating that the style applies paragraph formatting, or a character symbol (a), indicating that the style applies character formatting. If both characters display to the right of a style, the style applies both paragraph and character formatting. In addition to displaying styles that apply formatting, the Styles window also includes a Clear All style that clears all formatting from selected text.

Activity 2.11   Insert the Date, Time, and Quick Parts

Insert the current date and/or time into a document with options at the Date and Time dialog box. The Date and Time dialog box contains a list of date and time options in the *Available formats* list box. If the *Update automatically* check box at the Date and Time dialog box does not contain a check mark, the date and/or time are inserted in the document as text that can be edited in the normal manner. You can also insert the date and/or time as a field in a document. The advantage to inserting the date or time as a field is that you can automatically update the field by pressing the F9 function key. Insert the date and/or time as a field by inserting a check mark in the *Update automatically* check box before you select an option from the *Available formats* list box. Word also contains a Quick Parts button with options for inserting predesigned building blocks to help you build a document. Building blocks include cover pages, headers and footers, page numbers, tables, text boxes, and watermarks, which are all located at the Building Blocks Organizer dialog box.

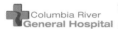 Columbia River General Hospital

What You Will Do   While reviewing the draft version of Columbia River General Hospital's document containing information on creating and maintaining medical records, you decide to insert the date and time and identify the document as a draft.

Tutorial
Inserting the Date and Time

Tutorial
Inserting and Sorting Building Blocks

1. Open **CRGHLegal.docx** and then save it with the name **2-CRGHLegal**.

2. Press Ctrl + End to move the insertion point to the end of the document.

3. Type Date: and then press the spacebar.

4. Click the Insert tab and then click the Date & Time button 📅 in the Text group.

5. At the Date and Time dialog box, click the third option from the top in the *Available formats* list box. (Your date will vary from what you see below.)

6. Click the *Update automatically* check box to insert a check mark and then click OK to close the dialog box.

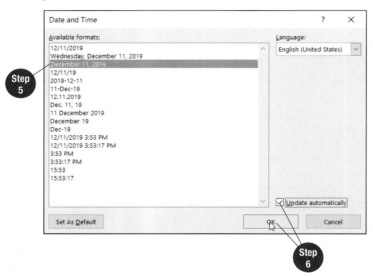

7. Press Shift + Enter, type Time:, and then press the spacebar.

8. Click the Date & Time button.

In Brief

Display Date and Time Dialog box
1. Click Insert tab.
2. Click Date and Time button.

Display Building Blocks Organizer Dialog Box
1. Click Insert tab.
2. Click Quick Parts button.
3. Click *Building Blocks Organizer.*

9 At the Date and Time dialog box, click the option that will insert the time in numbers with the hour, minutes, and seconds (for example, *3:53:56 PM*). Make sure the *Update automatically* check box contains a check mark and then click OK to close the dialog box.

This option may be the fourteenth or fifteenth from the top in the *Available formats* list box.

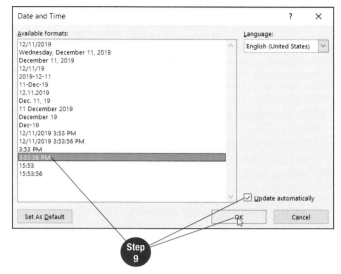

Step 9

10 Print the document.

11 To identify the document as a draft, insert a building block with the word *DRAFT* as a watermark (a lightened image behind the text). To begin, click the Quick Parts button in the Text group on the Insert tab and then click *Building Blocks Organizer* at the drop-down list.

Step 11

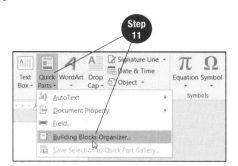

12 At the Building Blocks Organizer dialog box, click the *Gallery* column heading.

This sorts the building blocks alphabetically by gallery.

Step 12

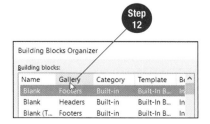

13 Scroll to the end of the list box, click *DRAFT 1*, and then click the Insert button.

> You may not see the entire name of the quick part in the list box, but if you click the first part of the name, the full name of the quick part will display in the lower right corner of the dialog box below the preview section.

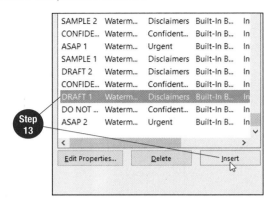

14 To begin inserting a predesigned cover page quick part, press Ctrl + Home to move the insertion point to the beginning of the document, click the Quick Parts button in the Text group on the Insert tab, and then click *Building Blocks Organizer* at the drop-down list.

15 At the Building Blocks Organizer dialog box, click the *Semaphore* cover page option in the list box and then click the Insert button.

> After you click *Semaphore*, check the Gallery column to make sure it contains the text *Cover Page*.

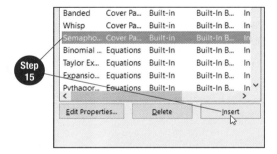

16 Click in the *[DATE]* placeholder text to select it, click the arrow at the right of the placeholder, and then click the Today button at the drop-down list.

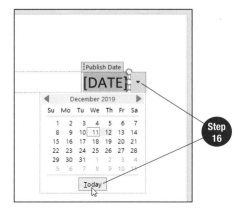

17 Click in the *[DOCUMENT TITLE]* placeholder text and then type Creating and Maintaining Medical Records.

18 Select the title *Creating and Maintaining Medical Records* and then change the font size to 36 points.

19 Click in the *[DOCUMENT SUBTITLE]* placeholder text and then type Legal Department.

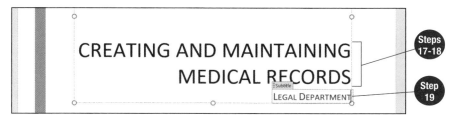

20 Click the text below the title (might be a personal name or a school name), click the placeholder tab, and then type your first and last names.

21 Click in the *[COMPANY NAME]* placeholder text and then type Columbia River General Hospital.

22 Click in the *[Company address]* placeholder text, click the placeholder tab, and then press the Delete key.

> Clicking a placeholder tab selects that object.

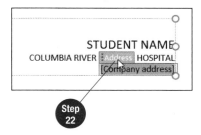

23 Press Ctrl + End to move the insertion point to the end of the document, click anywhere in the time text, and then press F9 to update the time.

> Pressing F9, the Update Field key, updates the time. You can also update the time by clicking the Update tab above the selected time.

24 Save, print, and then close **2-CRGHLegal.docx**.

> **Check Your Work** ▸ Compare your work with the model answer to ensure that you have completed the activity correctly.

In Addition

Sorting Data in the Building Blocks Organizer

The Building Blocks Organizer dialog box provides a single location where you can view all of the pre-designed building blocks available in Word. You can sort the building blocks in the dialog box alphabeti-cally by clicking the column headings. For example, to sort building blocks alphabetically by name, click the *Name* column heading.

Features Summary

Feature	Ribbon Tab, Group	Button, Option	Keyboard Shortcut
1.5 line spacing	Home, Paragraph		Ctrl + 5
align left	Home, Paragraph		Ctrl + L
align right	Home, Paragraph		Ctrl + R
bold	Home, Font	B	Ctrl + B
borders	Home, Paragraph		
bullets	Home, Paragraph		
center	Home, Paragraph		Ctrl + E
change case	Home, Font	Aa	Shift + F3
clear all formatting	Home, Font		
date	Insert, Text		Shift + Alt + D
decrease indent	Home, Paragraph		Ctrl + Shift + M
double line spacing	Home, Paragraph		Ctrl + 2
font	Home, Font		Ctrl + Shift + F
font color	Home, Font	A	
Font dialog box	Home, Font		Ctrl + D
font size	Home, Font		Ctrl + Shift + P
Format Painter	Home, Clipboard		Ctrl + Shift + C
hanging indent			Ctrl + T
highlight	Home, Font		
increase indent	Home, Paragraph		Ctrl + M
italics	Home, Font	I	Ctrl + I
justify	Home, Paragraph		Ctrl + J
line and paragraph spacing	Home, Paragraph		
numbering	Home, Paragraph		
Paragraph dialog box	Home, Paragraph		

continues...

Feature	Ribbon Tab, Group	Button, Option	Keyboard Shortcut
remove hanging indent			Ctrl + Shift + T
shading	Home, Paragraph		
single line spacing	Home, Paragraph		Ctrl + 1
spacing after paragraphs	Layout, Paragraph		
spacing before paragraphs	Layout, Paragraph		
styles	Home, Styles		
style sets	Design, Document Formatting		
subscript	Home, Font	X₂	
superscript	Home, Font	x²	
symbols	Insert, Symbols	Ω	
Tabs dialog box	Home, Paragraph OR Layout, Paragraph	, Tabs	
theme colors	Design, Document Formatting		
theme fonts	Design, Document Formatting	A	
themes	Design, Document Formatting	Aa	
underline	Home, Font	U ▾	Ctrl + U

Workbook Section study tools and assessment activities are available in the Workbook pages of the ebook. These resources are designed to help you further develop and demonstrate mastery of the skills learned in this section.

Word

Formatting and Enhancing a Document

Data Files Before beginning section work, copy the WordMedS3 folder to your storage medium and then make WordMedS3 the active folder.

Skills

- Find and replace text and formatting
- Reveal formatting
- Cut, copy, and paste text
- Use the Clipboard task pane to copy and paste items
- Change page margins and orientation
- Customize the page and page background
- Insert page numbers, headers, and footers

- Insert a page break and a section break
- Create and modify columns
- Insert, size, and move images
- Insert, size, and move WordArt
- Insert the contents of one file into another file
- Insert and customize shapes and text boxes
- Prepare an envelope
- Prepare labels

Precheck Check your current skills to help focus your study of the skills taught in this section.

Activities Overview

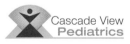

Edit, format, and reorganize a child development assessment form; format and add visual appeal to a monthly newsletter; enhance the appearance of a parenting class flyer; format and add visual appeal to a patient confidentiality document; prepare an envelope and mailing labels; prepare a notice and two announcements; and format a document on Fifth disease.

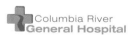

Format and add visual appeal to a document on writing and maintaining medical records.

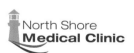

Prepare an envelope and mailing labels, format and add visual appeal to a document on fibromyalgia, and flip and copy shapes to create a clinic notice.

Model Answers Preview the model answers for an overview of the activities you will complete in each section.

Activity 3.1 Finding and Replacing Text

Use the Find and Replace feature to find specific text and replace it with other text. For example, you can create a template for an agreement by using a generic name throughout the document. You can then find and replace the generic name with a real name later on. To avoid having to constantly re-type a long phrase that occurs often in a document, you can type an abbreviation instead and then find and replace the abbreviations with the full phrase when you are finished. You can also find and replace certain formatting. These options are available at the Find and Replace dialog box with the Replace tab selected.

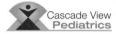

What You Will Do   Sydney Larsen, the office manager at Cascade View Pediatrics, has asked you to proofread the Assessment of Child Development form that parents fill out before each well-child appointment. Your review identifies some spelling and grammar errors that you will correct using the Find and Replace feature.

Tutorial
Finding and Replacing
Text

1. Open **CDAssessment.docx** and then save it with the name **3-CDAssessment**.

2. After looking over the document, you realize that *development* is misspelled as *developement* throughout the document. You decide to use the Find and Replace feature to correct this spelling error. To begin, click the Replace button in the Editing group on the Home tab.

3. At the Find and Replace dialog box with the Replace tab selected, type developement in the *Find what* text box and then press the Tab key.

    Pressing the Tab key moves the insertion point to the *Replace with* text box.

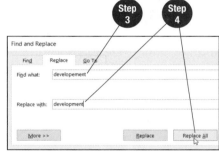

4. Type development in the *Replace with* text box and then click the Replace All button toward the bottom of the dialog box.

    Clicking the Replace All button replaces all occurrences of the text in the document. If you want control over which instances in a document are replaced, use the Find Next and Replace buttons to move through the document and replace or skip over each instance individually.

5. At the message telling you that three replacements were made, click OK.

6. Click the Close button to close the Find and Replace dialog box.

7. Looking at the document, you realize that *well-baby* should be replaced with *well-child*. To begin, display the Find and Replace dialog box by clicking the Replace button in the Editing group.

8. At the Find and Replace dialog box with the Replace tab selected, type well-baby in the *Find what* text box.

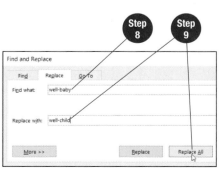

9. Press the Tab key, type well-child in the *Replace with* text box, and then click the Replace All button.

10. At the message telling you that two replacements were made, click OK.

11 Click the Close button to close the Find and Replace dialog box.

12 Select the title, *ASSESSMENT OF CHILD DEVELOPMENT*, change the font to 16-point Candara, apply bold formatting, change the alignment to center, and then add 12 points of spacing after the paragraph.

13 Select the subtitle *Ages Newborn to Three Years*, change the font to 14-point Candara, apply bold formatting, change the alignment to center, and then add 9 points of spacing after the paragraph.

14 Change the font of the headings *Child Development – Talking* and *Child Development – Hearing* to 12-point Candara and then apply bold formatting.

15 Save **3-CDAssessment.docx**.

Check Your Work Compare your work with the model answer to ensure that you have completed the activity correctly.

In Addition

Exploring Options at the Expanded Find and Replace Dialog Box

The Find and Replace dialog box contains a variety of check boxes with options you can choose for completing a find and replace. To display these options, click the More button at the bottom of the dialog box. This causes the Find and Replace dialog box to expand as shown at the right. The options are described in the table below.

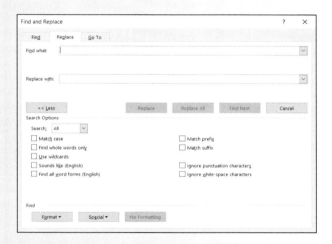

Option	Action
Match case	Exactly match the case of the search text. For example, if you search for *Book*, Word will stop at *Book* but not *book* or *BOOK*.
Find whole words only	Find a whole word, not a part of a word. For example, if you search for *her*, Word will stop at *her* but not *there*, *here*, or *hers*.
Use wildcards	Search for wildcards, special characters, or special search operators. For example, search for le*s, and Word finds *less*, *leases*, and *letters*.
Sounds like	Match words that sound alike but are spelled differently, such as *know* and *no*.
Find all word forms	Find all forms of the word entered in the *Find what* text box. For example, if you search for *hold*, Word will stop at *held* and *holding*.
Match prefix	Find only those words that begin with the letters in the *Find what* text box. For example, if you enter *per*, Word will stop at words such as *perform* and *perfect* but skip over words such as *super* and *hyperlink*.
Match suffix	Find only those words that end with the letters in the *Find what* text box. For example, if you search for *ly*, Word will stop at words such as *accurately* and *quietly* but skip over words such as *catalyst* and *lyre*.
Ignore punctuation characters	Ignore punctuation within characters. For example, if you enter *US* in the *Find what* text box, Word will stop at *U.S.*
Ignore white-space characters	Ignore spaces between letters. For example, if you enter *F B I* in the *Find what* text box, Word will stop at *FBI*.

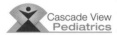

Activity 3.2 Revealing Formatting; Finding and Replacing Formatting

Display formatting applied to specific text in a document at the Reveal Formatting task pane. Display this task pane by pressing Shift + F1. The Reveal Formatting task pane displays font, paragraph, and section formatting that has been applied to the selected text or the text in which the insertion point is positioned. As mentioned in Activity 3.1, you can use options at the Find and Replace dialog box with the Replace tab selected to search for specific formatting or for text with specific formatting applied and replace it with different formatting. Click the More button to expand the options in the Find and Replace dialog box. Use the Format button at the expanded dialog box to specify the type of formatting to find and also the type of replacement formatting.

Cascade View Pediatrics

What You Will Do After reviewing the Assessment of Child Development form, you decide that the headings would look better in a different font and font color. To display the formatting applied to specific text, you will use the Reveal Formatting task pane. You will then use Find and Replace to change the font formatting.

Tutorial
Finding and Replacing Formatting

1 With **3-CDAssessment.docx** open, press Ctrl + Home to move the insertion point to the beginning of the document and then press Shift + F1.

Pressing Shift + F1 displays the Reveal Formatting task pane with information on the formatting applied to the title. Generally, a black triangle precedes *Font* and *Paragraph* and a white triangle precedes *Section* in the *Formatting of selected text* section. Clicking a black triangle hides items displayed below a heading and clicking a white triangle reveals them. Some items in the Reveal Formatting task pane are hyperlinks. For example, click the FONT hyperlink to display the Font dialog box. Use these hyperlinks to make changes to the document formatting.

2 Click anywhere in the paragraph of text below the subtitle and look at the Reveal Formatting task pane to determine the formatting.

3 Click anywhere in the heading *Child Development – Talking* and then notice the formatting applied to it.

4 Close the Reveal Formatting task pane by clicking the Close button in the upper right corner of the task pane.

5 You decide to change the font formatting of all text in 12-point Candara bold to 13-point Cambria bold in a dark blue font color. Start by positioning the insertion point at the beginning of the document and then clicking the Replace button in the Editing group on the Home tab.

6 At the Find and Replace dialog box, press the Delete key. (This deletes any text that displays in the *Find what* text box.)

7 Click the More button. (If a check mark displays in the *Find all word forms* check box, click to remove it.)

8 Click the Format button at the bottom of the dialog box and then click *Font* at the drop-down list.

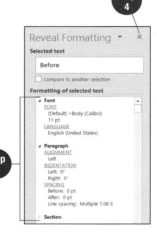

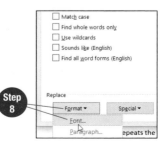

9 At the Find Font dialog box, change the font to *Candara*, the font style to *Bold*, and the size to *12*. Click OK to close the dialog box.

10 At the Find and Replace dialog box, press the Tab key and then press the Delete key. (This removes any text in the *Replace with* text box.)

11 Click the Format button at the bottom of the dialog box and then click *Font* at the drop-down list.

12 At the Replace Font dialog box, change the font to Cambria, the font style to Bold, the size to 13, and the font color to Dark Blue. Click OK to close the dialog box.

> To change the font size to *13*, select the existing text in the *Size* text box and then type 13.

13 At the Find and Replace dialog box, click the Replace All button. At the message telling you that the search of the document is complete and two replacements were made, click OK.

14 With the Find and Replace dialog box open and the insertion point positioned in the *Find what* text box, click the No Formatting button near the bottom of the dialog box. Press the Tab key to move the insertion point to the *Replace with* text box and then click the No Formatting button. (This deletes any font formatting that displays in the *Find what* and *Replace with* text boxes.)

15 With the Find and Replace dialog box open, find all text set in 12-point Calibri bold and replace it with 11-point Cambria bold in Dark Blue.

> Twelve replacements should be made.

16 At the Find and Replace dialog box with the insertion point positioned in the *Find what* text box, click the No Formatting button. Press the Tab key and then click the No Formatting button. Click the Less button and then click the Close button.

17 Select the title, *ASSESSMENT OF CHILD DEVELOPMENT*, and the subtitle *Ages Newborn to Three Years* and then change the font to 16-point Cambria and apply the Dark Blue font color. (Make sure bold formatting is still applied to the title and subtitle.)

18 Save **3-CDAssessment.docx**.

Check Your Work Compare your work with the model answer to ensure that you have completed the activity correctly.

In Addition

Comparing Formatting

Along with displaying formatting applied to text, you can use the Reveal Formatting task pane to compare formatting of two text selections to determine what is different. To compare formatting, display the Reveal Formatting task pane and then select the first instance of formatting to be compared. Click the *Compare to another selection* check box to insert a check mark and then select the second instance of formatting to compare. Any differences between the two selections will display in the *Formatting differences* list box.

Cutting, Copying, and Pasting Text; Using Paste Special

With the Cut, Copy, and Paste buttons in the Clipboard group on the Home tab, you can move and/or copy words, sentences, or entire sections of text to other locations in a document. You can cut and paste text or copy and paste text within the same document or between documents. Specify the formatting of pasted text with the Paste Options button or options at the Paste Special dialog box.

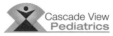
Cascade View Pediatrics

What You Will Do   After consulting with Deanna Reynolds, the child development specialist at Cascade View Pediatrics, Sydney Larsen has asked you to reorganize the Assessment of Child Development form and include additional information from other sources.

Tutorial
Cutting, Copying, and Pasting Text

Tutorial
Using the Paste Options Button

Tutorial
Using Paste Special

1 With **3-CDAssessment.docx** open, move the *Child Development – Hearing* section above the *Child Development – Talking* section. Begin by selecting from the beginning of the *Child Development – Hearing* heading to the end of the document.

2 Click the Cut button ✂ in the Clipboard group on the Home tab.

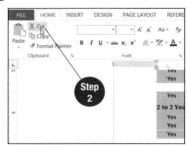

This places the text in a location called the Clipboard.

3 Position the insertion point at the beginning of the heading *Child Development – Talking* and then click the Paste button 📋 in the Clipboard group on the Home tab.

A Paste Options button 📋 (Ctrl) ▼ displays below the pasted text. Click this button to display a drop-down gallery of buttons. Use these buttons to specify the formatting of the pasted text. By default, the Keep Source Formatting button (first button from the left) is selected. With this button selected, text is pasted with the formatting from the source document. You can also click the Merge Formatting button (middle button) to merge formatting with the destination formatting or click the Keep Text Only button (third button) to paste only the text and not the formatting.

4 Copy text from another document and paste it in the Assessment of Child Development document. To begin, open **CDSpecialistQuestions.docx**.

5 Select the line containing the text *Child's Name:* _____ and the two lines of text below it and then click the Copy button 📋 in the Clipboard group.

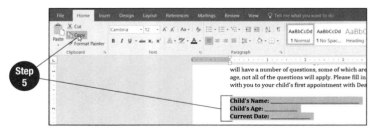

6 Click the Word button on the taskbar and then click the **3-CDAssessment.docx** thumbnail.

7 Position the insertion point at the end of the first paragraph of text (the paragraph that begins *Before you bring your child to the next*) and then press the Enter key two times.

Cut and Paste Text
1. Select text.
2. Click Cut button.
3. Position insertion point.
4. Click Paste button.

Copy and Paste Text
1. Select text.
2. Click Copy button.
3. Position insertion point.
4. Click Paste button.

Use Paste Special Dialog Box
1. Cut or copy text.
2. Click Paste button arrow.
3. Click *Paste Special*.
4. Click format in *As* list box.
5. Click OK.

8 Click the Paste button in the Clipboard group.

9 Click the Paste Options button in the lower right corner of the pasted text and then click the Merge Formatting button.

> The copied text and the heading below it should be separated by one blank line (a double space).

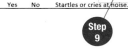

10 Click the Word button on the taskbar and then click the **CDSpecialistQuestions.docx** thumbnail.

11 Move the insertion point to the end of the document and then select the heading *Additional Information* and the paragraph of text below it.

12 Click the Copy button in the Clipboard group.

13 Click the Word button on the taskbar and then click the **3-CDAssessment.docx** thumbnail.

14 Move the insertion point to the end of the document and then press the Enter key two times. (The insertion point should be positioned a double space below the last line of text.)

15 Paste the copied text into the document without the formatting by clicking the Paste button arrow and then clicking *Paste Special* at the drop-down list.

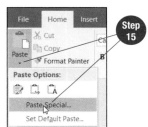

16 At the Paste Special dialog box, click *Unformatted Text* in the *As* list box and then click OK.

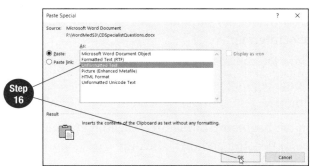

17 Set the heading *Additional Information* in 11-point Cambria and then apply bold formatting and the Dark Blue font color.

18 Save **3-CDAssessment.docx**.

Check Your Work Compare your work with the model answer to ensure that you have completed the activity correctly.

In Addition

Moving and Copying Text with the Mouse

You can move selected text using the mouse. To do this, select the text with the mouse and then move the I-beam pointer inside the selected text until the I-beam pointer turns into an arrow pointer. Click and hold down the left mouse button, drag the arrow pointer (with a gray box attached) to the location where you want to insert the selected text, and then release the mouse button. Copy and move selected text by following similar steps, but hold down the Ctrl key while dragging with the mouse. When you hold down the Ctrl key, a box containing a plus symbol displays near the gray box attached to the arrow pointer.

Activity 3.4   Using the Clipboard Task Pane

Using the Clipboard task pane, you can collect up to 24 different items and then paste them in various locations in a document. Display the Clipboard task pane by clicking the Clipboard group task pane launcher on the Home tab. Cut or copy an item and the item displays in the Clipboard task pane. If the item is text, the first 50 characters display. Paste an item by positioning the insertion point at the desired location and then clicking the item in the Clipboard task pane. Once all desired items have been inserted, click the Clear All button in the upper right corner of the task pane.

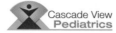
Cascade View
Pediatrics

What You Will Do   Sydney Larsen wants you to include additional information from the Child Development Specialist Questionnaire in the Assessment of Child Development form. You will use the Clipboard task pane to copy sections of text from the questionnaire and paste them into the form.

Tutorial
Using the Clipboard
Task Pane

1   Make sure **3-CDAssessment.docx** and **CDSpecialistQuestions.docx** are open.

2   Make **CDSpecialistQuestions.docx** active and then display the Clipboard task pane by clicking the Clipboard group task pane launcher on the Home tab. If items display in the Clipboard task pane, click the Clear All button in the upper right corner of the task pane.

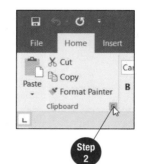
Step 2

3   Select from the beginning of the *Family Health History* heading to the blank line just above the next heading (*Feeding/Oral Behavior*) and then click the Copy button in the Clipboard group.

  Notice how the copied item appears in the Clipboard task pane.

4   Select from the beginning of the *Feeding/Oral Behavior* heading to the blank line just above the *Sleep* heading and then click the Copy button.

5   Select from the beginning of the *Sleep* heading to the blank line just above the *Your Child's Health* heading and then click the Copy button.

6   Select from the beginning of the *Feelings and Moods* heading to the blank line just above the *Additional Information* heading and then click the Copy button.

7   Click the Word button on the taskbar and then click the **3-CDAssessment.docx** thumbnail.

8   Click the Clipboard group task pane launcher to display the Clipboard task pane.

9   Move the insertion point to the blank line immediately above the heading *Additional Information* near the end of the document and then press the Enter key.

10   In the Clipboard task pane, click the item representing *Feelings and Moods*.

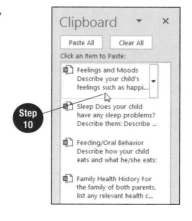
Step 10

11   Click the Paste Options button that displays below the pasted text and then click the Merge Formatting button.

In Brief

Use Clipboard Task Pane
1. Click Clipboard group task pane launcher.
2. Select text.
3. Click Copy button.
4. Select and copy any additional items.
5. Position insertion point.
6. Click item in Clipboard task pane.
7. Paste any other items from Clipboard task pane.
8. Click Clear All button.
9. Close task pane.

12 With the insertion point positioned on the blank line immediately above the heading *Additional Information*, click the item in the Clipboard task pane representing *Feeding/Oral Behavior*.

13 Click the Paste Options button and then click the Merge Formatting button.

14 With the insertion point positioned on the blank line immediately above the heading *Additional Information*, paste the item representing *Sleep*.

15 Click the Paste Options button and then click the Merge Formatting button.

16 Click the Clear All button in the upper right corner of the Clipboard task pane.

17 Close the Clipboard task pane by clicking the Close button in the upper right corner of the task pane.

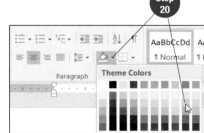

18 Click the Word button on the taskbar, click the **CDSpecialistQuestions.docx** thumbnail, and then close the document.

This displays **3-CDAssessment.docx**.

19 Set the headings *Feelings and Moods*, *Feeding/Oral Behavior*, and *Sleep* in 11-point Cambria bold and then apply the Dark Blue font color.

20 Select the title, *ASSESSMENT OF CHILD DEVELOPMENT*, and the subtitle *Ages Newborn to Three Years*, click the Shading button arrow, and then click the *Blue, Accent 5, Lighter 60%* option (ninth column, third row in the *Theme Colors* section).

21 Apply Blue, Accent 5, Lighter 80% shading to the headings *Child Development – Hearing* and *Child Development – Talking*.

22 Save **3-CDAssessment.docx**.

Check Your Work Compare your work with the model answer to ensure that you have completed the activity correctly.

In Addition

Using Clipboard Task Pane Options

Click the Options button at the bottom of the Clipboard task pane and a pop-up menu displays with five options as shown at the right. Insert a check mark before the options you want active. For example, you can choose to display the Clipboard task pane automatically when you cut or copy text, display the Clipboard task pane by pressing Ctrl + C two times, cut and copy text without displaying the Clipboard task pane, display the Office Clipboard icon on the taskbar when the Clipboard is active, or display a status message near the taskbar when copying items to the Clipboard. If the last option is selected, a message such as 2 of 24 - Clipboard displays at the right side of the taskbar.

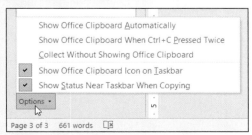

Activity 3.5   Customizing the Page Setup

In Word, a page contains default formatting such as a page size of 8.5 inches by 11 inches; top, bottom, left, and right margins of one inch; portrait page orientation; and a page break after approximately 9 inches of content on a page. You can change these defaults with buttons in the Page Setup group on the Layout tab. Change the default margins in a document with the Margins button. With the Orientation button, you can change the orientation from the default portrait to landscape. Use the Size button in the Page Setup group to specify a paper size.

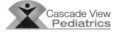 Cascade View Pediatrics

What You Will Do   To further improve the Assessment of Child Development form, you will change the document margins, orientation, and page size and then improve the appearance of the document by applying a theme and changing the theme colors.

Tutorial
Changing Margins

Tutorial
Changing Page
Orientation

Tutorial
Changing Paper Size

1 With **3-CDAssessment.docx** open, click the Layout tab, click the Margins button in the Page Setup group, and then click the *Office 2003 Default* option.

> The *Office 2003 Default* option changes the left and right margins to 1.25 inches, which is the default setting for Word 2003.

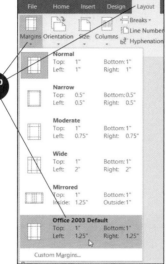

2 Change the page orientation by clicking the Orientation button in the Page Setup group on the Layout tab and then clicking *Landscape* at the drop-down list.

> Word considers a page in portrait orientation to be 8.5 inches wide and 11 inches tall. Word considers a page in landscape orientation to be 11 inches wide and 8.5 inches tall. You can also change page orientation at the Page Setup dialog box with the Margins tab selected.

3 With the document in landscape orientation, you decide to make changes to the margins. To begin, click the Margins button in the Page Setup group on the Layout tab and then click the text *Custom Margins* at the bottom of the drop-down list.

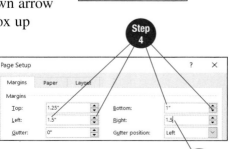

4 At the Page Setup dialog box with the Margins tab selected, click the *Bottom* measurement box down arrow until *1"* displays. Click the *Left* measurement box up arrow until *1.5"* displays.

> You can also change a margin by selecting the measurement and then typing the new measurement.

5 Select the current number in the *Right* measurement box and then type 1.5.

6 Click OK to close the Page Setup dialog box.

In Brief

Change Margins
1. Click Layout tab.
2. Click Margins button.
3. Click margins option.

Change Orientation
1. Click Layout tab.
2. Click Orientation button.
3. Click orientation option.

Change Page Size
1. Click Layout tab.
2. Click Size button.
3. Click size option.

7 You decide to experiment with paper size. Click the Size button in the Page Setup group and then click the *Legal* option at the drop-down list.

Your drop-down list may display differently than what you see in the image below.

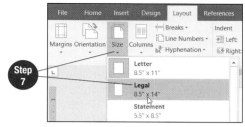

8 Scroll through the document and notice how it is affected by changing the page size to Legal. Return the document to the default page size by clicking the Size button in the Page Setup group and then clicking *Letter* at the drop-down list.

9 Return the margins to the default setting by clicking the Margins button and then clicking *Normal* at the drop-down list.

10 Return to portrait orientation by clicking the Orientation button and then clicking *Portrait* at the drop-down list.

11 Apply a theme to the document by clicking the Design tab, clicking the Themes button in the Document Formatting group, scrolling down the drop-down gallery, and then clicking the *Parallax* option.

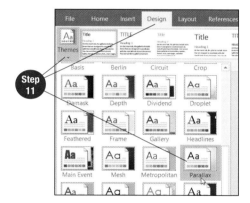

12 Click the Colors button in the Document Formatting group and then click *Blue II* at the drop-down gallery.

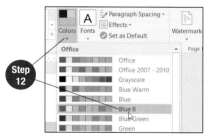

13 Save **3-CDAssessment.docx**.

Check Your Work Compare your work with the model answer to ensure that you have completed the activity correctly.

In Addition

Applying Landscape Orientation

Can you imagine some instances in which you might use a landscape orientation? Suppose you are preparing a company's annual report and you need to include a couple of tables that have several columns of text. If you use the default portrait orientation, the columns will need to be quite narrow, possibly so narrow that reading becomes difficult. Changing the orientation to landscape results in three more inches of usable space. If you choose to use landscape orientation on one page, you are not committed to using it for the entire document. You can use portrait and landscape in the same document. To do this, select the text, display the Page Setup dialog box, click the desired orientation, and then change the *Apply to* option to *Selected text*.

Customizing the Page and Page Background

The Page Background group on the Design tab contains buttons for inserting a watermark, changing the page color, and inserting a page border. In an activity in Section 1, you applied a watermark to a document using options at the Building Blocks Organizer dialog box, but you can also apply a watermark with the Watermark button in the Page Background group on the Design tab. In a project in Section 2, you applied a page border to a document by clicking the Borders button, but you can also apply a page border by using the Page Borders button in the Page Background group. The Pages group on the Insert tab contains buttons for inserting a cover page, a blank page, and a page break.

Cascade View Pediatrics

What You Will Do   To improve the appearance of the Assessment of Child Development document, you will apply page color and a page border. You will insert a cover page at the beginning of the document and identify the document as a draft by inserting a watermark.

Tutorial
Inserting and Removing a Watermark

Tutorial
Applying Page Background Color

Tutorial
Inserting a Page Border

Tutorial
Inserting and Removing a Page Break

Tutorial
Inserting and Removing a Cover Page

1. With **3-CDAssessment.docx** open, press Ctrl + Home.

2. Insert a watermark by clicking the Design tab, clicking the Watermark button 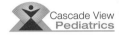 in the Page Background group, scrolling down the drop-down list, and then clicking the *DRAFT 1* option.

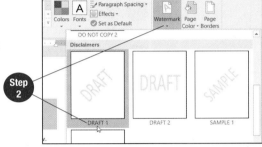

3. Apply a page color to the document by clicking the Page Color button in the Page Background group and then clicking the *Turquoise, Accent 3, Lighter 80%* option (seventh column, second row in the *Theme Colors* section).

   Page color only appears when viewing a document on the screen. The color does not print.

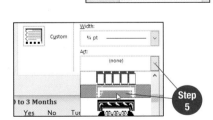

4. Click the Page Borders button in the Page Background group.

5. At the Borders and Shading dialog box with the Page Border tab selected, click the *Art* option box arrow. Scroll down the list of page borders and then click the art border option shown at the right. Click OK to close the dialog box.

6. Move the insertion point to the beginning of the heading *Feelings and Moods* and then insert a hard page break by clicking the Insert tab and then clicking the Page Break button in the Pages group.

   You can also insert a hard page break with the keyboard shortcut Ctrl + Enter or by clicking the Layout tab, clicking the Breaks button in the Page Setup group, and then clicking *Page* at the drop-down list.

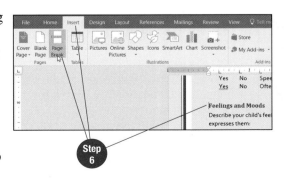

7. Save and then print **3-CDAssessment.docx**. (The page background color does not print.)

8. After looking at the printed document, you decide to make some changes. Remove the page color by clicking the Design tab, clicking the Page Color button in the Page Background group, and then clicking *No Color*.

9. Remove the page border by clicking the Page Borders button, clicking *None* in the *Setting* section of the Borders and Shading dialog box, and then clicking OK.

10. Delete the page break you inserted by positioning the insertion point on the blank line a double space below the line of text in the *2 to 3 Years* section at the bottom of page 2 and then pressing the Delete key two times.

11. Press Ctrl + Home to move the insertion point to the beginning of the document.

12. Insert a cover page by clicking the Insert tab, clicking the Cover Page button in the Pages group, scrolling down the drop-down list, and then clicking the *Whisp* option.

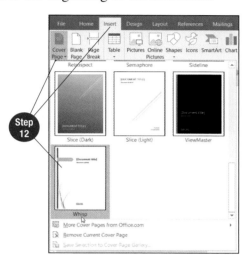

13. Click the *[Date]* placeholder text, click the arrow at the right of the placeholder, and then click the Today button to insert the current date.

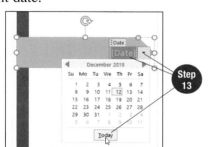

14. Click the *[Document title]* placeholder text and then type Assessment of Child Development.

15. Click the *[Document subtitle]* placeholder text and then type Ages Newborn to Three Years.

16. Click the *[COMPANY NAME]* placeholder text and then type Cascade View Pediatrics.

17. Select the name that displays above *CASCADE VIEW PEDIATRICS* and then type your first and last names.

18. Save **3-CDAssessment.docx**.

Check Your Work ▷ Compare your work with the model answer to ensure that you have completed the activity correctly.

In Addition

Inserting a Blank Page

The Pages group on the Insert tab contains a Blank Page button. Click this button to insert a blank page at the position of the insertion point. Inserting a blank page can be useful as a placeholder in a document when you want to insert an illustration, graphic, or figure.

Insert page numbers in a document with the Page Number button or in a header or footer. Click the Page Number button in the Header & Footer group on the Insert tab and a drop-down list displays with options for inserting page numbers at the top or bottom of the page or in the page margins, removing page numbers, and formatting page numbers. Text that appears at the top of every page is called a header and text that appears at the bottom of every page is referred to as a footer. Headers and footers are common in manuscripts, text-books, reports, and other publications. Insert a predesigned header in a document with the Header button in the Header & Footer group on the Insert tab. Insert a predesigned footer in the same manner as a header. Predesigned headers and footers contain formatting that you can customize.

Cascade View
Pediatrics

What You Will Do   Put the finishing touches on the Assessment of Child Development document by adding a header, footer, and page numbers.

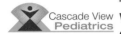
Tutorial
Inserting and Removing Page Numbers

Tutorial
Inserting and Removing a Predesigned Header and Footer

Tutorial
Editing a Header and Footer

1 With **3-CDAssessment.docx** open, move the insertion point to the beginning of the title *ASSESSMENT OF CHILD DEVELOPMENT* at the top of the second page (*not* on the cover page).

When a document contains a cover page, you generally insert elements such as page numbers, headers, and footers on the first page *after* the cover page.

2 Insert numbers at the bottom of each page by clicking the Insert tab, clicking the Page Number button in the Header & Footer group, and then pointing to *Bottom of Page*.

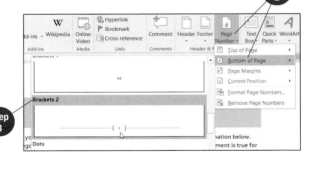

3 At the gallery of predesigned page numbers, scroll down and then click the *Brackets 2* option.

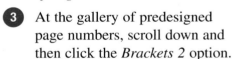

4 Double-click in the body of the document and then scroll through the document, observing how the page numbers display toward the bottom of each page except the cover page.

5 Remove page numbering by clicking the Insert tab, clicking the Page Number button in the Header & Footer group, and then clicking *Remove Page Numbers* at the drop-down list.

6 Insert a header in the document by clicking the Header button in the Header & Footer group, scrolling down the drop-down list, and then clicking the *Motion (Even Page)* option.

Notice how the document title you entered in the cover page is inserted in the header.

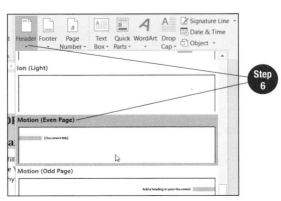

In Brief

Insert Page Numbers
1. Click Insert tab.
2. Click Page Number button.
3. Point to location.
4. Click page number option.

Insert Header
1. Click Insert tab.
2. Click Header button.
3. Click header option.

Insert Footer
1. Click Insert tab.
2. Click Footer button.
3. Click footer option.

7 Double-click in the body of the document.

> This makes the document active and dims the header.

8 Insert a footer in the document by clicking the Insert tab, clicking the Footer button in the Header & Footer group, scrolling down the drop-down list, and then clicking the *Motion (Odd Page)* option.

> Notice how the date you entered in the cover page is automatically inserted in the footer.

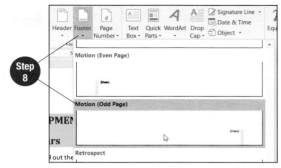

9 Click the Close Header and Footer button ☒ to close the footer pane and then scroll through the document, observing how the header and footer appear on each page except the cover page.

10 Save and then print **3-CDAssessment.docx**.

11 Remove the header by clicking the Insert tab, clicking the Header button in the Header & Footer group, and then clicking *Remove Header* at the drop-down list.

12 Edit the footer by clicking the Footer button in the Header & Footer group and then clicking *Edit Footer* at the drop-down list.

13 Select the date in the footer, change the font to 10-point Calibri, and then apply bold formatting.

14 Double-click in the document.

15 Remove the Draft watermark by clicking the Design tab, clicking the Watermark button, and then clicking *Remove Watermark* at the drop-down list.

16 Insert a page break at the beginning of the heading *Feelings and Moods*.

17 Save, print, and then close **3-CDAssessment.docx**.

Check Your Work — Compare your work with the model answer to ensure that you have completed the activity correctly.

In Addition

Creating Your Own Header or Footer

Create your own header or footer using the *Edit Header* or *Edit Footer* options from the corresponding button drop-down list. For example, to create a header, click the Insert tab, click the Header button, and then click *Edit Header* at the drop-down list. This opens the header pane and displays the Header & Footer Tools Design tab with buttons and options for editing the header. Make the desired edits to the header with options on the tab and then close the header pane by clicking the Close Header and Footer button in the Close group on the Header & Footer Tools Design tab. Complete similar steps to create your own footer.

To increase the ease with which a person can read and understand groups of words (referred to as the readability of a document), consider setting the text in a document in newspaper columns. Newspaper columns contain text that flows up and down on the page. Create columns with the Columns button in the Page Setup group on the Layout tab or with options at the Columns dialog box. If you want to apply column formatting to only a portion of a document, insert a section break in the document with options at the Breaks button drop-down list.

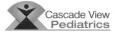
Cascade View Pediatrics

What You Will Do Sydney Larsen has asked you to format the monthly newsletter for Cascade View Pediatrics into columns and to apply formatting to improve the appearance of the newsletter.

Tutorial
Inserting and Deleting a Section Break

Tutorial
Formatting Text into Columns

1. Open **CVPNewsltr.docx** and then save it with the name **3-CVPNewsltr**.

2. Position the insertion point at the beginning of the first heading, *Pediatrician Joins CVP*.

3. Insert a continuous section break by clicking the Layout tab, clicking the Breaks button in the Page Setup group, and then clicking *Continuous* in the *Section Breaks* section.

   A continuous section break separates the document into sections but does not insert a page break. Continuous section breaks are not visible in Print Layout view. Click one of the other three options in the *Section Breaks* section of the Breaks button drop-down list to insert a section break that begins a new page.

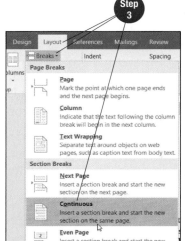

4. Click the View tab and then click the Draft button in the Views group.

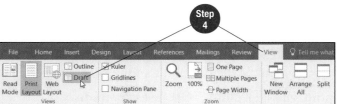

5. With the insertion point positioned below the section break, format the text below the section break into three columns by clicking the Layout tab, clicking the Columns button in the Page Setup group, and then clicking *Three* at the drop-down list.

   Formatting text into columns automatically changes the view to Print Layout view.

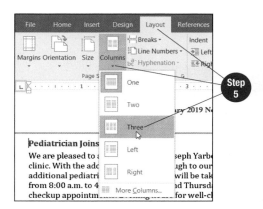

In Brief

Insert Continuous Section Break
1. Click Layout tab.
2. Click Breaks button.
3. Click *Continuous* in *Section Breaks* section.

Format Text into Columns
1. Click Layout tab.
2. Click Columns button.
3. Click number of columns.

Display Columns Dialog Box
1. Click Layout tab.
2. Click Columns button.
3. Click *More Columns*.

6 As you view the document, you notice that the three columns are pretty narrow, so you decide to set the text in two columns with a line between them. To do this, click in the heading *Pediatrician Joins CVP* and then display the Columns dialog box by clicking the Columns button in the Page Setup group and then clicking *More Columns* at the drop-down list.

7 At the Columns dialog box, click *Two* in the *Presets* section.

8 Slightly decrease the spacing between the two columns by clicking the *Spacing* measurement box down arrow in the *Width and spacing* section.

> Make sure *0.4"* displays in the *Spacing* measurement box.

9 Make sure a check mark displays in the *Equal column width* check box. If not, click the check box to insert a check mark.

> This option, when activated, makes the two columns the same width.

10 Click the *Line between* check box to insert a check mark.

> Turning on the *Line between* option inserts a line between the two columns. The *Preview* section of the dialog box provides a visual representation of this.

11 Click OK to close the Columns dialog box.

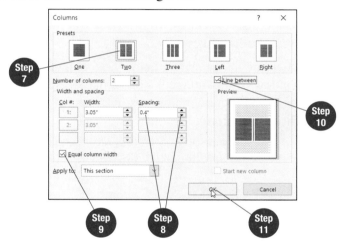

12 Press Ctrl + End to move the insertion point to the end of the document. Balance the two columns by clicking the Breaks button in the Page Setup group and then clicking *Continuous* in the *Section Breaks* section.

13 Save, print, and then close **3-CVPNewsltr.docx**.

> **Check Your Work** Compare your work with the model answer to ensure that you have completed the activity correctly.

In Addition

Changing Column Width

One method for changing column width in a document is to drag the column marker on the horizontal ruler. To change the width (and also the spacing) of columns of text, position the arrow pointer on the left or right edge of a column marker on the horizontal ruler until the pointer turns into a double-headed arrow pointing left and right.

Click and hold down the left mouse button, drag the column marker to the left or right to make the column wider or narrower, and then release the mouse button. Press and hold down the Alt key while dragging the column marker to display measurements on the horizontal ruler.

Inserting, Sizing, Moving, and Formatting an Image

Insert an image, such as a picture or clip art, in a document with buttons in the Illustrations group on the Insert tab. Click the Pictures button to display the Insert Picture dialog box containing image files located on the computer or click the Online Pictures button to search online images such as pictures and clip art. Format an inserted image with buttons and options on the Picture Tools Format tab. This tab is active when an image is selected.

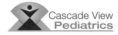
Cascade View Pediatrics

What You Will Do   Deanna Reynolds has asked you to enhance a document she created for her parenting classes. You decide to add clip art images to the document and apply some additional formatting to enhance the appearance.

Tutorial
Inserting, Sizing, and Positioning an Image

Tutorial
Formatting an Image

1 Open **CVPClasses.docx** and then save it with the name **3-CVPClasses**.

2 You know that adding images to a document can make it more engaging for readers, so you decide to insert an image of a parent and child. To begin, display the Insert Pictures window by clicking the Insert tab and then clicking the Online Pictures button 🖼 in the Illustrations group.

3 At the Insert Pictures window, click in the search box, type toddler parent, and then press the Enter key.

4 Click the image shown below and then click the Insert button at the bottom of the window. If this image is not available, click the Pictures button on the Insert tab. At the Insert Picture dialog box, navigate to the WordMedS3 folder and then double-click *toddler.png*.

The image displays selected (with sizing handles around it) in the document and the Picture Tools Format tab displays as shown in Figure W3.1.

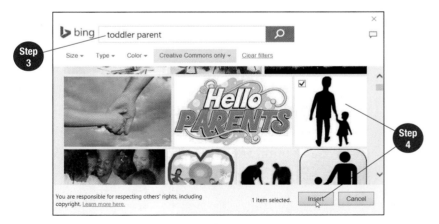

Figure W3.1 Picture Tools Format Tab

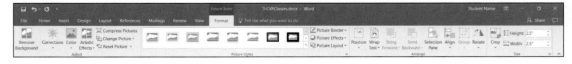

5 With the image selected, click the Wrap Text button 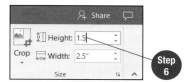 in the Arrange group on the Picture Tools Format tab and then click *Tight* at the drop-down list.

Step 5

6 Click in the *Shape Height* measurement box in the Size group, type 1.5, and then press the Enter key.

> When you change the height measurement, the width measurement is automatically changed to maintain the proportions of the image.

Step 6

7 Change the color of the image by clicking the Color button 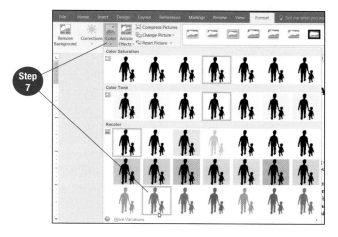 in the Adjust group and then clicking the blue option in the second column, third row in the *Recolor* section.

Step 7

Step 8

8 Add a shadow effect to the image by clicking the *Reflected Rounded Rectangle* option in the Picture Styles group (fifth option).

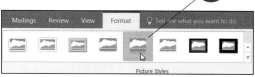

9 Move the image by positioning the mouse pointer on the image until the pointer displays with a four-headed arrow attached, holding down the mouse button, dragging the image so it is positioned as shown in Figure W3.2 on page 83, and then releasing the mouse button.

10 Click outside the image to deselect it.

11 Position the insertion point at the beginning of the bulleted list.

12 Click the Insert tab and then click the Pictures button in the Illustrations group.

Step 12

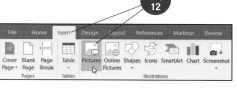

13 At the Insert Picture dialog box, navigate to the WordMedS3 folder and then double-click *parentchild.png*.

14 With the image selected, click the Wrap Text button in the Arrange group and then click *Square* at the drop-down list.

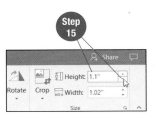
Step 15

15 Click the *Shape Height* measurement box down arrow in the Size group until *1.1"* displays in the box.

16 Add a shadow effect to the image by clicking the More Picture Styles button that displays at the right side of the picture style thumbnails in the Picture Styles group and then clicking the *Center Shadow Rectangle* option.

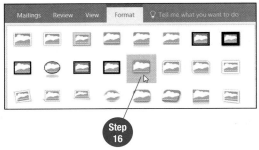
Step 16

17 Rotate the image by clicking the Rotate button in the Arrange group and then clicking *Flip Horizontal* at the drop-down gallery.

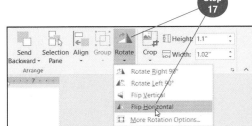
Step 17

18 Change the color of the image by clicking the Color button in the Adjust group and then clicking the blue option in the sixth column, second row in the *Recolor* section.

19 Move the image by positioning the arrow pointer on the image until the pointer displays with a four-headed arrow attached, holding down the left mouse button, dragging the image so it is positioned as shown in Figure W3.2, and then releasing the mouse button.

20 Click outside the image to deselect it.

21 Move the insertion point to the end of the document and then insert the Cascade View Pediatrics logo. To begin, click the Insert tab and then click the Pictures button in the Illustrations group.

22 At the Insert Picture dialog box, navigate to the WordMedS3 folder on your storage medium and then double-click *CVPLogo.jpg*.

23 With the image selected in the document, click the Wrap Text button in the Arrange group and then click *Tight* at the drop-down list.

24 With the image still selected, hold down the Shift key and then drag one of the corner sizing handles to reduce the size of the logo so it displays as shown in Figure W3.2. Move the logo to the position shown in the figure.

> Holding down the Shift key while increasing or decreasing the size of an image maintains the proportions of the image.

25 Save, print, and then close **3-CVPClasses.docx**.

CASCADE VIEW PEDIATRICS
Basic Parenting Course

Presented by Deanna Reynolds
Child Development Specialist

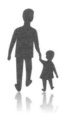

Parenting is a full-time job and wondering about your child's behaviors and your responsibilities as a parent are normal. You may have asked yourself:

- What can I do when my child misbehaves?
- Is my child's development and behavior "normal"?
- What is the difference between punishment and discipline?
- How can I improve the way I communicate with my child?
- How can I help my child learn to make good choices?

Deanna Reynolds, Child Development Specialist at Cascade View Pediatrics, will cover these questions as well as others in a four-week course designed to help you better handle the challenges of parenting.

When ....Monday and Wednesday
Beginning..Monday, March 7
Ending..Wednesday, March 30
Time..7:00 p.m. to 8:30 p.m.
Where ....Cascade View Pediatrics
Location ....Suite 150, Room 3
Cost $85

For more information on this important parenting course and to sign up for the class, call (503) 555-7753. You can also read more about the course and register online by visiting the Cascade View Pediatrics website at http://ppi-edu.net/cvp.

Check Your Work Compare your work with the model answer to ensure that you have completed the activity correctly.

In Addition

Formatting an Image with Buttons on the Picture Tools Format Tab

Images inserted in a document can be formatted in a variety of ways, which might include adding fill color and border lines, increasing or decreasing the brightness or contrast, choosing a wrapping style, and cropping the image. Format an image with buttons on the Picture Tools Format tab as shown in Figure W3.1. With buttons in the Adjust group, you can correct the brightness and contrast of the image; change the image color; change to a different image; reset the image to its original size, position, and color; and compress the image.

Compress an image to reduce resolution or discard extra information to save room on the hard drive or reduce download time. Use buttons in the Picture Styles group to apply a predesigned style, insert a picture border, or apply a picture effect. The Arrange group contains buttons for positioning the image, wrapping text around the image, and aligning and rotating the image. Use options in the Size group to crop the image and specify the height and width of the image.

Creating and Modifying WordArt Text; Inserting a File

Use the WordArt feature to distort or modify text to conform to a variety of shapes. Consider using WordArt to create a company logo, letterhead, flyer title, or heading. When WordArt is selected, the Drawing Tools Format tab displays. Use options on this tab to change the font, style, and alignment of text; use different fill patterns and colors; customize border lines; and add shadow and three-dimensional effects. You can size and move selected WordArt text as desired. In some situations, you may want to insert the contents of one file into another. Do this at the Insert File dialog box, which you display by clicking *Text from File* at the Object button drop-down list in the Text group on the Insert tab.

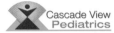
Cascade View Pediatrics

What You Will Do   The Health Insurance Portability and Accountability Act of 1996 (HIPAA) requires that healthcare providers adopt and adhere to policies and procedures that protect the patient's privacy regarding disclosure of sensitive health information. Cascade View Pediatrics has established clear guidelines for patient confidentiality. Sydney Larsen has asked you to compile a document with information on patient confidentiality and enhance the document with WordArt for more impact.

Tutorial
Insert a File

Tutorial
Inserting, Sizing, and Positioning WordArt

Tutorial
Formatting WordArt

1. Open **CVPHIPAA.docx** and then save it with the name **3-CVPHIPAA**.

2. Press Ctrl + End to move the insertion point to the end of the document.

3. Insert a file into the current document by clicking the Insert tab, clicking the Object button arrow 🗗 in the Text group, and then clicking *Text from File* at the drop-down list.

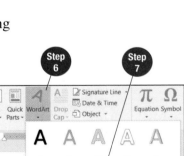
Step 3

4. At the Insert File dialog box, navigate to the WordMedS3 folder on your storage medium and then double-click *CVPRules.docx*.

5. Select the paragraphs of text in the document (excluding the title) and then insert bullets by clicking the Bullets button in the Paragraph group on the Home tab.

Step 6   Step 7

6. Move the insertion point to the beginning of the document and then insert WordArt by clicking the Insert tab and then clicking the WordArt button 🅐 in the Text group.

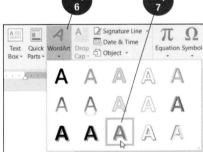

7. At the WordArt button drop-down list, click the blue WordArt option in the third column, third row.

8. Type Important.

> This inserts the WordArt text *Important* in the document, selects the WordArt text box, and displays the Drawing Tools Format tab. (See the In Addition on the next page for more information.)

9. Increase the width of the WordArt text by clicking in the *Shape Width* measurement box in the Size group on the Drawing Tools Format tab, typing 5, and then pressing the Enter key.

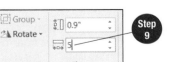
Step 9

10 Change the shape of the WordArt by clicking the Text Effects button 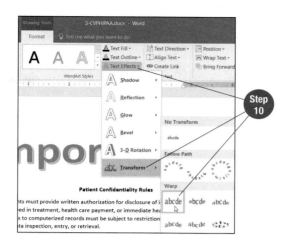 in the WordArt Styles group on the Drawing Tools Format tab, pointing to *Transform* at the drop-down list, and then clicking the *Square* option (first column, first row in the *Warp* section).

11 Click the Text Fill button arrow in the WordArt Styles group on the Drawing Tools Format tab and then click the *Gold, Accent 4* option at the drop-down gallery (eighth column, first row in the *Theme Colors* section).

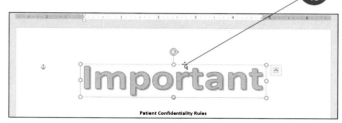

12 Click the Text Outline button arrow in the WordArt Styles group and then click the *Blue* option in the *Standard Colors* section of the drop-down gallery.

13 Position the WordArt text so it is centered between the left and right margins. To do this, position the mouse pointer on the WordArt text until the pointer displays with a four-headed arrow attached. Hold down the left mouse button, drag the WordArt text to the desired position, and then release the mouse button.

14 Click outside the WordArt text box to deselect it.

15 Save **3-CVPHIPAA.docx**.

Check Your Work Compare your work with the model answer to ensure that you have completed the activity correctly.

In Addition

Using the Drawing Tools Format Tab

When WordArt is selected, the Drawing Tools Format tab displays as shown below. Use options in the Insert Shapes group to draw a shape or text box. With options in the Shape Styles group, you can apply a predesigned style, change the shape fill color and the shape outline color, and apply shape effects. Change the style of the WordArt text with options in the WordArt Styles group, apply text formatting to WordArt with options in the Text group, specify the layering of the WordArt text with options in the Arrange group, and identify the height and width of the WordArt text box with measurement boxes in the Size group.

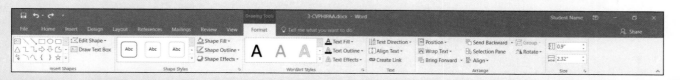

Inserting and Customizing Shapes and Text Boxes

The Shapes button in the Illustrations group on the Insert tab contains a number of shape options for drawing shapes in a document including lines, rectangles, basic shapes, block arrows, flow chart shapes, stars, banners, and callouts. Click a shape and the mouse pointer displays as crosshairs. Position the crosshairs where you want the shape positioned and then click the left mouse button or click and hold down the left mouse, drag to create the shape, and then release the mouse button. This inserts the shape in the document and also displays the Drawing Tools Format tab. Use buttons on this tab to format, arrange, and size a shape. Use the Text Box button in the Text group on the Insert tab to create a text box or insert a predesigned text box in a document.

Cascade View Pediatrics

What You Will Do To further enhance the patient confidentiality rules document and to emphasize the priority of maintaining confidentiality, you decide to add a shape containing text at the bottom of the document and a text box containing a brief statement within the body of the text.

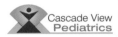 **Tutorial**
Inserting, Sizing, and Positioning a Shape and Line

Tutorial
Formatting a Shape and Line

Tutorial
Inserting a Text Box

Tutorial
Formatting a Text Box

1. With **3-CVPHIPAA.docx** open, press Ctrl + End to move the insertion point to the end of the document.

2. Click the Insert tab, click the Shapes button in the Illustrations group, and then click the banner option in the first column, second row in the *Stars and Banners* section.

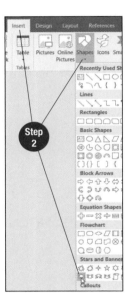

3. Position the mouse pointer (displays as crosshairs) below the text at approximately the 1-inch mark on the horizontal ruler and the 6.5-inch mark on the vertical ruler. Hold down the left mouse button, drag down and to the right until the banner is approximately 5 inches wide and 1.5 inches high, and then release the mouse button.

   This inserts the shape in the document and makes the Drawing Tools Format tab active.

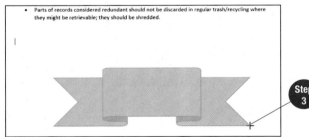

4. Apply a shape style by clicking the More Shape Styles button at the right of the thumbnails in the Shape Styles group and then clicking the yellow style option in the fifth column, fourth row in the *Theme Styles* section.

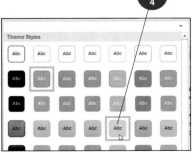

5. Click in the *Shape Height* measurement box in the Size group, type 1.5, and then press the Enter key.

6. Click in the *Shape Width* measurement box, type 5, and then press the Enter key.

7 With the shape selected, type Patient confidentiality is a top priority at Cascade View Pediatrics!

> The typed text is automatically inserted in the selected shape.

8 Select the text you just typed, change the font size to 16 points, turn on bold formatting, and then change the font color to Blue.

9 Press Ctrl + Home to move the insertion point to the beginning of the document and then insert a predesigned text box. Begin by clicking the Text Box button in the Text group on the Insert tab and then clicking the *Austin Quote* option at the drop-down list.

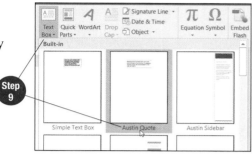

> Predesigned text boxes are listed in alphabetical order.

10 Click the Position button in the Arrange group and then click the *Position in Middle Right with Square Text Wrapping* option (third column, second row in the *With Text Wrapping* section).

11 Type the following text in the text box: It is important that patients must provide written authorization for disclosure of information to others.

12 Click in the *Shape Width* measurement box in the Size group, type 2.6, and then press the Enter key.

13 Click the Shape Fill button arrow and then click *Blue, Accent 1, Lighter 80%* at the drop-down gallery (fifth column, second row in the *Theme Colors* section).

14 Click the Shape Effects button in the Shape Styles group, point to *Bevel*, and then click the first option in the first column, first row in the *Bevel* section.

15 Click the Text Fill button arrow and then click *Blue, Accent 1, Darker 50%* at the drop-down gallery (fifth column, sixth row in the *Theme Colors* section).

16 Deselect the text box by clicking outside the text box.

17 Save, print, and then close **3-CVPHIPAA.docx**.

> **Check Your Work** ▶ Compare your work with the model answer to ensure that you have completed the activity correctly.

In Addition

Drawing Lines

The Shapes button drop-down list contains a number of options for drawing lines in a document. Click the *Curve* option in the *Lines* section to draw curved lines by clicking at the beginning position, dragging to the location where you want the curve to appear, and then clicking the mouse button again. Continue in this manner until you have drawn all the desired curved lines. Click the *Freeform* option in the *Lines* section to draw freeform in a document. When you want to stop drawing, double-click the left mouse button. You can also use the *Scribble* option to draw freeform in a document.

Activity 3.12   Preparing an Envelope

Word automates the creation of envelopes with options at the Envelopes and Labels dialog box with the Envelopes tab selected. At this dialog box, type a delivery address and a return address. If you open the Envelopes and Labels dialog box in a document containing a name and address, that name and address are inserted automatically as the delivery address. If you enter a return address, Word will ask you before printing if you want to save the new return address as the default return address. Click the Yes button if you want to use the return address for future envelopes or click the No button if you will use a different return address for future envelopes.

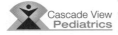
Cascade View Pediatrics

What You Will Do   Deanna Reynolds has asked you to mail a Basic Parenting Course flyer to Lowell Quasim, Education Coordinator at Columbia River General Hospital.

Tutorial
Preparing an Envelope

① Press Ctrl + N to display a blank document.

> You can also display a blank document by clicking the File tab, clicking the *New* option, and then clicking the *Blank document* template. Another method is to insert the New button on the Quick Access Toolbar and then click the button to display a blank document. To insert the New button on the Quick Access Toolbar, click the Customize Quick Access Toolbar button at the right side of the toolbar and then click *New* at the drop-down list.

② Click the Mailings tab and then click the Envelopes button 🔲 in the Create group.

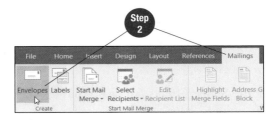

③ At the Envelopes and Labels dialog box with the Envelopes tab selected, type the following name and address in the *Delivery address* text box. (Press the Enter key at the end of each line except the last line [contains the city name, state, and ZIP code.])

> Mr. Lowell Quasim
> Education Coordinator
> Columbia River General Hospital
> 4550 Fremont Street
> Portland, OR 97045

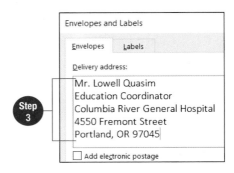

4 Click in the *Return address* text box and then type the following name and address, pressing the Enter key at the end of each line except the last one. (If any text displays in the *Return address* text box, select and then delete it before you begin typing.)

> Deanna Reynolds
> Cascade View Pediatrics
> 350 North Skagit
> Portland, OR 97505

5 Click the Add to Document button.

Clicking the Add to Document button inserts the envelope in the document. You can also send the envelope directly to the printer by clicking the Print button.

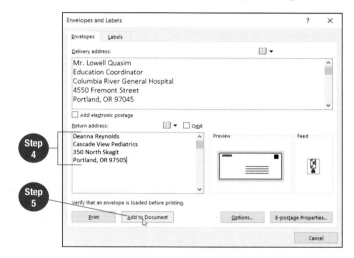

6 At the message asking if you want to save the new return address as the default address, click No.

7 Save the document with the name **3-CVPEnv**.

8 Print and then close **3-CVPEnv.docx**. *Note: Manual feed of the envelope into the printer may be required. Please check with your instructor before printing.*

Check Your Work — Compare your work with the model answer to ensure that you have completed the activity correctly.

In Addition

Customizing Envelopes

You can customize an envelope with options at the Envelope Options dialog box shown at the right. Display this dialog box by clicking the Options button in the Envelopes and Labels dialog box with the Envelopes tab selected. At the Envelope Options dialog box, you can change the envelope size, change the font for the delivery and return addresses, and specify the positioning of the addresses in relation to the left and top edges of the envelope.

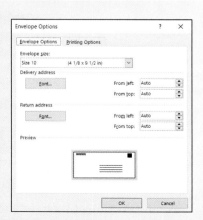

Activity 3.13 Preparing Mailing Labels

Use Word's Labels feature to print text on mailing labels, file labels, disc labels, and other types of labels. You can create labels for printing on a variety of predefined sheets of labels, which you can purchase at an office supply store. With the Labels feature, you can create a sheet of mailing labels with the same name and address or image, or you can enter a different name and address on each label. Create labels with options at the Envelopes and Labels dialog box with the Labels tab selected.

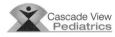
Cascade View Pediatrics

What You Will Do   You will create a sheet of return-address mailing labels containing the Cascade View Pediatrics name and address. You will also create mailing labels for sending the Basic Parenting Course flyer to various professionals and clinics in the area and create labels for the new Cascade View Pediatrics office in Lake Oswego.

Tutorial
Creating Mailing Labels with the Same Name and Address and an Image

Tutorial
Creating Mailing Labels with Different Names and Addresses

1. Press Ctrl + N to display a blank document.

2. Click the Mailings tab and then click the Labels button in the Create group.

3. Type the following information in the *Address* text box. (Press the Enter key at the end of each line except the last line.)

   Cascade View Pediatrics
   350 North Skagit
   Portland, OR 97505

4. Click the Options button.

5. At the Label Options dialog box, click the *Label vendors* option box arrow and then click *Avery US Letter* at the drop-down list.

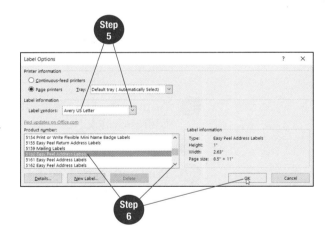

6. Scroll down the *Product number* list box, click *5160 Easy Peel Address Labels* in the list box, and then click OK to close the dialog box.

7. Click the New Document button at the Envelopes and Labels dialog box.

8. Save the document with the name **3-CVPLabels**.

9. Print and then close **3-CVPLabels.docx**.

   The number of labels printed on the page varies depending on the label selected at the Label Options dialog box.

10. Click the Mailings tab and then click the Labels button in the Create group.

11. At the Envelopes and Labels dialog box, click the New Document button.

12. In the first label, type the first name and address shown in Figure W3.3. Press the Tab key two times to move the insertion point to the next label and then type the second name and address shown in Figure W3.3. Continue in this manner until you have typed all of the names and addresses shown in the figure.

13. Save the document with the name **3-CVPContactLabels**.

14 Print and then close **3-CVPContactLabels.docx**.

15 At the blank document, create mailing labels for the Lake Oswego office of Cascade View Pediatrics using an image. Begin by clicking the Insert tab and then clicking the Pictures button in the Illustrations group.

16 At the Insert Picture dialog box, navigate to the WordMedS3 folder on your storage medium and then double-click ***CVPLakeOswegoLabel.png***.

17 With the label image selected, click the Position button in the Arrange group on the Picture Tools Format tab and then click the *Position in Top Center with Square Text Wrapping* option (second column, first row in the *With Text Wrapping* section).

18 With the image still selected, click the Mailings tab and then click the Labels button.

19 At the Envelopes and Labels dialog box, make sure the Avery US Letter label number 5160 is selected and then click the New Document button.

> When you click the New Document button, the label image is inserted in each label in the page and inserted in a new document.

20 Save the document and name it **3-CVPLakeOswegoLabels**.

21 Print and then close **3-CVPLakeOswegoLabels.docx**.

22 Close the document containing the label image without saving it.

Figure W3.3 Mailing Labels for Step 12

Paul Watanabe
Division Street Clinic
5330 Division Street
Portland, OR 97255

Nora Reeves
Community Counseling
1235 North 122nd Avenue
Portland, OR 97230

Dr. Thomas Wickstrom
Columbia Mental Health Center
550 Columbia Boulevard
Portland, OR 97305

Christina Fuentes
Parenting Services
210 Martin Luther King Way
Portland, OR 97403

Check Your Work — Compare your work with the model answer to ensure that you have completed the activity correctly.

In Addition

Customizing Labels

Click the Options button at the Envelopes and Labels dialog box with the Labels tab selected and the Label Options dialog box displays as shown at the right. At this dialog box, choose the type of printer, the desired label vendor, and the product number. This dialog box also displays information about the selected label such as type, height, width, and paper size. When you select a label, Word automatically determines the label margins. To customize these default settings, click the Details button at the Label Options dialog box.

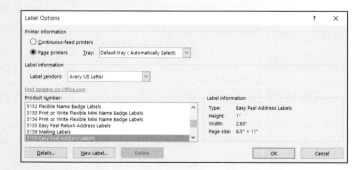

Features Summary

Feature	Ribbon Tab, Group	Button, Option	Keyboard Shortcut
blank page	Insert, Pages		
Clipboard task pane	Home, Clipboard		
columns	Layout, Page Setup		
Columns Dialog Box	Layout, Page Setup	, *More Columns*	
continuous section break	Layout, Page Setup	, *Continuous*	
copy selected text	Home, Clipboard		Ctrl + C
cover page	Insert, Pages		
cut selected text	Home, Clipboard		Ctrl + X
Envelopes and Labels dialog box with Envelopes tab selected	Mailings, Create		
Envelopes and Labels dialog box with Labels tab selected	Mailings, Create		
Find and Replace dialog box with Replace tab selected	Home, Editing		Ctrl + H
footer	Insert, Header & Footer		
header	Insert, Header & Footer		
insert file	Insert, Text	, *Text from File*	
Insert Picture dialog box	Insert, Illustrations		
Insert Pictures window	Insert, Illustrations		
page background color	Design, Page Background		
page border	Design, Page Background		
page break	Insert, Pages		Ctrl + Enter
page margins	Layout, Page Setup		
page number	Insert, Header & Footer		
page orientation	Layout, Page Setup		
Page Setup dialog box	Layout, Page Setup		
page size	Layout, Page Setup		
paste selected text	Home, Clipboard		Ctrl + V

continues...

Feature	Ribbon Tab, Group	Button, Option	Keyboard Shortcut
Paste Special dialog box	Home, Clipboard	, *Paste Special*	
Reveal Formatting task pane			Shift + F1
shapes and lines	Insert, Illustrations		
text box	Insert, Text		
watermark	Design, Page Background		
WordArt	Insert, Text		

Workbook Section study tools and assessment activities are available in the Workbook pages of the ebook. These resources are designed to help you further develop and demonstrate mastery of the skills learned in this section.

Word

Formatting with Special Features

Skills

- Create, edit, and modify merged documents
- Sort and filter records in a data source
- Merge envelopes
- Create, format, and modify tables
- Create a form for handwritten entries

Data Files Before beginning section work, copy the WordMedS4 folder to your storage medium and then make WordMedS4 the active folder.

- Create a form and save it as a template
- Fill in and print a form document
- Edit a form template
- Create and fill in a form with a drop-down list field

Precheck Check your current skills to help focus your study of the skills taught in this section.

Activities Overview

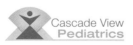 Cascade View Pediatrics

Prepare a main document reminding parents to schedule a well-child checkup appointment and create a data source using the Mail Merge feature, edit the main document and input text during a merge, and create and format a calendar.

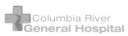 Columbia River General Hospital

Prepare a main document advising clients of upcoming parent education classes and create a data source using the Mail Merge feature, merge envelopes, and prepare a template document for gathering information on secondary payer information.

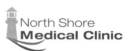 North Shore Medical Clinic

Sort and filter data source records by ZIP code and by last name, filter records in a data source and then print a letter for patients living in Lake Oswego, prepare and print merged envelopes, insert a table in a fact sheet on caffeine and then format the table, create a patient post-operative call sheet using tables, prepare a template document for updating patient information, prepare a main document advising patients of childbirth education classes and create a data source using the Mail Merge feature, create and format a medical questionnaire, create and format a table containing information on airfare from Portland to Chicago, create a treadmill test form, and prepare a pre-op questions document.

Model Answers Preview the model answers for an overview of the activities you will complete in each section.

95

Activity 4.1 Merging Documents

If you need to mail the same basic letter to a number of clients or customers, consider using the Mail Merge feature to make the job easier and to make the letter more personalized. Generally, performing a mail merge requires two documents—the data source file and the main document. The data source file contains the variable information about each client or customer that will be inserted into the main document. Before creating a data source file, determine what type of correspondence you will be creating and the type of information you will need to include. Variable information in a data source file is saved as a record. A record contains all of the information for one unit (for example, a person, family, customer, client, or business). A series of fields compose a record, and a series of records compose a data source file. Use buttons on the Mailings tab to create main documents and data source files for merging.

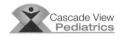

What You Will Do Your supervisor, Sydney Larsen, has asked you to create both a main document reminding parents to schedule a well-child checkup appointment and a data source file containing parent and patient information.

Tutorial
Creating a Data Source File

Tutorial
Creating a Main Document

Tutorial
Previewing and Merging Documents

1 At a blank document, click the Mailings tab, click the Select Recipients button 🔲 in the Start Mail Merge group, and then click *Type a New List* at the drop-down list.

> This displays the New Address List dialog box with predesigned fields. You can use these predesigned fields and/or create your own custom fields.

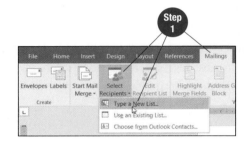

2 Delete the fields you do not need. Begin by clicking the Customize Columns button at the bottom of the dialog box.

> The predesigned fields cover most of the fields you need for your data source file, but you decide to delete seven of the predesigned fields and insert two of your own.

3 At the Customize Address List dialog box, click *First Name* in the *Field Names* list box and then click the Delete button.

4 At the message asking if you are sure you want to delete the field, click Yes.

5 Complete steps similar to those in Steps 3 and 4 to delete the following fields from the *Field Names* list box: *Company Name*, *Address Line 2*, *Country or Region*, *Home Phone*, *Work Phone*, and *E-mail Address*.

6 Click the Add button.

> If the New Address List dialog box does not contain fields for all the variable information you need to include, create your own custom field.

7 At the Add Field dialog box, type Child and then click OK.

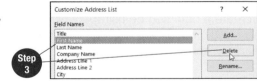

8 Click OK to close the Customize Address List dialog box.

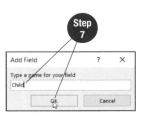

9 At the New Address List dialog box with the insertion point positioned in the *Title* field, type Mr. and Mrs. and then press the Tab key.

Pressing the Tab key moves the insertion point to the *Last Name* field. Press the Tab key to move the insertion point to the next field and press Shift + Tab to move the insertion point to the previous field.

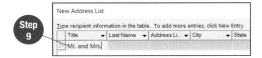

10 Type Nordyke and then press the Tab key. Type 12330 South 32nd and then press the Tab key. Type Portland and then press the Tab key. Type OR and then press the Tab key. Type 97233 and then press the Tab key. Type Lillian and then press the Tab key.

11 With the insertion point positioned in the *Title* column, complete steps similar to those in Steps 9 and 10 to enter the information for the three other patients shown in Figure W4.1.

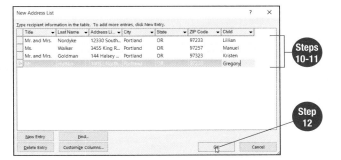

12 After entering all of the patient information in Figure W4.1, click OK to close the New Address List dialog box.

After typing Gregory for the Mr. Hutton record, do not press the Tab key. If you do, a new blank client record will be created. To remove a blank record, click the Delete Entry button and then click Yes at the message.

13 At the Save Address List dialog box, navigate to your WordMedS4 folder. Click in the *File name* text box, type 4-CVPPatients, and then press the Enter key.

Figure W4.1 Patient Information

Title	Mr. and Mrs.	*Title*	Ms.
Last Name	Nordyke	*Last Name*	Walker
Address Line 1	12330 South 32nd	*Address Line 1*	3455 King Road
City	Portland	*City*	Portland
State	OR	*State*	OR
ZIP Code	97233	*ZIP Code*	97257
Child	Lillian	*Child*	Manuel
Title	Mr. and Mrs.	*Title*	Mr.
Last Name	Goldman	*Last Name*	Hutton
Address Line 1	144 Halsey Street	*Address Line 1*	10032 North 23rd
City	Portland	*City*	Portland
State	OR	*State*	OR
ZIP Code	97323	*ZIP Code*	97230
Child	Kristen	*Child*	Gregory

14 At the blank document, click the Home tab and then click the *No Spacing* style in the Styles group. Press the Enter key six times, type February 4, 2019 as shown in Figure W4.2, and then press the Enter key four times.

15 Insert the address block field by clicking the Mailings tab and then clicking the Address Block button ▤ in the Write & Insert Fields group.

16 At the Insert Address Block dialog box, click OK.

This inserts the necessary field code to insert the client name and address in the letter.

17 Press the Enter key two times and then click the Greeting Line button ▤ in the Write & Insert Fields group.

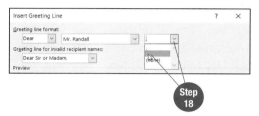

18 At the Insert Greeting Line dialog box, click the arrow in the option box containing the comma (appears to the right of the option box containing *Mr. Randall*) and then click the colon at the drop-down list.

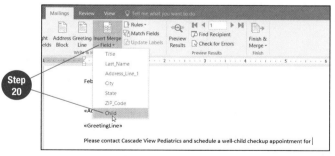

19 Click OK to close the dialog box.

20 Press the Enter key two times and then begin to type the letter shown in Figure W4.2. Stop when you get to the location of the *Child* field. Insert the field by clicking the Insert Merge Field button arrow ▤ and then clicking *Child* at the drop-down list.

21 Type the remainder of the letter as shown in Figure W4.2. *Note: Type your initials in place of the* **xx** *toward the end of the letter.*

22 When you are finished typing the letter, merge the letter with the records in the data source. Begin by clicking the Finish & Merge button ▤ in the Finish group on the Mailings tab and then clicking *Edit Individual Documents* at the drop-down list.

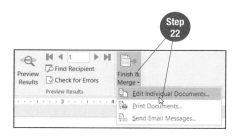

February 4, 2019

«AddressBlock»

«GreetingLine»

Please contact Cascade View Pediatrics and schedule a well-child checkup appointment for «Child». At Cascade View Pediatrics, we recommend that children are seen by a pediatrician at the ages of 2 weeks and 2, 4, 6, 12, 18, and 24 months. Your child may require immunizations so plan at least 60 minutes for the appointment.

Your child's well-child appointment consists of a routine physical examination; vision, hearing, and speech screening; testing for anemia and lead poisoning; and immunizations. Additional services may include development testing, nutrition and social assessment, and guidance and parenting education.

To schedule a well-child appointment, please call our clinic at (503) 555-7700 or stop by our clinic at 350 North Skagit.

Sincerely,

Sydney Larsen
Office Manager

xx
4-Well-ChildMainDoc.docx

23 At the Merge to New Document dialog box, make sure *All* is selected and then click OK.

> The letters are merged with the records and displayed in a new document.

24 Save the merged letters in the normal manner with the name **4-Well-ChildApptLtrs**.

25 Print and then close **4-Well-ChildApptLtrs.docx**.

> Four letters will print.

26 Save the main document in the normal manner with the name **4-Well-ChildMainDoc**.

27 Close **4-Well-ChildMainDoc.docx**.

Check Your Work — Compare your work with the model answer to ensure that you have completed the activity correctly.

In Addition

Using the Mail Merge Wizard

The Mail Merge feature includes a Mail Merge wizard to guide you through the merge process. To access the Wizard, click the Mailings tab, click the Start Mail Merge button in the Start Mail Merge group, and then click *Step-by-Step Mail Merge Wizard* at the drop-down list.

The first of six Mail Merge task panes displays at the right side of the screen. Complete tasks at one pane and then display the next. The options in each task pane may vary depending on the type of merge you are performing.

Activity 4.2 Editing Merged Documents; Inputting Text during a Merge

When you complete a mail merge, you create a data source file and a main document. The data source file is associated with the main document. If you need to edit the main document, open it in the normal manner and make the required changes. To make changes to the data source file, click the Edit Recipient List button in the Start Mail Merge group on the Mailings tab. Changes you make to the data source file are saved automatically. To save edits made to the main document, you must do so manually. In some situations, you may not want to store all variable information in the data source file. If you want to input certain variable information directly into the main document during a merge, insert a fill-in field at the appropriate location in the main document.

What You Will Do Sydney Larsen has asked you to customize the well-child checkup appointments letters to include an area to identify the specific type of appointment.

Tutorial
Editing a Data Source File

Tutorial
Inputting Text during a Merge

1. Open **4-Well-ChildMainDoc.docx**. If a message displays telling you that opening the document will run an SQL command, click Yes.

2. Click the Mailings tab.

3. Edit the first paragraph so it displays as shown in Figure W4.3. To insert the *Child* field, click the Insert Merge Field button arrow in the Write & Insert Fields group and then click *Child* at the drop-down list. Do not type the text *(Checkup)*. You will insert this as a fill-in field in the next step.

4. To insert a fill-in field for *(Checkup)*, click the Rules button 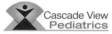 in the Write & Insert Fields group and then click *Fill-in* at the drop-down list.

> Insert a fill-in field in those locations in a main document where you want to enter specific information during a merge.

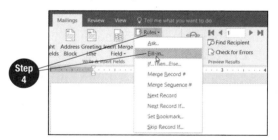

5. At the Insert Word Field: Fill-in dialog box, type Insert specific well-child checkup appointment in the *Prompt* text box and then click OK.

> The text you type in the *Prompt* text box will display during a merge to indicate what information the user should type.

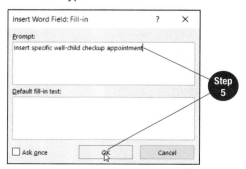

Figure W4.3 Edited Paragraph

According to our records, «Child» is due for (Checkup). Please contact Cascade View Pediatrics and schedule the well-child checkup appointment. Your child may require immunizations so plan at least 60 minutes for the appointment.

6 At the Microsoft Word dialog box with *Insert specific well-child checkup appointment* displayed in the upper left corner, type (Checkup) and then click OK. Type or edit the remainder of the paragraph so it displays as shown in Figure W4.3.

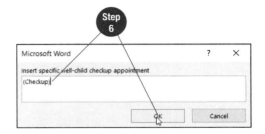

7 You need to edit some of the records in the data source. To begin, click the Edit Recipient List button in the Start Mail Merge group.

8 At the Mail Merge Recipients dialog box, click the file name *4-CVPPatients.mdb* in the *Data Source* list box and then click the Edit button below the list box.

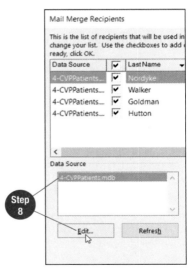

9 At the Edit Data Source dialog box, click any character in the address *3455 King Road* (in the record for Ms. Walker) and then type 6795 32nd Street.

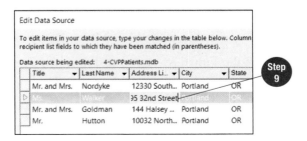

10 In the same record, click any character in the ZIP code *97257* and then type *97239*.

11 Click the New Entry button and then type the following in the specified fields:

Title	Mrs.
Last Name	Milovich
Address Line 1	19443 144th Place
City	Portland
State	OR
ZIP Code	97340
Child	Paulina

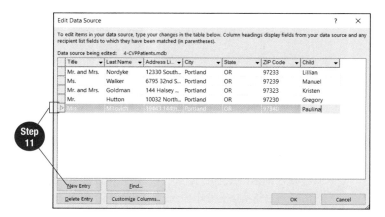

Step 11

12 Delete the record for Mr. Hutton by clicking the gray square at the left of the record for Mr. Hutton and then clicking the Delete Entry button.

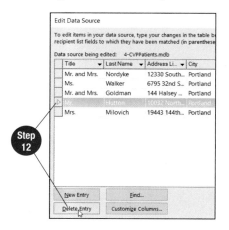

Step 12

13 At the message asking if you want to delete the entry, click Yes.

14 At the Edit Data Source dialog box, click OK. At the message asking if you want to update your recipient list, click Yes.

15 Click OK to close the Mail Merge Recipients dialog box.

16 Click the Finish & Merge button in the Finish group on the Mailings tab and then click *Edit Individual Documents* at the drop-down list.

17 At the Merge to New Document dialog box, make sure *All* is selected and then click OK.

In Brief

Edit Data Source
1. Open main document.
2. Click Mailings tab.
3. Click Edit Recipient List button.
4. Click data source file name in *Data Source* list box.
5. Click Edit button.
6. Make changes at Edit Data Source dialog box.
7. Click OK.
8. Click Yes.
9. Click OK.

18 When Word merges the main document with the first record, the text *(Checkup)* is selected in the document and a dialog box displays with the message *Insert specific well-child checkup appointment*. At this dialog box, type her two-week checkup and then click OK.

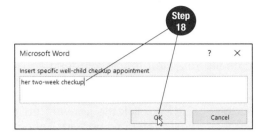

19 At the next dialog box, type his 18-month checkup (over *her two-week checkup*) and then click OK.

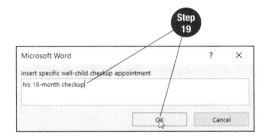

20 At the next dialog box, type her 12-month checkup and then click OK.

21 At the next dialog box, type her four-month checkup and then click OK.

22 Save the merged letters in the normal manner in the WordMedS4 folder on your storage medium and name the document **4-Well-ChildEditedLtrs**.

23 Print and then close **4-Well-ChildEditedLtrs.docx**.

> Four letters will print.

24 Save and then close **4-Well-ChildMainDoc.docx**.

> **Check Your Work**   Compare your work with the model answer to ensure that you have completed the activity correctly.

In Addition

Editing a Data Source Using the Mail Merge Wizard

In addition to editing a data source by opening the main document and then clicking the Edit Recipient List button, you can edit a data source by using the Mail Merge wizard. To do so, open a main document, click the Mailings tab, click the Start Mail Merge button, and then click the *Step-by-Step Mail Merge Wizard* option. This series of actions causes the Mail Merge wizard to open at the third step. At this step, click the Edit recipient list hyperlink. At the Mail Merge Recipients dialog box, click the data source file name in the *Data Source* list box, click the Edit button, and then make the necessary edits to the fields in the records at the Edit Data Source dialog box.

Activity 4.3   Sorting Records in a Data Source

To organize records in a data source, you can sort them in ascending or descending order. To do this, click the Mailings tab, click the Select Recipients button, and then click *Use an Existing List*. At the Select Data Source dialog box, navigate to the folder that contains the data source file you want to use and then double-click the file. Click the Edit Recipient List button in the Start Mail Merge group on the Mailings tab and the Mail Merge Recipients dialog box displays. Click a column heading to sort data in ascending order by that field. To perform additional sorts, click the arrow at the right of a field column heading and then click the sort order. You can refine a sort with options at the Filter and Sort dialog box.

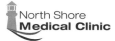
North Shore
Medical Clinic

What You Will Do   Lee Elliott has asked you to sort data source records by last name, city, and ZIP code.

Tutorial
Sorting Records in a
Data Source File

1. Open **NSMCMainDoc.docx**. If a message displays telling you that opening the document will run an SQL command, click Yes.

   If a message displays telling you that Word cannot find the data source, proceed to Step 2.

2. Click the Mailings tab, click the Select Recipients button in the Start Mail Merge group, and then click *Use an Existing List* at the drop-down list. At the Select Data Source dialog box, navigate to the WordMedS4 folder on your storage medium and then double-click **NSMCPatientsDS.mdb**.

3. Sort records alphabetically in the data source attached to this main document. To begin, click the Edit Recipient List button in the Start Mail Merge group on the Mailings tab.

4. At the Mail Merge Recipients dialog box, click the *Last Name* column heading.

   This sorts the last names in ascending alphabetical order.

5. Scroll to the right to display the *City* field, click the arrow at the right of the *City* column heading, and then click *Sort Descending* at the drop-down list.

   This sorts the city names in descending alphabetical order.

6. Sort by ZIP code and then by last name. To begin, click the <u>Sort</u> hyperlink in the *Refine recipient list* section.

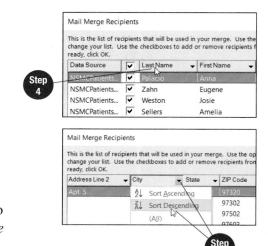

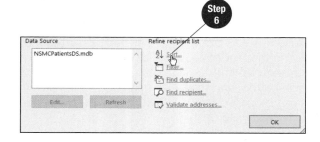

In Brief

Sort Records in a Data Source File
1. Click Mailings tab.
2. Click Select Recipients button.
3. Click *Use an Existing List*.
4. Double-click file.
5. Click Edit Recipient List button.
6. At Mail Merge Recipients dialog box, sort by specific field by clicking field column heading.
7. Click OK.

7 At the Filter and Sort dialog box with the Sort Records tab selected, click the *Sort by* option box arrow and then click *ZIP Code* at the drop-down list.

   You will need to scroll down the list to display *ZIP Code*.

8 Make sure *Last Name* displays in the *Then by* option box.

9 Click OK to close the Filter and Sort dialog box.

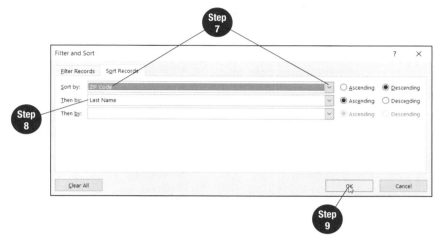

10 Click OK to close the Mail Merge Recipients dialog box.

11 Preview each letter by clicking the Preview Results button in the Preview Results group on the Mailings tab and then clicking the Next Record button in the Preview Results group. Keep clicking the Next Record button until the last letter (the tenth letter) displays.

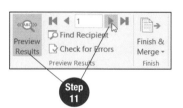

12 Click the Finish & Merge button in the Finish group on the Mailings tab and then click *Edit Individual Documents* at the drop-down list.

13 At the Merge to New Document dialog box, make sure *All* is selected and then click OK.

14 Save the merged letters document with the name **4-NSMCApptLtrs**.

15 Print only the first page of **4-NSMCApptLtrs.docx**.

16 Close **4-NSMCApptLtrs.docx**.

17 Close **NSMCMainDoc.docx** without saving the changes.

Check Your Work Compare your work with the model answer to ensure that you have completed the activity correctly.

In Addition

Clearing Sort Data

If you sort data in a data source file by clicking a column heading, the sort information will display when you open the Filter and Sort dialog box. Also, if you identify fields for sorting at the Filter and Sort dialog box, that information will display the next time you open the dialog box. To complete a new sort at the Filter and Sort dialog box, first click the Clear All button in the lower left corner of the dialog box to remove any existing sort information.

Activity 4.4   Filtering Records

Once you have created a main document and a data source file to produce personalized letters, situations may arise in which you want to merge the main document with only certain records in the data source. For example, you may want to send a letter to patients living in a particular city or patients seeing a specific doctor. Filtering allows you to identify records that meet specific criteria and include only those records in the merge. One method for filtering records is to display the Mail Merge Recipients dialog box and then insert or remove check marks next to specific records. If you only need to select a few records, start by clicking the check box at the right of the *Data Source* column heading. This removes the check marks from all of the check boxes, making it easier for you to select only those few records that you need.

North Shore Medical Clinic

Tutorial
Selecting Specific
Records for Merging

What You Will Do   You need to send a letter to only those patients living in Lake Oswego. Select the appropriate records and then merge and print the patient letters.

1   Open **NSMCMainDoc.docx**. If a message displays telling you that opening the document will run an SQL command, click Yes.

> If a message displays telling you that Word cannot find the data source, proceed to Step 2.

2   Click the Mailings tab, click the Select Recipients button in the Start Mail Merge group, and then click *Use an Existing List* at the drop-down list. At the Select Data Source dialog box, navigate to the WordMedS4 folder on your storage medium and then double-click **NSMCPatientsDS.mdb**.

3   Click the Mailings tab, if necessary, and then click the Edit Recipient List button in the Start Mail Merge group.

4   At the Mail Merge Recipients dialog box, click the check box at the right of the *Data Source* column heading.

> This removes the check mark from the check box preceding each record.

5   Select the records of those individuals coming to the clinic for dermatology reasons by clicking the check boxes preceding the names *Zahn*, *Sellers*, *Higgins*, *Koehler*, and *Coburn*.

6   Click OK to close the Mail Merge Recipients dialog box.

7   Click the Preview Results button and then click the Next Record and/or Previous Record buttons to view the merged letters.

8   Select the records of those patients living in the city of Lake Oswego. Begin by clicking the Edit Recipient List button in the Start Mail Merge group.

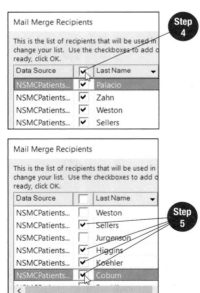

In Brief

Filter Records
1. Open main document.
2. Click Mailings tab.
3. Click Edit Recipient List button.
4. At Mail Merge Recipients dialog box, select specific records by inserting/removing check marks.
5. Click OK.

9 At the Mail Merge Recipients dialog box, click the check box at the right of the *Data Source* column heading.

> This removes the check mark from the check box preceding each record.

10 Click the check boxes preceding the patient names *Koehler* and *Lockard* to insert check marks.

11 Click OK to close the Mail Merge Recipients dialog box.

12 View the merged letter and then click the Previous Record button to view the other merged letter.

13 Send the merged letters directly to the printer by clicking the Finish & Merge button in the Finish group on the Mailings tab and then clicking *Print Documents* at the drop-down list.

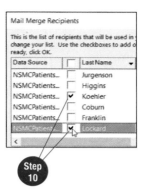

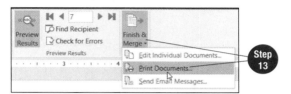

14 Click OK at the Merge to Printer dialog box and then click OK at the Print dialog box.

> Two letters will print.

15 Close **NSMCMainDoc.docx** without saving the changes.

Check Your Work — Compare your work with the model answer to ensure that you have completed the activity correctly.

In Addition

Filtering Records Using the Filter and Sort Dialog Box

Using check boxes to select specific records is useful in a data source that contains a limited number of records, but it may not be practical when you are working with a larger data source. When a data source contains many different records, filter records with options at the Filter and Sort dialog box with the Filter Records tab selected, as shown below. Display this dialog box by clicking the Filter hyperlink in the *Refine recipient list* section of the Mail Merge Recipients dialog box. When you select a field from the *Field* drop-down list, Word automatically inserts *Equal to* in the *Comparison* option box, but you can make other comparisons. Clicking the *Comparison* option box arrow causes a drop-down list to display with these additional options: *Not equal to, Less than, Greater than, Less than or equal, Greater than or equal, Is blank, Is not blank, Contains,* and *Does not contain*. Use one of these options to create a filter equation. For example, select all customers with a ZIP code higher than 97439 by clicking *ZIP Code* at the *Field* drop-down list, clicking *Greater than* at the *Comparison* drop-down list, and then typing 97439 in the *Compare to* text box.

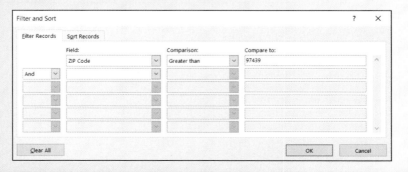

Activity 4.5   Preparing and Merging Envelopes

When you create a letter as a main document and then merge it with a data source file, you will most likely need properly addressed envelopes in which to send the letters. Create and print envelopes with options on the Mailings tab.

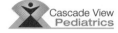

What You Will Do   Before mailing letters to clinic patients, you need to prepare and print the envelopes.

Tutorial
Merging Envelopes

1 At a blank document, click the Mailings tab, click the Start Mail Merge button, and then click *Envelopes* at the drop-down list.

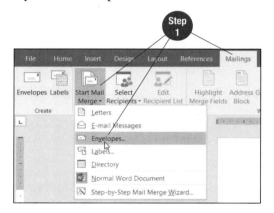

2 At the Envelope Options dialog box, make sure the envelope size is set to *10* and then click OK.

3 Click the Select Recipients button in the Start Mail Merge group and then click *Use an Existing List* at the drop-down list.

4 At the Select Data Source dialog box, navigate to the WordMedS4 folder on your storage medium and then double-click the *4-CVPPatients.mdb* file you created in Activity 4.1 in the *Select Data Source* list box.

> Notice that an Access icon displays before *4-CVPPatients.mdb*, indicating that it is an Access database file.

5 In the document window, click the approximate location in the envelope where the recipient's name and address will appear.

> This causes a box with a dashed gray border to display. If you do not see this box, try clicking a different location in the envelope.

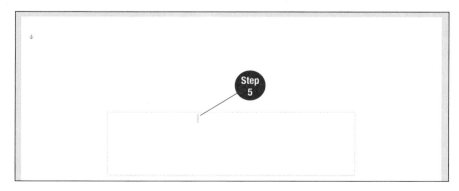

6 Click the Address Block button in the Write & Insert Fields group.

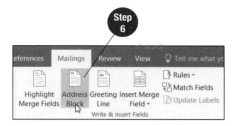

Step 6

7 At the Insert Address Block dialog box, click OK.

This inserts the field «AddressBlock» inside the box in the envelope.

8 Click the Finish & Merge button in the Finish group and then click *Edit Individual Documents* at the drop-down list.

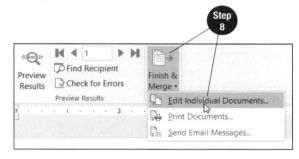

Step 8

9 At the Merge to New Document dialog box, make sure *All* is selected and then click OK.

10 Save the merged envelopes in the normal manner in the WordMedS4 folder on your storage medium and name the document **4-CVPPatientEnvs**.

11 Print **4-CVPPatientEnvs.docx**.

This document will print four envelopes. Check with your instructor about specific steps for printing envelopes. You may need to hand-feed envelopes into your printer.

12 Close **4-CVPPatientEnvs.docx**.

13 Save the envelope main document in the normal manner in the WordMedS4 folder and name it **4-CVPEnvMainDoc**.

14 Close **4-CVPEnvMainDoc.docx**.

Check Your Work Compare your work with the model answer to ensure that you have completed the activity correctly.

In Addition

Preparing a Directory Using the Mail Merge Feature

When merging letters, envelopes, or mailing labels, a new form is created for each record. For example, if a data source file containing eight records is merged with a letter main document, eight letters are created. If a data source file containing 20 records is merged with a mailing label main document, 20 labels are created. However, in some situations, you may want merged information to remain on the same page. This is useful, for example, when creating a directory or address list. To create a merged directory, click the Start Mail Merge button and then click *Directory* at the drop-down list. Create or identify an existing data source file and then insert the desired fields in the directory document. Set tabs if you want to insert the text in columns.

Creating a Table and Changing the Table Layout

Word's Table feature is useful for displaying data in columns and rows. This data may be text, values, and/or formulas. Create a table using the Table button on the Insert tab or with options at the Insert Table dialog box. Once you specify the desired numbers of rows and columns, Word displays the table and you are ready to enter information into the cells. A cell is the box created by the intersection of a column and a row. With the insertion point positioned in a table, two tabs are available for modifying and formatting the table—the Table Tools Design tab and the Table Tools Layout tab. Use options and buttons on the Table Tools Layout tab to perform such actions as selecting a table, row, or the entire table; inserting or deleting rows and/or columns; changing the height and width of rows and columns; and specifying text alignment in cells. You can also click the Properties button to display the Table Properties dialog box with options for vertically and horizontally centering a table on the page.

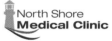
North Shore
Medical Clinic

What You Will Do Lee Elliott has asked you to edit a fact sheet on caffeine. You will open the fact sheet and then insert additional information about caffeine in a table for easy viewing. You will then increase and decrease the column widths, increase the height of a row, and apply formatting to both the entire table and specific cells within the table.

Tutorial
Creating a Table

Tutorial
Changing the Table Layout

Tutorial
Customizing Cells in a Table

1 Open **NSMCCaffeine.docx** and then save it with the name **4-NSMCCaffeine**. (If necessary, change the zoom to *100%*.)

2 Press Ctrl + End to move the insertion point to the end of the document.

3 Display the Insert Table dialog box by clicking the Insert tab, clicking the Table button in the Tables group, and then clicking *Insert Table* at the drop-down list.

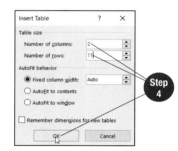

4 At the Insert Table dialog box, type 2 in the *Number of columns* measurement box, press the Tab key, type 11 in the *Number of rows* measurement box, and then click OK to close the dialog box.

5 Type the text in the cells as shown in Figure W4.4. Press the Tab key to move the insertion point to the next cell or press Shift + Tab to move the insertion point to the previous cell. To move the insertion point to different cells within the table using the mouse, click in the desired cell. After typing the last entry in the table, *20 mg*, do not press the Tab key. This action will insert another row. If this happens, immediately click the Undo button.

Figure W4.4 Step 5

Drink/Food	Amount of Caffeine
Brewed coffee	115 mg
Pepsi	38 mg
Coca-Cola	34 mg
Diet Coke	45 mg
Mountain Dew	55 mg
Tea (leaf or bag)	50 mg
Iced tea	70 mg
Cocoa beverage	4 mg
Milk chocolate	6 mg
Dark chocolate	20 mg

6 After typing the table, you realize that you need to include a column that identifies the specific amount of the drink or food. To do this, click in the cell containing the text *Amount of Caffeine*, click the Table Tools Layout tab, and then click the Insert Left button in the Rows & Columns group.

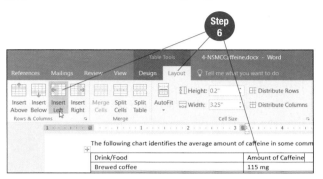

7 Click in the top cell of the new column, type Amount of Drink/Food, and then press the Down Arrow key. Type the amounts in the remaining cells as shown at the right. (Press the Down Arrow key to move to the next cell down.)

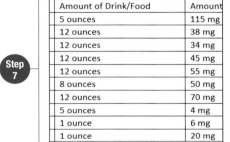

Amount of Drink/Food	Amount
5 ounces	115 mg
12 ounces	38 mg
12 ounces	34 mg
12 ounces	45 mg
12 ounces	55 mg
8 ounces	50 mg
12 ounces	70 mg
5 ounces	4 mg
1 ounce	6 mg
1 ounce	20 mg

8 Delete the *Cocoa beverage* row. To do this, click anywhere in the text *Cocoa beverage*, click the Table Tools Layout tab, click the Delete button in the Rows & Columns group, and then click *Delete Rows* at the drop-down list.

9 Insert a row above *Drink/Food* by clicking anywhere in the text *Drink/Food* and then clicking the Insert Above button in the Rows & Columns group.

10 With the new top row selected, merge the cells by clicking the Merge Cells button in the Merge group.

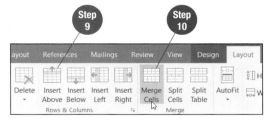

11 Type CAFFEINE CHART in the top row.

12 Select all cells in the table by clicking the table move handle in the upper left corner of the table (square with a four-headed arrow inside).

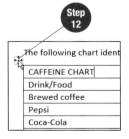

> You can also select all cells in a table by clicking the Table Tools Layout tab, clicking the Select button in the Table group, and then clicking *Select Table* at the drop-down list.

13 Click the Home tab, change the font to Cambria, change the font size to 12 points, and then click outside the table to deselect it.

14 Position the mouse pointer on the gridline between the first and second columns until the pointer turns into a double-headed arrow pointing left and right with a short double line in the middle. Click and hold down the left mouse button, drag to the left until the table column marker displays at the 1.5-inch mark on the horizontal ruler, and then release the mouse button.

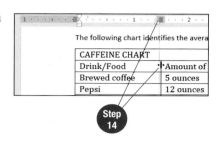

Step 14

15 Following the same procedure, drag the gridline between the second and third columns to the left until the table column marker displays at the 3.5-inch mark on the horizontal ruler.

16 Drag the gridline at the far right side of the table to the left until the table column marker displays at the 5.25-inch mark on the horizontal ruler.

17 Position the mouse pointer on the gridline between the first and second rows until the pointer turns into a double-headed arrow pointing up and down with a short double line in the middle. Hold down the left mouse button, drag down approximately 0.25 inch on the vertical ruler, and then release the mouse button.

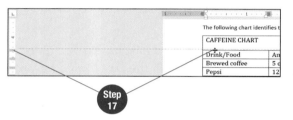

Step 17

18 Click in the top cell (contains the text *CAFFEINE CHART*), click the Select button in the Table group on the Table Tools Layout tab, and then click *Select Cell* at the drop-down list.

Step 18

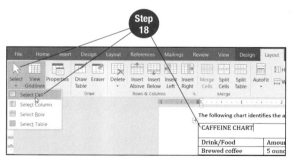

19 Apply character formatting by clicking the Home tab, clicking the Bold button in the Font group, clicking the *Font Size* option box arrow, and then clicking *16* at the drop-down gallery.

20 With the cell still selected, horizontally and vertically center the text in the cell by clicking the Table Tools Layout tab and then clicking the Align Center button in the Alignment group.

21 Increase the height of the top row by clicking the *Table Row Height* measurement box up arrow in the Cell Size group on the Table Tools Layout tab until *0.5″* displays.

Step 21   Step 20

In Brief

Insert Table
1. Click Insert tab.
2. Click Table button.
3. Drag in grid to select columns and rows.

OR

1. Click Insert tab.
2. Click Table button.
3. Click *Insert Table*.
4. Type number of columns.
5. Press Tab key.
6. Type number of rows.
7. Click OK.

Increase/Decrease Column/Row
1. Click Table Tools Layout tab.
2. Click in *Table Row Height* measurement box or *Table Column Width* measurement box.
3. Type measurement.
4. Press Enter.

OR

1. Position mouse pointer on gridline until it turns into double-headed arrow.
2. Click and hold down left mouse button, drag to new position, release mouse button.

22 Click in the cell containing the text *Drink/Food*.

23 Click the Select button in the Table group and then click *Select Row* at the drop-down list.

24 Apply bold formatting to the text in the row by pressing Ctrl + B and then click the Align Bottom Center button ▤ in the Alignment group on the Table Tools Layout tab.

25 Position the mouse pointer in the cell containing the first occurrence of the text *5 ounces*, click and hold down the left mouse button, drag down and to the right to the cell containing the text *20 mg*, and then release the mouse button.

26 With the cells selected, click the Align Bottom Center button in the Alignment group.

27 Click anywhere in the table to deselect the cells.

28 Center the table between the left and right margins. To begin, click the Properties button ▤ in the Table group on the Table Tools Layout tab.

29 At the Table Properties dialog box with the Table tab selected, click the *Center* option in the *Alignment* section.

30 Click OK to close the dialog box.

31 Save **4-NSMCCaffeine.docx**.

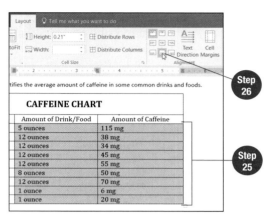

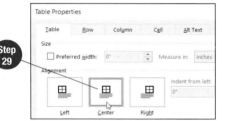

Check Your Work Compare your work with the model answer to ensure that you have completed the activity correctly.

In Addition

Other Methods for Creating a Table

You can also create a table using the Table button drop-down grid. To do so, click the Insert tab, click the Table button, drag the mouse pointer down and to the right until the desired number of columns and rows are selected and the numbers above the grid display the numbers of columns and rows, and then click the left mouse button. Another method for creating a table is to draw a table by clicking the Table button and then clicking *Draw Table* at the drop-down list. The mouse pointer display as a pencil. Drag in the document screen to create the desired number of columns and rows.

Selecting Cells with the Keyboard

Besides using the mouse, you can also select cells using the following keyboard shortcuts:

To select	Press
the next cell's contents	Tab
the preceding cell's contents	Shift + Tab
the entire table	Alt + 5 (on numeric keypad with Num Lock off)
adjacent cells	Hold Shift key and then press an arrow key repeatedly.
a column	Position insertion point in top cell of a column, hold down Shift key, and then press Down Arrow key until column is selected.

Activity 4.7 Changing the Table Design

The Table Tools Design tab contains a number of options for enhancing the appearance of a table. Use options in the Table Styles group to select a predesigned style that applies color and border lines to a table. Maintain further control over the predesigned style formatting applied to columns and rows with options in the Table Style Options group. Apply additional formatting to cells in a table with the Shading button in the Table Styles group and the Borders button in the Borders group. With options in the Borders group, you can customize the borders of cells in a table, display a list of predesigned border lines; change the line style, width, and color; add or remove borders; and apply the same border style formatting to other cells with the Border Painter button.

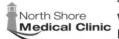
North Shore
Medical Clinic

Tutorial
Changing the Table Design

Tutorial
Sorting Text in a Table

What You Will Do   You will add final touches to the Caffeine Chart table by applying border, shading, and style formatting.

1. With **4-NSMCCaffeine.docx** open, click anywhere in the table and then select the entire table by clicking the table move handle in the upper left corner of the table.

2. With the table selected, click the Table Tools Design tab, click the Borders button arrow in the Borders group, and then click *Borders and Shading* at the drop-down list.

    This displays the Borders and Shading dialog box with the Borders tab selected.

3. At the Borders and Shading dialog box, click the *Grid* option in the *Setting* section, scroll down the *Style* list box, and then click the first thick/thin line option as shown at the right.

4. Click the *Color* option box arrow and then click the *Green, Accent 6, Darker 25%* option at the drop-down list (tenth column, fifth row in the *Theme Colors* section).

5. Click OK to close the Borders and Shading dialog box.

6. Select the second row in the table, click the Shading button arrow in the Table Styles group, and then click the *Gold, Accent 4, Lighter 80%* option at the drop-down list (eighth column, second row in the *Theme Colors* section).

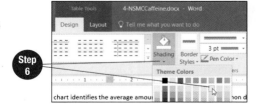

7. Save and then print **4-NSMCCaffeine.docx**.

8. Make sure the insertion point is positioned in the table and then apply a table style. Begin by clicking the More Table Styles button in the Table Styles group on the Table Tools Design tab.

    This displays a drop-down gallery of style choices.

9 Click the table style option in the second column, fourth row in the *Grid Tables* section.

> Notice the color and border style formatting and how applying the style changed the border and shading formatting you applied earlier.

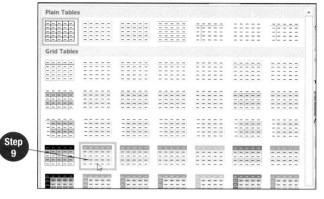

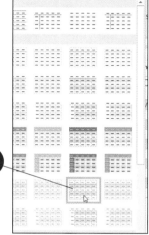

10 Experiment with an additional style by clicking the More Table Styles button in the Table Styles group and then clicking the table style option in the sixth column, sixth row in the *Grid Tables* section.

11 Change the formatting by clicking the *Header Row* check box in the Table Style Options group to remove the check mark and then clicking the *First Column* check box to remove the check mark.

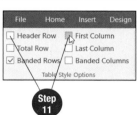

12 Applying the table styles removed the horizontal alignment of the table. Reapply this formatting by clicking the Table Tools Layout tab, clicking the Properties button, clicking the *Center* option in the *Alignment* section, and then clicking OK to close the dialog box.

13 Save, print, and then close **4-NSMCCaffeine.docx**.

> **Check Your Work** Compare your work with the model answer to ensure that you have completed the activity correctly.

In Addition

Sorting in a Table

Sort text in a table alphabetically, numerically, or by date with options at the Sort dialog box. Display this dialog box by positioning the insertion point in a cell in the table and then clicking the Sort button in the Data group on the Table Tools Layout tab. Make sure the column you want to sort is selected in the *Sort by* option box and then click OK. If the first row in the table contains data such as headings that you do not want to include in the sort, click the *Header row* option in the *My list has* section of the Sort dialog box. If you want to sort specific cells in a table, select the cells first and then click the Sort button.

Inserting a Row Using the Mouse

You can use the mouse to insert a row by moving the mouse pointer immediately left of the row above or below the location where you want the new row inserted. As you move the mouse pointer to the left side of a row, a plus symbol inside a circle displays along with thin, blue, double lines across the top or bottom of the row. Move the symbol and lines to the bottom of the row and then click the plus symbol and a new row is inserted below the current row. Move the symbol and lines to the top of the row and then click the plus symbol and a row is inserted above the current row.

Activity 4.8 Creating a Form for Handwritten Entries

Forms are a major part of a patient's medical records. They come in a variety of types in a medical office or hospital and include those that require patients to enter handwritten information and those that require a medical office assistant or hospital worker to enter information at the computer. When creating forms for entering handwritten information, consider using tables to improve readability.

North Shore Medical Clinic

What You Will Do   One of your job duties is to make follow-up calls to patients after they have received surgery. You realize that creating a form will improve the clarity and completeness of the information you gather from the patients. You decide to create a table in which you can handwrite the patients' responses to your questions as you conduct your follow-up calls.

1. Open **NSMCLtrhd.docx** and then save it with the name **4-NSMCCallRecord**.

2. Click the *No Spacing* style in the Styles group on the Home tab, change the font to 12-point Cambria, and then press the Enter key two times.

3. Create the form shown in Figure W4.5. To begin, type the title, POST-OPERATIVE CALL RECORD, select the text, change the paragraph alignment to center, and then apply bold formatting.

4. Press the Enter key two times and then change the paragraph alignment back to left.

5. Create a table with four rows and four columns by clicking the Insert tab, clicking the Table button, dragging the mouse pointer down and to the right until four rows and four columns are selected in the grid and *4x4 Table* displays above it, and then clicking the left mouse button.

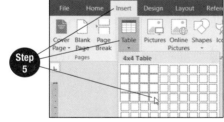

6. Type the text in the cells as shown in Figure W4.5. Bold and center the column heading text and apply Blue, Accent 1, Lighter 60% shading as shown.

7. After creating the first table, press Ctrl + End to move the insertion point below the table.

8. Press the Enter key and then type the text below the first table as shown in Figure W4.5.

9. Create the second table with four columns and six rows as shown in the figure.

10. Decrease or increase the size of the columns so they match what displays in the figure.

11. Type the text in the cells, bold and center the column heading text as shown in the figure, and then apply Blue, Accent 1, Lighter 60% shading as shown.

12. Press Ctrl + End to move the insertion point below the table and then press the Enter key.

13 Create the remaining two tables as shown in Figure W4.5.

14 Save, print, and then close **4-NSMCCallRecord.docx**.

Figure W4.5 Form for Handwritten Entries

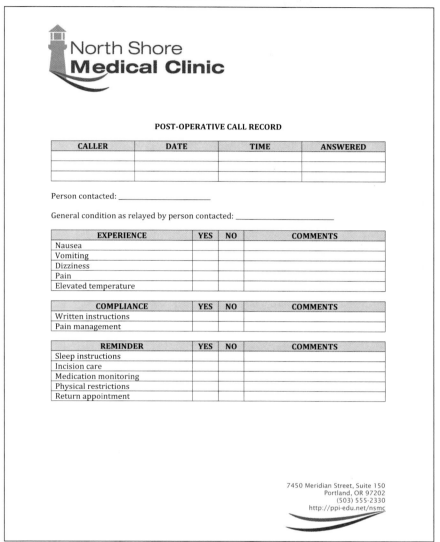

In Addition

Customizing Cell Size

When you first create a table, the column widths are equal, as are the row heights. You can customize the width of columns and the height of rows with buttons in the Cell Size group on the Table Tools Layout tab. Use the *Table Row Height* measurement box to increase or decrease the height of rows and use the *Table Column Width* measurement box to increase or decrease the width of columns. The Distribute Rows button distributes equally the height of selected rows and the Distribute Columns button distributes equally the width of selected columns. You can also change column width using the move table column markers on the horizontal ruler. To do this, position the mouse pointer on a column marker until the pointer turns into an arrow pointing left and right and then drag the marker to the desired position. Hold down the Shift key while dragging a column marker and the horizontal ruler remains stationary while the column marker moves. Hold down the Alt key while dragging a column marker and precise measurements display on the horizontal ruler.

Many hospitals and clinics purchase and use preprinted forms that are generally filled in by hand or using a computer. You can use Word to create your own forms, eliminating the need for preprinted ones. You can insert text boxes, check boxes, and drop-down lists. Forms created in Word are saved as templates so that when someone fills in the form, they are working on a copy of the form, not the original. The original is the template that is saved as a protected document. When a form is created from the protected template, information can be typed only in certain designated fields. Use options in the Controls group on the Developer tab to insert text content controls, check box content controls, or other form content controls into a form template document. Turn on the display of the Developer tab at the Word Options dialog box.

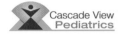
Cascade View
Pediatrics

What You Will Do   You are responsible for checking in patients as they arrive at the clinic and for updating their records, if necessary. You decide to create a form with fields that can be used to enter revised patient data at the computer.

Tutorial
Protecting a Form
Template

1 To begin creating a form, you first need to display the Developer tab. Begin by clicking the File tab and then clicking *Options*.

2 At the Word Options dialog box, click *Customize Ribbon* in the left panel.

3 In the list box at the right, click the *Developer* tab check box to insert a check mark and then click OK to close the Word Options dialog box.

The Developer tab displays to the right of the View tab on the ribbon.

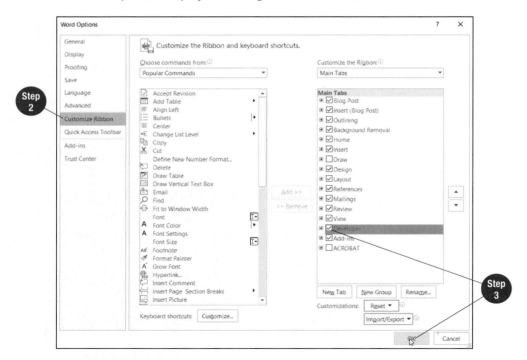

4 Open **CVPPatientForm.docx**.

5 Save CVPPatientForm.docx as a template. Begin by pressing the F12 key to display the Save As dialog box.

6 At the Save As dialog box, type XXX-UpdateTemplate in the *File name* text box (typing your initials in place of the *XXX*).

7 Click the *Save as type* option box and then click *Word Template (*.dotx)* at the drop-down list.

> Word automatically displays the Custom Office Templates folder in the Documents folder on the computer's hard drive.

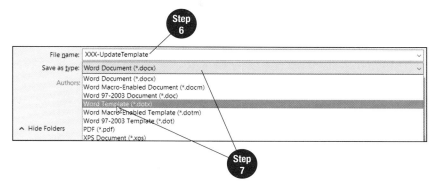

8 Click the Save button.

9 Position the mouse pointer to the right of the text *Patient Name:* and then click the left mouse button. This positions the insertion point one space to the right of the colon after *Patient Name:*.

10 Click the Developer tab and then click the Plain Text Content Control button [Aa] in the Controls group.

> This inserts a plain text content control with the text *Click or tap here to enter text*.

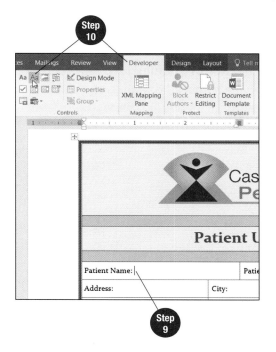

11 Insert plain text content control fields in the remaining cells as shown in Figure W4.6. To insert the check boxes in the *Check the appropriate box identifying with whom the patient lives.* section, click in the desired cell and then click the Check Box Content Control button 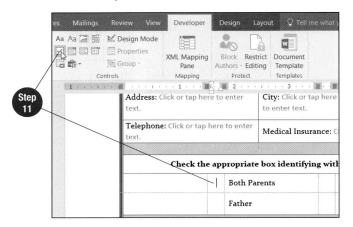 in the Controls group.

> As you type, content controls and text appear crowded and wrap to the next line. Data you enter into the form will replace the content control text.

12 Protect the template by clicking the Restrict Editing button 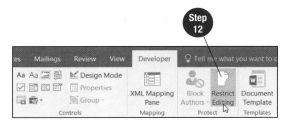 in the Protect group on the Developer tab.

13 At the Restrict Editing task pane, click the *Allow only this type of editing in the document* check box to insert a check mark, click the down-pointing arrow at the right of the option box in the *Editing restrictions* section, and then click *Filling in forms* at the drop-down list.

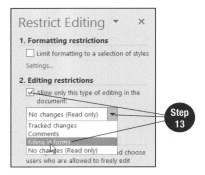

14 Click the Yes, Start Enforcing Protection button and then click OK at the Start Enforcing Protection dialog box. (Creating a password is optional.)

15 Close the Restrict Editing task pane by clicking the Close button in the upper right corner of the task pane.

16 Save, print, and then close **XXX-UpdateTemplate.dotx**.

Save a Form as a Template
1. Open document.
2. Press F12.
3. At Save As dialog box, change *Save as type* option to *Word Template (*.dotx)*.
4. Type document name.
5. Click Save button.

Display the Developer Tab
1. Click File tab.
2. Click *Options*.
3. Click *Customize Ribbon*.
4. Click *Developer tab* check box to insert check mark.
5. Click OK.

Protect a Template
1. Click Developer tab.
2. Click Restrict Editing button.
3. Click *Allow only this type of editing in the document* check box.
4. Click option box arrow in *Editing restrictions* section.
5. Click *Filling in forms*.
6. Click Yes, Start Enforcing Protection button.
7. Click OK.

Figure W4.6 Form Template

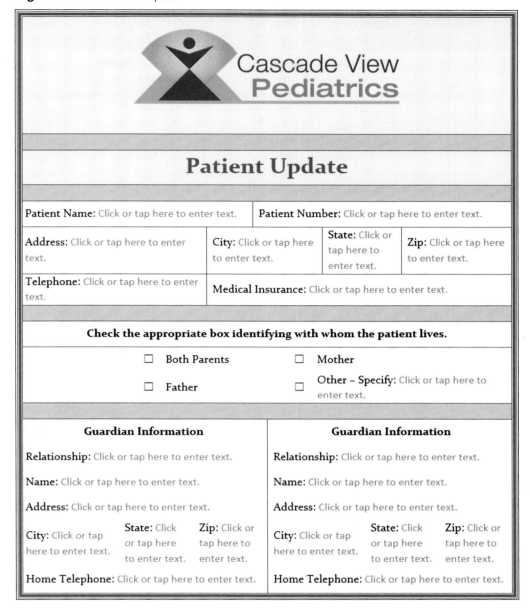

Check Your Work — Compare your work with the model answer to ensure that you have completed the activity correctly.

In Addition

Defining a Group

Another method for protecting a region in a form from being edited or deleted by a respondent is by defining a group using the Group button on the Developer tab. A group can contain text, tables, graphics, and content controls. When a group is defined, the respondent can enter information in the content controls but cannot edit the other text or items in the group. To define a group, select the text and content controls, click the Group button in the Controls group on the Developer tab, and then click the *Group* option at the drop-down list.

Saving a Template to a Storage Medium

If you are working on a computer in a public environment, you should save a backup of your template on your storage medium (such as a USB flash drive). That way, if the computer is reset on a regular basis, you can copy your template back to the Custom Office Templates folder.

Activity 4.10　Filling In and Printing a Form Document

After a form template has been created, grouped, and saved, it can be used to create a personalized form document. To begin, open a document based on the form template by clicking the File tab and then clicking the *New* option. At the New backstage area, click the *PERSONAL* option and then click the thumbnail representing the template. When a document based on a form template is opened, the insertion point is automatically positioned in the first content control. Enter the required text and then press the Tab key to select the placeholder text in the next content control. You can move the insertion point to a previous form field by pressing Shift + Tab. Fill in a check box form field by clicking the check box.

Cascade View Pediatrics

What You Will Do　A patient that is a minor child has arrived at the clinic for an appointment. You will enter the updated information for the patient and her parents using the Patient Update form.

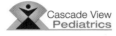
Tutorial
Filling in a Form with Content Controls

Tutorial
Printing a Form

1 Create a form with the **XXX-UpdateTemplate.dotx** template. To begin, click the File tab and then click the *New* option.

2 At the New backstage area, click the *PERSONAL* option.

3 Click the *XXX-UpdateTemplate* thumbnail.

> This opens a new document based on the form template.

4 Word displays the form document with the *Patient Name:* content control selected. Type the name Jolie Pearson, as shown at the right and in Figure W4.7.

5 Press the Tab key to move to the next content control.

6 Fill in the remaining information as shown in Figure W4.7. Press the Tab key to move the insertion point to the next content control and press Shift + Tab to move the insertion point to the previous content control. To insert an *X* in a check box, click the check box. If you insert an *X* by mistake, click the check box again to remove it.

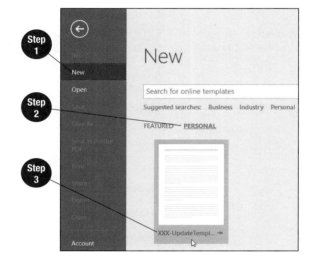

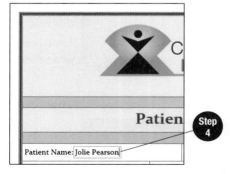

7 When the form is completed, save the document in the WordMedS4 folder on your storage medium and name it **4-CVPUpdate**.

8 Print and then close **4-CVPUpdate.docx**.

In Brief

**Open a Document
Based on a Template**
1. Click File tab.
2. Click *New*.
3. Click *PERSONAL*.
4. Click template
   thumbnail.

Figure W4.7 Filled-in Form

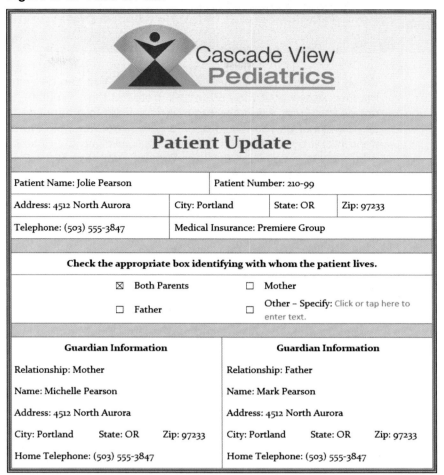

Cascade View **Pediatrics**

Patient Update

Patient Name: Jolie Pearson | Patient Number: 210-99

Address: 4512 North Aurora | City: Portland | State: OR | Zip: 97233

Telephone: (503) 555-3847 | Medical Insurance: Premiere Group

Check the appropriate box identifying with whom the patient lives.

☒ Both Parents ☐ Mother

☐ Father ☐ Other – Specify: Click or tap here to enter text.

Guardian Information

Relationship: Mother

Name: Michelle Pearson

Address: 4512 North Aurora

City: Portland State: OR Zip: 97233

Home Telephone: (503) 555-3847

Guardian Information

Relationship: Father

Name: Mark Pearson

Address: 4512 North Aurora

City: Portland State: OR Zip: 97233

Home Telephone: (503) 555-3847

Check Your Work — Compare your work with the model answer to ensure that you have completed the activity correctly.

In Addition

Customizing Plain Text Content Control Properties

To change options for a plain text content control, select the plain text content control and then click the Properties button in the Controls group on the Developer tab. This displays the Content Control Properties dialog box, shown at the right. At this dialog box, you can apply a title or tag to the content control, lock the content control, and apply formatting options.

Customizing Check Box Content Control Properties

You can customize check box content control options at the Content Control Properties dialog box, shown at the right. Display this dialog box by selecting a check box content control and then clicking the Properties button in the Controls group on the Developer tab. At the dialog box, you can specify options such as check box symbols and formatting options.

Editing a Form Template; Inserting a Drop-Down List Content Control

When creating a form template, the template text can be edited and saved in the normal manner. However, if you create and protect a form template, the text in the template cannot be changed. If you need to make changes to a template, open the template in the same manner as you would open a normal document in Word. With the template open, unprotect it by clicking the Developer tab, clicking the Restrict Editing button in the Protect group, and then clicking the Stop Protection button at the Restrict Editing task pane. Make the desired changes to the template and then protect the template again. Some fields in a form may require the person entering the information to choose from a list of specific options. Create this type of field by using the Drop-Down List Content Control button in the Controls group on the Developer tab. After inserting a drop-down list content control, click the Properties button in the Controls group and the Content Control Properties dialog box displays. Use options at this dialog box to type the options you want to include in the list. A drop-down list content control in a form displays as a content control placeholder with a down-pointing arrow at the right side of the box. When entering data in a form, click the down-pointing arrow and then click the desired option at the drop-down list.

Cascade View Pediatrics

What You Will Do   After using the Patient Update form a couple of times, you realize that you need to add additional fields. You will update the form template to include new content controls and change the *Medical Insurance* field to a drop-down form field since your clinic only accepts medical insurance from three healthcare providers.

Tutorial
Editing a Form
Template

Tutorial
Setting Content
Control Properties

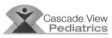

1. Press Ctrl + F12 to display the Open dialog box.

2. At the Open dialog box, click the *Documents* folder (if necessary) in the Navigation pane and then double-click the *Custom Office Templates* folder in the Content pane.

3. Double-click **XXX-UpdateTemplate.dotx** in the Content pane.

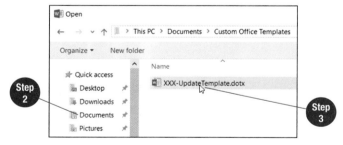

4. Unprotect the template document by clicking the Developer tab and then clicking the Restrict Editing button in the Protect group.

5. At the Restrict Editing task pane, click the Stop Protection button that displays toward the bottom.

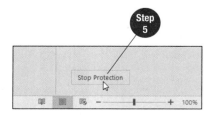

6 Insert a new row at the bottom of the table. To do this, click in one of the cells in the bottom row, click the Table Tools Layout tab, and then click the Insert Below button [icon] in the Rows & Columns group.

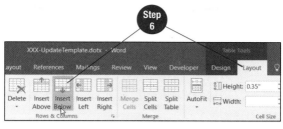

Step 6

7 Click in the first column of the new row, type Work Telephone:, and then press the spacebar.

8 Insert a plain text content control by clicking the Developer tab and then clicking the Plain Text Content Control button in the Controls group.

9 Press the Right Arrow key to deselect the content control, press the Tab key to move the insertion point to the new cell in the second column, type Work Telephone:, press the spacebar, and then insert a plain text content control.

10 To change the *Medical Insurance:* plain text content control to a drop-down content control, begin by clicking the plain text content control, clicking the content control tab, and then pressing the Delete key.

This removes the plain text content control from the cell.

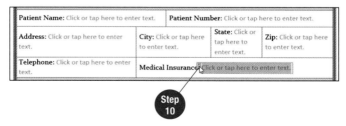

Step 7

Step 8

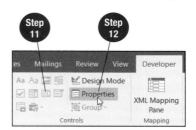

Step 10

11 Click the Drop-Down List Content Control button [icon] in the Controls group on the Developer tab.

12 Click the Properties button [icon] in the Controls group.

This displays the Content Control Properties dialog box.

Step 11

Step 12

13 At the Content Control Properties dialog box, click the Add button.

14 At the Add Choice dialog box, type Health Plus America in the *Display Name* text box and then click OK.

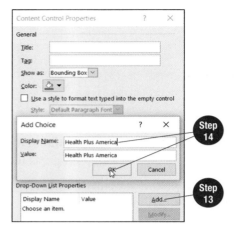

15 Click the Add button, type Premiere Group in the *Display Name* text box, and then click OK. Click the Add button, type Healthwise Cooperative, and then click OK. Click the Add button, type Self Insured, and then click OK.

16 Click OK to close the Content Control Properties dialog box.

17 Protect the template by clicking the Yes, Start Enforcing Protection button in the task pane and then clicking OK at the Start Enforcing Protection dialog box.

18 Close the Restrict Editing task pane.

19 Save and then close **XXX-UpdateTemplate.dotx**.

20 Click the File tab, click the *New* option, click the *PERSONAL* option, and then click the ***XXX-UpdateTemplate.dotx*** thumbnail.

21 Fill in the text and check boxes as shown in Figure W4.8. Press the Tab key to move to the next field or press Shift + Tab to move to the previous field. To fill in the drop-down form field, click the arrow at the right of the *Medical Insurance:* option box and then click *Healthwise Cooperative* at the drop-down list.

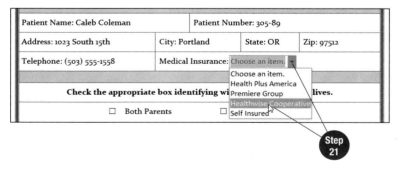

22 Save the completed form and name it **4-PatUpdate**.

23 Print and then close **4-PatUpdate.docx**.

Open a Form Template
1. Press Ctrl + F12.
2. Click *Documents* in
   Navigation pane.
3. Double-click *Custom
   Office Templates*
   folder.
4. Double-click template.

**Insert a Drop-Down
List Content Control**
1. Click Developer tab.
2. Click Drop-Down
   List Content Control
   button.

**Specify Drop-Down
List Content Control
Properties**
1. Select drop-down list
   content control.
2. Click Developer tab.
3. Click Properties
   button.
4. Click Add button.
5. Type choice.
6. Click OK.
7. Continue clicking Add
   button and typing
   choices.
8. Click OK.

Figure W4.8 Filled-in Form

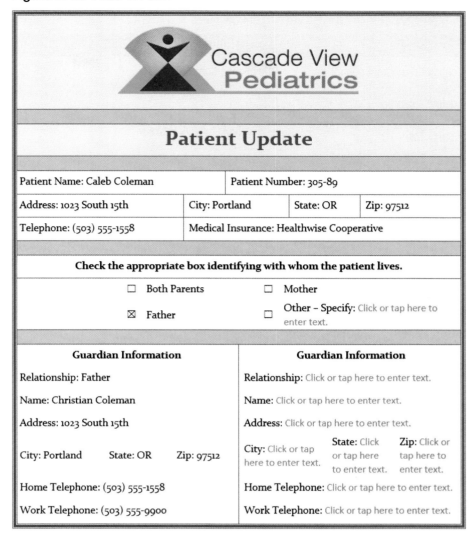

Check Your Work — Compare your work with the model answer to ensure that you have completed the activity correctly.

In Addition

Creating a Form with Legacy Tools

Click the Legacy Tools button in the Controls group on the Developer tab and a drop-down list displays with a number of fields you can insert in a form, including a text, check box, or drop-down list form field. The Text Form Field button in the Legacy Tools drop-down list is similar to the Plain Text Content Control button. To insert a text form field, position the insertion point in the desired location, click the Legacy Tools button in the Controls group on the Developer tab, and then click the Text Form Field button. This inserts a gray shaded box in the form. This shaded box is the location where data is entered when a person fills in the form.

Selecting an Option from a Drop-down List

When filling in a drop-down form field, make the field active and then either click the arrow at the right side of the form field or press Alt + Down Arrow on the keyboard. At the drop-down list that displays, click the desired choice. You may also use the Up or Down Arrow keys to navigate to the desired choice and then press the Enter key to select it.

Features Summary

Feature	Ribbon Tab, Group	Button	Option
check box content control	Developer, Controls	☑	
delete column	Table Tools Layout, Rows & Columns		*Delete Columns*
delete row	Table Tools Layout, Rows & Columns		*Delete Rows*
drop-down content control	Developer, Controls		
Insert Address Block dialog box	Mailings, Write & Insert Fields		
insert column	Table Tools Layout, Rows & Columns	OR	
Insert Greeting Line dialog box	Mailings, Write & Insert Fields		
insert merge field	Mailings, Write & Insert Fields		
insert row	Table Tools Layout, Rows & Columns	OR	
Insert Table dialog box	Insert, Tables		*Insert Table*
merge documents	Mailings, Finish		
plain text content control	Developer, Controls	Aa	
protect document	Developer, Protect		
select recipients	Mailings, Start Mail Merge		
start mail merge	Mailings, Start Mail Merge		
table	Insert, Tables		
Table Properties dialog box	Table Tools Layout, Table		
table styles	Table Tools Design, Table Styles		

Workbook   Section study tools and assessment activities are available in the Workbook pages of the ebook. These resources are designed to help you further develop and demonstrate mastery of the skills learned in this section.

Using Excel
in the Medical Office

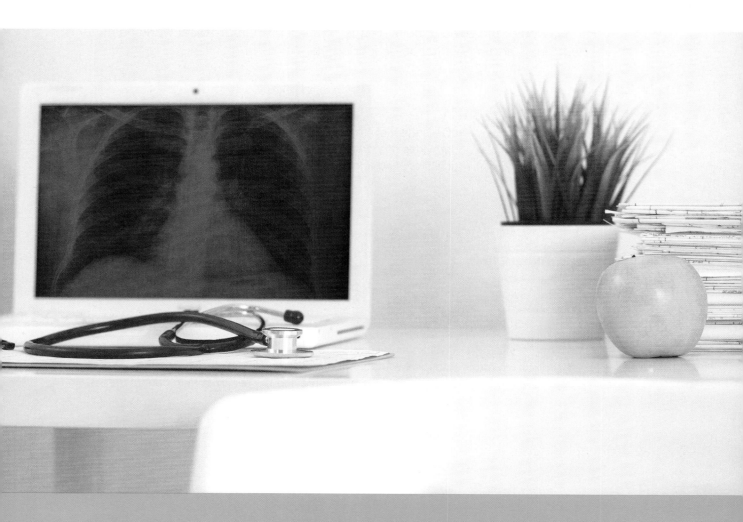

Introducing Excel 2016

Microsoft Excel 2016 is a popular choice among individuals and companies for presenting and analyzing data. Excel organizes information in columns and rows in a document called a worksheet. Once a worksheet has been created, you can perform analyses of hypothetical situations such as "What if medical supplies increase in price by 4%?" Changing a value in a worksheet causes Excel to automatically recalculate any other values dependent on the number you changed. In an instant, your question is answered.

In Section 1, you will create new worksheets by entering labels, values, and formulas. To improve your efficiency, you will learn to use tools such as the fill handle and special techniques for performing common tasks such as copying. Section 2 presents editing and formatting you can use to improve a worksheet's appearance and correct errors. Section 3 introduces function formulas; visual elements such as charts, images, and drawing objects; page layout and print options; and data management features for working with lists.

In each of the three Excel sections, you will prepare medical worksheets for two clinics and a hospital as described below.

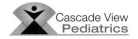

Cascade View Pediatrics is a full-service pediatric clinic that provides comprehensive primary pediatric care to infants, children, and adolescents.

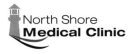

North Shore Medical Clinic is an internal medicine clinic dedicated to providing exceptional care to all patients. The physicians in the clinic specialize in a number of fields including internal medicine, family practice, cardiology, and dermatology.

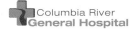

Columbia River General Hospital is an independent, not-for-profit hospital with the mission of providing high-quality, comprehensive care to patients and improving the health of members of the community.

Excel

Analyzing Data Using Excel

Skills

Data Files
Before beginning section work, copy the ExcelMedS1 folder to your storage medium and then make ExcelMedS1 the active folder.

- Create, save, print, and close a workbook
- Select cells
- Enter data
- Navigate and scroll
- Use the fill handle to enter a series
- Enter formulas
- Use the SUM function
- Copy formulas
- Improve the worksheet appearance

- Display cell formulas in a worksheet
- Sort a selection
- Use the Tell Me feature
- Use the Help feature
- Preview and print a worksheet
- Change the page orientation to landscape
- Create a new workbook using a template

Precheck
Check your current skills to help focus your study of the skills taught in this section.

Activities Overview

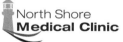
North Shore **Medical Clinic**

Create a payroll worksheet, browse a supplies inventory and standard exam room cost report, create an invoice, create a purchase order for medical supplies, and create an invoice for in-service training.

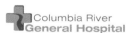
Columbia River **General Hospital**

Edit an executive management salary report, calculate funds needed for a professional development budget, and prepare a surgery cost report.

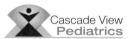
Cascade View **Pediatrics**

Complete an estimated travel expenses worksheet and calculate costs and registration fees for a medical seminar.

Model Answers
Preview the model answers for an overview of the activities you will complete in each section.

Activity 1.1 Creating, Saving, Printing, and Closing a Workbook

Excel is a spreadsheet application that is used to organize numerical and financial data and to analyze and evaluate information. Information is created in Excel in a worksheet and is saved in a file called a workbook. A workbook can contain several worksheets. Imagine a worksheet as a page with horizontal and vertical lines drawn in a grid to represent columns and rows. Data is entered into a cell, which is the intersection of a column and a row. Columns are lettered A to Z, AA to AZ, BA to BZ, and so on. The last column in a worksheet is labeled *XFD*. Rows are numbered 1, 2, 3, and so on. A column letter and a row number identify each cell. For example, A1 is the cell address for the intersection of column A with row 1. By default, an Excel workbook contains one worksheet labeled *Sheet1*. Additional sheets can be inserted as needed.

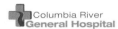 Columbia River General Hospital

What You Will Do   You have been asked to begin creating a weekly payroll report for Columbia River General Hospital by opening a blank workbook, entering data, printing the worksheet, and then closing the workbook and Excel.

Tutorial
Opening a Blank Workbook

Tutorial
Exploring the Excel Screen

Tutorial
Saving with a New Name

Tutorial
Closing a Workbook and Closing Excel

1 At the Windows 10 desktop, click the Start button.

2 At the Start menu, click the Excel 2016 tile.

> Depending on your system configuration, this step may vary.

3 At the Excel 2016 opening screen, click the *Blank workbook* template.

4 At the Excel screen, identify the various features by comparing your screen with the one shown in Figure E1.1. If necessary, maximize the Excel window. Depending on your screen resolution, what you see may vary slightly from what is shown in the figure. Refer to Table E1.1 for a description of the screen features.

Figure E1.1 Excel Worksheet Screen

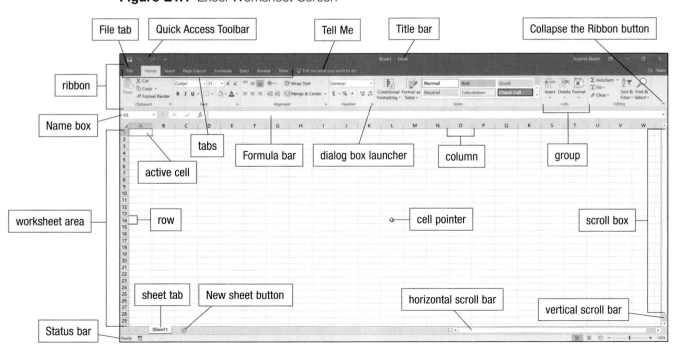

Table E1.1 Excel Screen Features and Descriptions

Feature	Description
active cell	location in the worksheet that will display typed data or that will be affected by a command
cell pointer	when you see this icon, select cells by clicking or dragging the mouse
Collapse the Ribbon button	click to remove the ribbon from the screen; double-click to redisplay the ribbon
dialog box or task pane launcher	click the down-pointing diagonal arrow in the bottom right corner of a group to open a dialog box or task pane with more options for that group
File tab	displays the backstage area that contains options for working with and managing files
Formula bar	displays the contents stored in the active cell
group	area on the ribbon, defined by separators, that contains similar buttons or features
Name box	displays the active cell address or the name assigned to the active cell
New sheet button	click to insert a new worksheet in the workbook
Quick Access Toolbar	contains buttons that allow commonly used commands to be executed with a single mouse click
ribbon	area containing tabs with commands and buttons divided into groups
scroll box	drag or click to scroll horizontally and vertically in a worksheet
sheet tab	identifies the worksheet in the workbook
Status bar	displays current mode, action messages, view buttons, and Zoom slider bar
tabs	contain commands and buttons organized into groups
Tell Me	used to look up a feature and provide options for using the feature
Title bar	displays workbook name followed by program name
vertical and horizontal scroll bars	used to view various parts of the worksheet beyond the current screen
worksheet area	contains cells used to create the worksheet

5 With cell A1 the active cell, type Payroll as the title for the new worksheet.

> When you type a new entry in a cell, the entry appears in the Formula bar as well as within the active cell in the worksheet area. To end a cell entry, press the Tab key or Enter key to move to another cell in the worksheet, or click the Enter button on the Formula bar.

6 Press the Enter key.

7 With cell A2 the active cell, type Week Ended: September 26, 2019 and then press the Enter key.

> The entry in cell A2 is overflowing into columns B, C, and D. You can allow a label to spill over into adjacent columns as long as you do not plan to enter other data in the overflow cells.

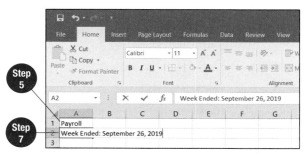

8 Click the File tab.

9 Click the *Print* option.

> The Print backstage area contains options, galleries, and buttons for printing the active worksheet.

10 Click the Print button.

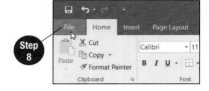

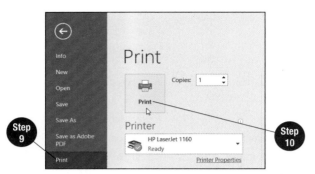

11 Click the File tab and then click the *Save As* option.

> To save a workbook with a new name (other than *Book1.xlsx*), use the *Save As* option. Saving a workbook with a different name is useful when you want to preserve the original file.

12 At the Save As backstage area, click the *Browse* option.

13 In the Navigation pane of the Save As dialog box, click the removable disk that contains the ExcelMedS1 folder.

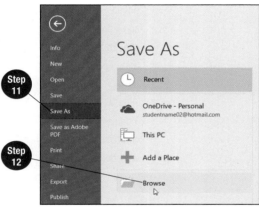

14 Double-click the *ExcelMedS1* folder in the Content pane.

15 Click in the *File name* text box.

16 Type the file name 1-Payroll and then click the Save button or press the Enter key.

> Press the F12 function key to display the Save As dialog box without displaying the Save As backstage area.

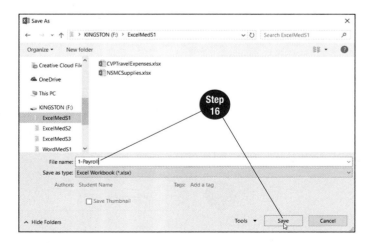

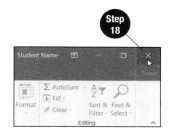

17 Click the File tab and then click the *Close* option to close the workbook.

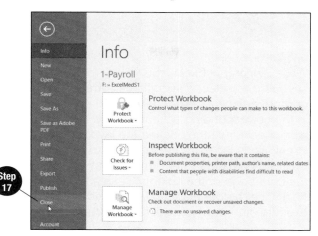

In Brief

Open Excel
1. Click Start button.
2. Click Excel 2016 tile.

Enter Data
1. Make cell active.
2. Type data.
3. Press Enter.

Print Workbook
1. Click File tab.
2. Click *Print*.
3. Click Print button.

Save Workbook with New Name
1. Click File tab.
2. Click *Save As*.
3. Click *Browse*.
4. Navigate to folder.
5. Click in *File name* text box.
6. Type workbook name.
7. Click Save or press Enter.

Close Workbook
1. Click File tab.
2. Click *Close*.

Close Excel
Click Close button.

18 Click the Close button to close Excel.

When no workbooks are open, Excel displays a blank gray screen.

Check Your Work Compare your work with the model answer to ensure that you have completed the activity correctly.

In Addition

Using AutoComplete

As you start to type a new entry in a cell, the AutoComplete feature in Excel will attempt to complete it for you. If the first few letters that you type match another entry in the column, Excel automatically fills in the remaining text. Press Tab, Enter, or one of the arrow keys to accept the suggested text, or continue typing the correct text. You can turn off AutoComplete at the Excel Options dialog box. Do this by clicking the File tab and then clicking *Options*. Click *Advanced* in the left panel, click the *Enable AutoComplete for cell values* check box to remove the check mark, and then click OK.

While working in Excel, you will be required to select cells in a worksheet. Use the mouse or keyboard to select a specific cell or a range of cells. A range of cells is a collection of two or more adjacent cells. A label is an entry in a cell that helps the reader relate to the values in the corresponding column or row. Labels are generally entered first when creating a new worksheet since they define the layout of the data in the columns and rows. By default, Excel aligns labels at the left edge of the column. A value is a number, formula, or function that can be used to perform calculations in the worksheet. By default, Excel aligns values at the right edge of the column. Take a few moments to plan or sketch out the layout of a new worksheet before entering labels and values. Think about the calculations you will need to execute, and how you will display the data so it will be easily understood and interpreted.

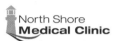

North Shore
Medical Clinic

What You Will Do   You need to calculate gross pay in the payroll worksheet for the hourly paid staff at North Shore Medical Clinic. Begin by entering labels and values.

> **Tutorial**
> Opening a Workbook from a Removable Disk

> **Tutorial**
> Selecting Cells

> **Tutorial**
> Entering Data

> **Tutorial**
> Saving with the Same Name

1 At the Windows 10 desktop, click the Start button and then click the Excel 2016 tile.

2 Click the <u>Open Other Workbooks</u> link at the bottom of the *Recent* list to display the Open backstage area.

> The Open backstage area contains options, buttons, and lists for opening workbooks saved on the computer, OneDrive, and other locations.

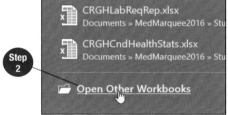

3 Click the *Browse* option.

4 At the Open dialog box, navigate to the folder in which you saved the *1-Payroll* workbook.

5 Click *1-Payroll.xlsx* in the Content pane and then click the Open button.

6 With cell A3 the active cell, press the Down Arrow key to make cell A4 active (surrounded by a thick green border).

> The arrow keys, along with other keys, are used to make different cells active. Refer to Table E1.2 for information on how to make a specific cell active using the keyboard.

Table E1.2 Keyboard Movement Commands

Press	To move to
Alt + Page Down	one screen to the right
Alt + Page Up	one screen to the left
Arrow keys	one cell up, down, left, or right
Ctrl + Home	first cell in worksheet (cell A1)
Ctrl + End	last cell in worksheet
Home	beginning of row
Page Down	down one screen
Page Up	up one screen

In Brief

Open from Removable Disk
1. Click File tab.
2. Click *Open*.
3. Click *Browse*.
4. Click removable disk.
5. Double-click folder.
6. Double-click workbook.

Select Cell
1. Position mouse pointer over cell.
2. Click in cell.
OR
Use arrow keys.

Enter Data
1. Make cell active.
2. Type data.
3. Press Enter.

Save Workbook with Same Name
Click Save button on Quick Access Toolbar.
OR
1. Click File tab.
2. Click *Save*.

7 Type Lancaster, press the Tab key, and then type Darrin.

Pressing the Tab key makes the cell to the right of the current cell.

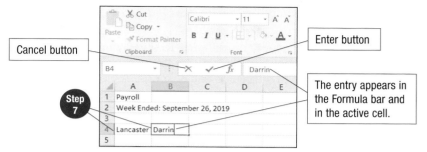

Cancel button

Enter button

The entry appears in the Formula bar and in the active cell.

Step 7

8 Click in cell J3 to make it active.

Use the mouse to select a specific cell by clicking in the desired cell when the mouse pointer displays as a white cross.

9 Type Total, press Alt + Enter, type Hours, and then press the Enter key.

Pressing Alt + Enter inserts a line break in the cell, forcing text to the next line. The row height will automatically adjust to accommodate the two lines of text.

10 Enter the remaining labels as shown below by making the appropriate cell active, typing the label, and then using the mouse or keyboard to make the next cell active. (Do not complete the labels for the days of the week beyond *Sun*, as this will be completed in the next activity.

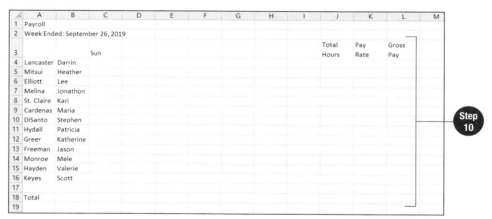

Step 10

11 Click the Save button 🖫 on the Quick Access Toolbar.

Clicking the Save button on the Quick Access Toolbar saves the workbook with the same name, which overwrites the original file with the changes made in this activity.

Check Your Work — Compare your work with the model answer to ensure that you have completed the activity correctly.

In Addition

Selecting Multiple Cells

A range of adjacent or nonadjacent cells is selected using the keyboard and/or mouse by clicking in the first cell and holding down the left mouse button, dragging into the last cell, and then releasing the mouse button. Adjacent cells are selected using the keyboard by making the first cell in the range active, pressing and holding down the Shift key, pressing the arrow in the desired direction until the last cell is selected, and then releasing the Shift key. To select nonadjacent cells, press and hold down the Ctrl key, click in the desired cells, and then release the Ctrl key.

Activity 1.3   Navigating and Scrolling

Excel provides a variety of methods to quickly navigate a worksheet as you enter and edit data. The Name box (displays to the left of the Formula bar) and the Go To dialog box are used to navigate to a specific cell or range. A worksheet can also be navigated using keyboard shortcuts, such as Ctrl + Home. Worksheets can contain data that extends past the worksheet area. Change what cells are visible by scrolling horizontally and vertically in the worksheet. To scroll, use the horizontal and vertical scroll bars that display on the bottom right and right edge of the window. The scroll bars contain scroll buttons that are used to move the view by one column or row. The scroll bars also contain scroll boxes that can be clicked and dragged to change which cells are visible. The mouse wheel will also vertically scroll in a worksheet, making it more efficient to move up and down.

North Shore Medical Clinic

What You Will Do   You need to demonstrate that you can navigate the payroll worksheet using keyboard shortcuts, the Go To dialog box, and the Name box. You also need to demonstrate that you can scroll in the payroll worksheet.

Tutorial

Navigating and Scrolling

1. With **1-Payroll.xlsx** open, press Ctrl + Home.

   Pressing Ctrl + Home makes cell A1 the active cell.

2. Press the Page Down key.

   Each time you press the Page Down key, you move the active cell down one screen.

3. Press the Page Up key.

   Each time you press the Page Up key, you move the active cell up one screen.

4. Click the Find & Select button in the Editing group on the Home tab and then click *Go To* at the drop-down list.

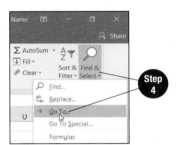

5. At the Go To dialog box, type L3 in the *Reference* text box and then click OK or press the Enter key.

   Using Go To moved the position of the active cell to L3.

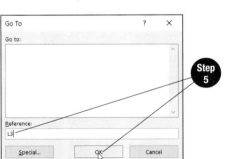

6. Use the Up, Down, Left, and Right Arrow keys on the keyboard to practice moving the active cell around the worksheet.

   Pressing and holding down a directional arrow key causes the screen to scroll very quickly. Table E1.2 in the previous activity illustrates more keyboard movement commands.

In Brief

Navigate to Cell with Go To
1. Click Find & Select button.
2. Click *Go To*.
3. Type cell reference.
4. Click OK.

Navigate to Cell with Name Box
1. Click in Name box.
2. Type cell reference.
3. Press Enter.

7 Click in the Name box located to the left of the Formula bar, above cell A1.

Clicking in the Name box will highlight the current cell reference.

8 Type J3 and then press the Enter key.

Make sure you press the Enter key after typing a cell reference in the Name box, otherwise no action will occur.

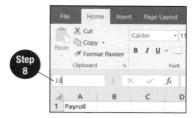

9 Position the mouse pointer on the scroll arrow at the right edge of the horizontal scroll bar and then click the left mouse button a few times to scroll to the right edge of the worksheet.

10 Position the mouse pointer on the horizontal scroll box, click and hold down the left mouse button, drag the scroll box to the left edge of the horizontal scroll bar, and then release the mouse button.

The width or height of the scroll box indicates the proportional amount of the used cells in the worksheet that are visible in the current window. The position of the scroll box within the scroll bar indicates the relative location of the visible cells within the remainder of the worksheet.

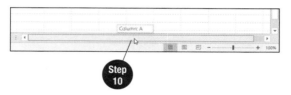

11 If possible, use the mouse wheel to scroll down in the worksheet area. Otherwise, click the Scroll Down button a few times to scroll down in the worksheet area.

12 Press Ctrl + Home to make cell A1 active.

13 Save **1-Payroll.xlsx**.

In Addition

Entering Scroll Lock Mode

Historically, computers generally only had a keyboard as an input device. The mouse wasn't popular in the infancy of personal computing, so all commands and actions were accomplished on the keyboard. For example, scrolling in an application would require the user to turn on scroll lock and then use keys such as the arrow keys to scroll in the application. This functionality still exists in Excel and may be a more efficient way for some users to scroll in a worksheet. Turn on scroll lock mode by pressing the Scroll Lock key. The status bar will display the words Scroll Lock when the feature is enabled. Once scroll lock mode is on, use the following commands to scroll in the worksheet.

Keys	Scroll Lock Action
Arrow keys	scrolls one column or row in the direction of the arrow keys used
Page keys	scrolls one screen up or down
Home key	makes the top left cell in the screen active
End key	makes the bottom right cell in the screen active

Activity 1.4   Using the Fill Handle

When a cell is active, a thick green border surrounds it and a small green square displays in the bottom right corner of the border. This green square is called the fill handle. The fill handle is an AutoFill feature in Excel that enters repetitive, series, or patterned data. For example, you can type the first day of a week in a cell and then use the fill handle to populate the adjacent cells with the remaining days of the week. The entries that are automatically inserted in the adjacent cells are dependent on the contents of the active cell, which is called the source cell. Use the fill handle by making the source cell active, clicking the fill handle and holding down the left mouse button, dragging the pointer into the desired cell, and then releasing the mouse button.

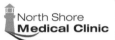
North Shore
Medical Clinic

What You Will Do   Finish entering the data in the payroll worksheet using the fill handle to enter repetitive and series data.

1   With **1-Payroll.xlsx** open, click in cell C3 to make it the active cell.

You will use the fill handle in cell C3 to automatically enter the remaining days of the week in cells D3 through I3.

2   Point to the fill handle in cell C3. The cell pointer changes from a large white cross to a thin black cross.

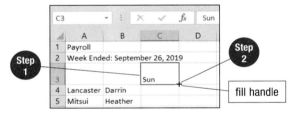

3   Click and hold down the left mouse button, drag the pointer to cell I3, and then release the left mouse button.

The entries *Mon* through *Sat* appear in cells D3 through I3. As you drag the pointer to the right, a green border surrounds the selected cells and a ScreenTip appears below the pointer indicating the label or value that will be inserted. When you release the left mouse button, the cells remain selected and the Auto Fill Options button appears.

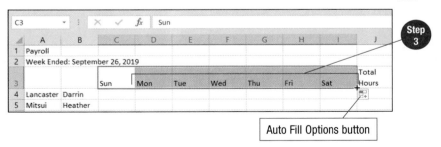

4   Click in cell F4 to make it the active cell.

5   Type 8 and then click the Enter button on the Formula bar.

6   Click the fill handle in cell F4, hold down the left mouse button, drag the pointer down into cell F16, and then release the mouse button.

This time the active cell contained a value. The value *8* is copied to the adjacent cells.

7 Enter the remaining values for employee hours as shown below. Use the fill handle where duplicate values appear in adjacent cells to enter the data as efficiently as possible.

	A	B	C	D	E	F	G	H	I	J
1	Payroll									
2	Week Ended: September 26, 2019									
3			Sun	Mon	Tue	Wed	Thu	Fri	Sat	Total Hours
4	Lancaster	Darrin	8	5	6	8	5	0	8	
5	Mitsui	Heather	0	8	6	8	7	5	0	
6	Elliott	Lee	8	8	0	8	7	7	0	
7	Melina	Jonathon	8	8	0	8	7	8	0	
8	St. Claire	Kari	0	8	0	8	8	7	0	
9	Cardenas	Maria	0	0	0	8	8	7	8	
10	DiSanto	Stephen	8	0	0	8	8	7	8	
11	Hydall	Patricia	8	0	0	8	8	7	8	
12	Greer	Katherine	8	6	8	8	0	0	8	
13	Freeman	Jason	0	5	8	8	6	0	8	
14	Monroe	Mele	5	6	8	8	0	8	0	
15	Hayden	Valerie	6	4	8	8	0	8	0	
16	Keyes	Scott	7	6	8	8	0	8	0	
17										
18	Total									

Step 7

8 Make cell K4 the active cell, type 15.25, and then press the Enter key.

9 Position the cell pointer over cell K4, click and hold down the left mouse button, drag down to cell K16, and then release the mouse button.

> A group of two or more adjacent cells is referred to as a range. Select a range of cells when you want to perform an action on more than one cell at once.

10 With the Home tab active, click the Fill button ⬇ in the Editing group and then click *Down* at the drop-down list.

11 Click in any cell in the worksheet to deselect the range.

12 Save **1-Payroll.xlsx**.

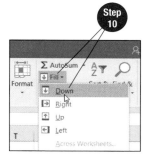

Step 10

Check Your Work Compare your work with the model answer to ensure that you have completed the activity correctly.

In Addition

Using the Fill Handle to Enter a Pattern

The fill handle is versatile and can be used to enter a series of values, dates, times, or other labels as a pattern. The pattern is established based on the cells you select before dragging the fill handle. In the worksheet shown below, the cells in columns C through J were all populated using the fill handle. In each row, the first two cells in columns A and B were selected and then the fill handle was dragged to column J.

Using the Auto Fill Options Button

Use the Auto Fill Options button drop-down list to control how a series is entered. After dragging the fill handle, the Auto Fill Options button displays at the end of the series. Pointing at the button causes it to expand and display an arrow. Click the arrow and then select the desired fill action in the drop-down list. By default, *Fill Series* is selected. Click the *Copy Cells* option to repeat the value in the first cell.

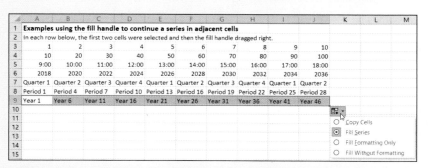

A formula is entered into a cell to perform mathematical calculations in a worksheet. All formulas in Excel begin with the equals sign (=) as the first character. After the equals sign, the cell addresses that contain the values you want to calculate are entered between mathematical operators. The mathematical operators are + (addition), − (subtraction), * (multiplication), / (division), and ^ (exponentiation). An example of a valid formula is =A3*B3. In this formula, the value in cell A3 is multiplied by the value in cell B3 and the result is placed in the formula cell. By including the cell address in the formula rather than typing the actual value, you can utilize the powerful recalculation feature in Excel. If you change a cell's content, the result of the formula is automatically recalculated so that all values are current.

North Shore
Medical Clinic

What You Will Do   You will use two methods to enter formulas to calculate total hours and gross pay for the first two medical office assistants listed in the payroll worksheet for North Shore Medical Clinic.

Tutorial
Entering Formulas
Using the Keyboard

Tutorial
Entering Formulas
Using the Mouse

Tutorial
Determining the Order
of Operations

1 With **1-Payroll.xlsx** open, make cell J4 the active cell.

Begin a formula by making the cell active in which you want the result to appear.

2 Type =c4+d4+e4+f4+g4+h4+i4 and then press the Enter key.

The values in cells C4 through I4 are added and the result, *40*, is displayed in cell J4. You can type cell column letters in a formula in uppercase or lowercase letters. If you type lowercase column letters in a formula, Excel will convert the letters to uppercase when you press the Enter key or click the Enter button on the Formula bar.

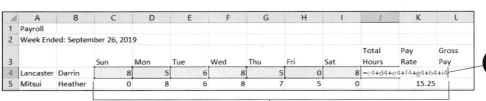

Cell references are color-coded to the originating cell for quick reference and error checking.

3 Press the Up Arrow key to make cell J4 the active cell.

Notice that the result of the formula displays in the worksheet area and the formula used to calculate the result displays in the Formula bar.

4 Make cell J5 the active cell, type the formula =c5+d5+e5+f5+g5+h5+i5, and then press the Enter key.

Seem like too much typing? A more efficient way to add a series of cells is available. This method will be introduced in the next activity after you learn the pointing method for entering formulas.

5 Make cell L4 active.

To calculate gross pay, you need to multiply the total hours by the pay rate. In Steps 6 through 10, you will enter this formula using the pointing method.

6 Type an equals sign (=).

7 Click in cell J4.

A moving dashed border (called a marquee) displays around cell J4, indicating that it is the cell included in the formula, and the cell address is added to the formula cell (L4) with a blinking insertion point after the reference. The word *Point* displays at the left side of the Status bar.

8 Type an asterisk (*), which is the multiplication operator.

The marquee surrounding cell J4 disappears and cell J4 is color-coded to match the cell reference *J4* within the formula cell.

9 Click in cell K4.

A marquee displays around the cell and the cell address is added to the formula in cell L4. Both the cell and the reference display in the same color.

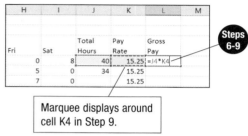

Marquee displays around cell K4 in Step 9.

10 Click the Enter button on the Formula bar.

The result, *610*, is displayed in cell L4. In Activity 1.6, you will learn how to display two decimal places for cells containing dollar values.

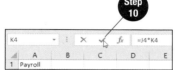

11 Click in cell K4, type 15.75, and press the Enter key.

When the value in cell K4 was changed, the result of the formula in cell L4 recalculated.

12 Save **1-Payroll.xlsx**.

Check Your Work Compare your work with the model answer to ensure that you have completed the activity correctly.

In Addition

Order of Operations

If you include several operators in a formula, Excel calculates the result using the order of operations as follows: negations (e.g., -1) first, then percents (%), then exponentiations (^), then multiplication and division (* and /), and finally addition and subtraction (+ and −). If a formula contains more than one operator at the same level of precedence—for example, both an addition and a subtraction operation—Excel calculates the equation from left to right. To change the order of operations, include parentheses around the part of the formula you want calculated first.

Formula	Calculation
=B5*C5/D5	Both operators are at the same level of precedence—Excel would multiply the value in B5 times the value in C5 and then divide the result by the value in D5.
=B5+B6+B7*C10	Multiplication takes precedence over addition, so Excel would first multiply the value in B7 times the value in C10. Excel would then take the value in B5 and add to it the value in B6 and then add the result of the multiplication.
=(B5+B6+B7)*C10	Because of the parentheses, Excel would first add the values in B5 through B7 then multiply this sum by the value in C10.

Activity 1.6 Using the SUM Function

The formulas to calculate the hours worked by the first two employees were lengthy. A more efficient way to calculate the total hours for Darrin Lancaster in cell J4 would be to enter the formula =SUM(C4:I4). This formula includes one of Excel's built-in functions, called SUM. A function is a preprogrammed formula. The structure of a formula utilizing a function begins with the equals sign (=), followed by the name of the function, and then the argument. Argument is the term given to the values identified within parentheses. In the example provided, the argument C4:I4 contains the starting cell and the ending cell separated by a colon (:). Since the SUM function is used frequently, an AutoSum button is available on the Home tab.

North Shore Medical Clinic

What You Will Do Lee Elliott, North Shore Medical Clinic's office manager, wants you to use a more efficient method of payroll calculation, so you will use the SUM function to calculate the hours worked.

Tutorial

Entering Formulas Using the AutoSum Button

1 With **1-Payroll.xlsx** open, make cell J4 the active cell and then press the Delete key.

> This deletes the cell contents. Although there was nothing wrong with the formula in cell J4, you are deleting it so that the formulas in the completed worksheet will be consistent.

2 Click the AutoSum button Σ in the Editing group on the Home tab. (Do not click the AutoSum button arrow.)

> A marquee surrounds cells C4 through I4 and a ScreenTip appears below the formula cell indicating the correct format for the SUM function. Excel enters the formula =SUM(C4:I4) in cell J4. The suggested range C4:I4 is selected within the formula so that you can highlight a different range with the mouse if the suggested range is not correct.

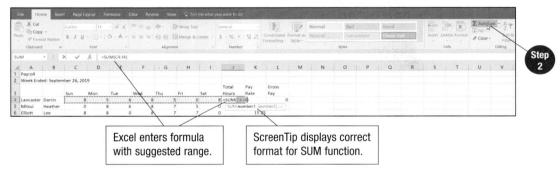

Excel enters formula with suggested range.

ScreenTip displays correct format for SUM function.

Step 2

3 Press the Enter key.

> Since the range Excel suggested is the correct range, you can finish the formula by pressing the Enter key or by clicking the Enter button on the Formula bar.

4 With cell J5 the active cell, press the Delete key to delete the existing formula in the cell.

5 Click the AutoSum button. When Excel displays the formula =SUM(C5:I5), press the Enter key.

6 With cell J6 the active cell, click the AutoSum button.

> This time the range of cells Excel is suggesting to add (J4:J5) is the wrong range. When you click the AutoSum button, Excel looks for multiple values in the cells immediately above the active cell. In this case, multiple values appear above cell J6, so Excel inserts J4:J5 as the range in the SUM formula.

7 Position the cell pointer over cell C6, click and hold down the left mouse button, drag the pointer to the right to cell I6, and then release the mouse button.

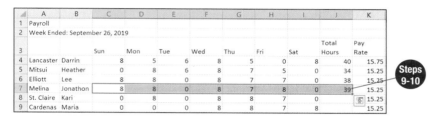

Steps 6-7

8 Press the Enter key.

Now that you have seen how the AutoSum button operates, you already know that the suggested range for the next employee's total hours will be incorrect. In Step 9, you will select the range of cells *first* to avoid the incorrect suggestion.

9 Position the cell pointer over cell C7, click and hold down the left mouse button, drag the pointer to cell J7, and then release the mouse button.

Notice that you are including J7, the cell that will display the result, in the range of cells.

10 Click the AutoSum button.

The result, *39*, appears in cell J7.

Steps 9-10

11 Click cell J7 and then look at the formula the SUM function created in the Formula bar: *=SUM(C7:I7)*.

Since Excel created the correct SUM formula from a range of selected cells, you decide to try calculating total hours for more than one employee in one step using the method in Steps 9 and 10 but with an expanded range.

12 Position the cell pointer over cell C8, click and hold down the left mouse button, drag the pointer down and to the right to cell J16, and then release the mouse button.

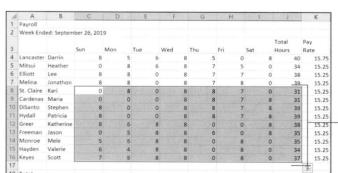

Steps 12-13

13 Click the AutoSum button.

14 Starting with J8 and ending with J16, click each of the cells to confirm that the correct formulas appear in the Formula bar.

15 Save **1-Payroll.xlsx**.

Check Your Work Compare your work with the model answer to ensure that you have completed the activity correctly.

Activity 1.7 Copying Formulas

Many times you may create a worksheet in which several formulas are basically the same. For example, in the payroll worksheet, the formula to total the hours for Darrin Lancaster is =SUM(C4:I4), the formula for Heather Mitsui is =SUM(C5:I5), and so on. The only differences between the two formulas are the row numbers. Whenever formulas are this similar, you can use the Copy and Paste feature or the fill handle to copy the formula from one cell to another. The cell containing the original formula is called the *source*, and the cell(s) to which the formula is copied is called the *destination*. When the formula is pasted, Excel automatically changes column letters or row numbers to reflect the destination location. By default, Excel assumes *relative addressing*, which means that cell addresses update relative to the destination.

North Shore Medical Clinic

Tutorial
Copying Formulas

What You Will Do   To simplify your completion of the payroll worksheet, you will copy formulas using two methods: Copy and Paste and the fill handle.

1 With **1-Payroll.xlsx** open, make cell L4 active.

> This cell contains the formula =J4*K4 to calculate the gross pay for Darrin Lancaster. You will copy this formula to the remaining cells in column L to complete the *Gross Pay* column.

2 Click the Copy button in the Clipboard group on the Home tab. (Make sure to click the button rather than the button arrow.)

> A moving marquee surrounds the active cell, indicating that the source contents have been copied to the Clipboard, which is a temporary storage location. The content being copied is the formula =J4*K4—not the value *630*.

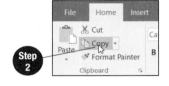

3 Select the range L5:L16. To do this, position the cell pointer over cell L5, click and hold down the left mouse button, drag the pointer down to cell L16, and then release the mouse button.

marquee indicating source range

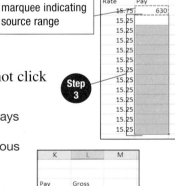

4 Click the Paste button in the Clipboard group. (Do not click the button arrow.)

> Excel pastes the formula into the selected cells and displays the results. The Paste Options button (Ctrl) appears. Clicking this button will display a drop-down list with various alternatives for pasting the data. The marquee remains around the source cell and the destination cells remain highlighted. The marquee disappears as soon as you start another activity or press the Esc key.

5 Press the Esc key to remove the marquee and the Paste Options button, click cell L5, and then look at the entry in the Formula bar: =J5*K5.

> The row number in the source formula was increased by one to reflect the destination. The actions you completed in Steps 1 through 4 are called *relative copying*.

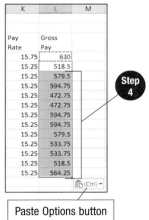

Paste Options button

6 Use the Down Arrow key to check the remaining formulas in column L.

In Brief

Copy Formula
1. Make source cell active.
2. Click Copy button.
3. Select destination cell(s).
4. Click Paste button.

Copy Formula with Fill Handle
1. Make source cell active.
2. Click and hold down fill handle.
3. Drag into last cell.
4. Release mouse button.

7 Make cell C18 active.

8 Click the AutoSum button and then click the Enter button in the Formula bar.

> The SUM function inserts the formula *=SUM(C4:C17)*. Next, you will copy the formula using the fill handle.

9 Drag the fill handle in cell C18 right to cell L18.

> When the active cell contains a formula, dragging the fill handle causes Excel to copy the formula and change cell references relative to each destination location.

	A	B	C	D	E	F	G	H	I	J	K	L
1	Payroll											
2	Week Ended: September 26, 2019											
3			Sun	Mon	Tue	Wed	Thu	Fri	Sat	Total Hours	Pay Rate	Gross Pay
4	Lancaster	Darrin	8	5	6	8	5	0	8	40	15.75	630
5	Mitsui	Heather	0	8	6	8	7	5	0	34	15.25	518.5
6	Elliott	Lee	8	8	0	8	7	7	0	38	15.25	579.5
7	Melina	Jonathon	8	8	0	8	7	8	0	39	15.25	594.75
8	St. Claire	Kari	0	8	0	8	8	7	0	31	15.25	472.75
9	Cardenas	Maria	0	0	0	8	8	7	8	31	15.25	472.75
10	DiSanto	Stephen	8	0	0	8	8	7	8	39	15.25	594.75
11	Hydall	Patricia	8	0	0	8	8	7	8	39	15.25	594.75
12	Greer	Katherine	8	6	8	8	0	0	8	38	15.25	579.5
13	Freeman	Jason	0	5	8	8	6	0	8	35	15.25	533.75
14	Monroe	Mele	5	6	8	8	0	8	0	35	15.25	533.75
15	Hayden	Valerie	6	4	8	8	0	8	0	34	15.25	518.5
16	Keyes	Scott	7	6	8	8	0	8	0	37	15.25	564.25
17												
18	Total		66	64	52	104	64	72	48	470	198.75	7187.5
19												

Step 9

Need Help?

If the results do not appear in D18 through L18, you probably dragged the cell pointer instead of the fill handle. Click cell C18 and try again, making sure you drag using the thin black cross.

10 Make cell K18 the active cell and then press the Delete key.

> The sum of the *Pay Rate* column is not useful information.

11 Make cell D18 the active cell and look at the entry in the Formula bar: *=SUM(D4:D17)*.

> The column letter in the source formula was changed to reflect the destination.

12 Use the Right Arrow key to check the formulas in the remaining columns.

13 Save **1-Payroll.xlsx**.

Check Your Work Compare your work with the model answer to ensure that you have completed the activity correctly.

In Addition

Understanding Copy and Paste versus Fill

What is the difference between copying and pasting and using the fill handle? When you use the Copy button, the contents of the source cell(s) are placed in the Clipboard. The data will remain in the Clipboard and can be pasted several times in the current worksheet, into any other worksheet that is open, or into an open file in another application. Use the Copy and Paste buttons when the formula is to be inserted more than once or into nonadjacent cells. Use the fill handle when the formula is only being copied to adjacent cells.

Activity 1.8 Improving Worksheet Appearance; Displaying Formulas; Sorting

Basic formatting should be applied to even the simplest worksheets to ensure that the information they contain is easy to understand. Some of the most basic formatting options in Excel are number, alignment, and font formatting, all of which are located on the Home tab. Apply formatting to a cell by first making it active and then using the buttons and options on the Home tab to format the cell. Formatting can also be applied to ranges of cells, which saves the time you would spend to individually format each cell. When you have finished building the worksheet, it is a good idea to verify the accuracy of the formulas you have entered. The worksheet could contain formulas that are correct in structure but not mathematically correct for the situation. For example, the wrong range in a SUM formula, or parentheses missing from a multi-operator formula may cause an incorrect result. One method of reviewing formulas for accuracy is to display formulas in the cells of a worksheet. To display formulas in cells, click the Formulas tab and then click the Show Formulas button in the Formula Auditing group. You can also display formulas with the keyboard shortcut Ctrl + `. Data in Excel can be rearranged by sorting rows in ascending order or descending order. You can select a single column or define a custom sort to specify multiple columns that determine the sort order.

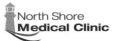
North Shore Medical Clinic

What You Will Do   To confirm the accuracy of your calculations in the payroll worksheet, you will enter proof formulas to test the worksheet and then use two formatting options to improve the worksheet's appearance. Finally, you will sort the worksheet in ascending order by last name.

Tutorial
Displaying Formulas

Tutorial
Merging and Centering Cells

1 With **1-Payroll.xlsx** open, select the range L4:L18.

> In column L, the amount of digits displayed after the decimal point is inconsistent. Since the *Gross Pay* column represents money, you will format these cells to display a dollar symbol and show two digits past the decimal point.

2 Click the Accounting Number Format button $ · in the Number group on the Home tab. (Do not click the button arrow.)

> The Accounting format adds a dollar sign, a comma in the thousands place, and two digits after the decimal point for each value in the selection.

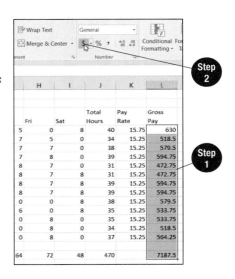

3 Select the range K4:K16 and then click the Accounting Number Format button.

4 Select the range A1:L1.

5 Click the Merge & Center button in the Alignment group.

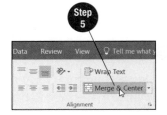

6 Select the range A2:L2 and then click the Merge & Center button.

7 Select the range C3:L3.

Display Formulas
1. Click Formulas tab.
2. Click Show Formulas button.

OR

Press Ctrl + `.

8 Click the Align Right button ≣ in the Alignment group on the Home tab.

> The data labels are now aligned above the data below them, making identifying values in the worksheet easier.

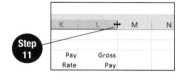

Step 8

Step 10

9 Select the range A18:L18.

10 Click the Bold button in the Font group.

> The *Total* row is now bolded, making identifying the totals for each column easier.

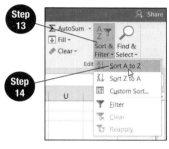

11 If the value in L18 displays as pound symbols (########), AutoFit column L so the number value is completely visible by double-clicking the border between the column L and column M headers.

Step 11

12 Select the range A4:L16.

> You are selecting the range before performing the sort since you do not want to include the cells above and below the list of names in the sort.

Step 13

Step 14

13 Click the Sort & Filter button ⬇ in the Editing group on the Home tab.

14 Click *Sort A to Z* at the drop-down list.

15 Click in any cell to deselect the range.

16 Click the Formulas tab.

17 Click the Show Formulas button 🔢 in the Formula Auditing group.

> The cells in the worksheet are automatically expanded and cells that contain formulas now display the formula in the worksheet area.

Step 17

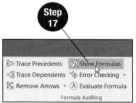

18 Click the File tab, click the *Print* option, and then click the Print button.

> The worksheet will print on three pages with cell formulas visible.

19 Press Ctrl + ` to turn off the display of formulas.

> The ` symbol is the grave symbol. On the keyboard, it is usually located on the key immediately to the left of the number 1 key.

20 Save **1-Payroll.xlsx**.

Check Your Work   Compare your work with the model answer to ensure that you have completed the activity correctly.

In Addition

Displaying Formulas at the Excel Options Dialog Box

In addition to the Show Formulas button on the Formulas tab and the keyboard shortcut, you can also display formulas at the Excel Options dialog box. Display this dialog box by clicking the File tab and then clicking *Options*. At the Excel Options dialog box, click *Advanced* in the left panel, click the *Show formulas in cells instead of their calculated results* check box in the *Display options for this worksheet* section to insert a check mark, and then click OK.

Activity 1.9   Using the Tell Me and Help Features

A new feature in Excel 2016 is the Tell Me feature, which displays on the ribbon to the right of the tabs. The Tell Me feature provides information as well as guidance on how to perform a function. As you type a search phrase in the *Tell Me* text box, a drop-down list displays with options that are refined as you continue typing—a feature referred to as word-wheeling. The drop-down list will have options for completing the function, displaying the top three help links most related to the search, or displaying the Help task pane. The Help task pane can be opened through the Tell Me feature or by pressing the F1 function key on the keyboard. You can also display the Help task pane by hovering the mouse pointer over certain buttons on the ribbon and then clicking the *Tell me more* hyperlink in the ScreenTip that displays. The Help task pane displays with information about the button feature.

North Shore Medical Clinic

Tutorial
Using the Tell Me Feature

Tutorial
Using the Help Feature

What You Will Do   After reviewing the payroll worksheet, you think the first two title rows would look better if the text were enlarged. You will use the Tell Me feature to do this.

1 With **1-Payroll.xlsx** open, make the range A1:A2 active.

To increase the font size of the title rows above the columns in the worksheet, you decide to use the Tell Me feature.

2 Click in the *Tell Me* text box.

The *Tell Me* text box is located on the ribbon to the right of the View tab and contains the text *Tell me what you want to do*. When you click in the text box, the last five functions entered will display in a drop-down list.

3 Type font in the *Tell Me* text box.

A drop-down list displays with options such as *Font*, *Font Size*, *Theme Fonts*, and *Font Color*.

4 Position the mouse pointer on the arrow at the right of the *Font Size* option in the drop-down list.

5 At the side menu that displays, click *14*.

The size of the text in cells A1 and A2 is increased to 14 points.

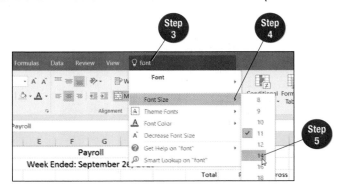

6 Display the Help task pane by pressing the F1 function key.

7 At the Help task pane, click in the search text box, type preview worksheet, and then press the Enter key.

8 At the Help task pane, click the <u>Preview worksheet pages before you print</u> hyperlink.

Since Microsoft Office Online is updated frequently, your search results list may vary. The hyperlink may have a slightly different title or position within the list.

9 Read the information and then close the Help task pane by clicking the Close button in the upper right corner of the task pane.

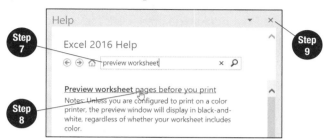

10 Position the mouse pointer on the Font Color button in the Font group on the Home tab and then read the information that displays in the ScreenTip.

11 Click the <u>Tell me more</u> hyperlink in the ScreenTip and then read the information that displays in the Help task pane.

12 Close the Help task pane.

13 If necessary, select the cells A1:A2, click the Font Color button arrow, and then click *Blue, Accent 1, Darker 25%* at the drop-down gallery (fifth column, fifth row in the *Theme Colors* section).

14 Save **1-Payroll.xlsx**.

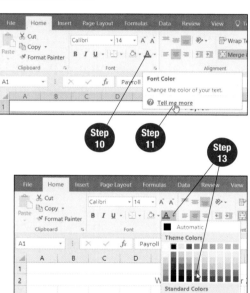

Check Your Work ▸ Compare your work with the model answer to ensure that you have completed the activity correctly.

In Addition

Using the Smart Lookup Task Pane

The Tell Me drop-down list also includes a *Smart Lookup* option. Clicking the *Smart Lookup* option will display the Smart Lookup task pane as shown on the right. This task pane provides information on the function from a variety of sources on the Internet. The Smart Lookup task pane can also be accessed with the Smart Lookup button [icon] in the Insights group on the Review tab, or by selecting text, right-clicking the selected text, and then clicking *Smart Lookup* at the shortcut menu.

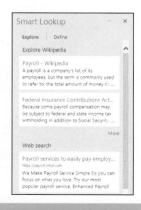

Print a worksheet so that you have a paper copy, also called a hard copy, to file or to attach to a report. Large, complex worksheets are often easier to proofread and check on a paper copy. Display the Print backstage area to preview the worksheet and modify print options. To display the Print backstage area, click the File tab and then click the *Print* option. At the Print backstage area, a preview of how the worksheet will look when printed displays at the right side. The center of the Print backstage area is divided into three sections: *Print*, *Printer*, and *Settings*. Use the galleries available in each category to modify print options. Use the Print backstage area to preview the worksheet before printing. This will help avoid wasted paper by letting you verify in advance whether the entire worksheet will fit on one page, as well as preview and/or change other print options. Once you have selected all of the desired printing options, click the Print button in the *Print* section to print the worksheet.

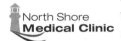

What You Will Do   The payroll worksheet is finished. You want to preview the worksheet and then print a copy for the office manager.

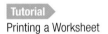

Printing a Worksheet

1 With **1-Payroll.xlsx** open, make cell A24 the active cell and then type the student information your instructor has directed for printouts. For example, type your last name, press the Tab key, type your first name, and then press the Enter key.

> Make sure you have checked with your instructor as to whether you should include other identifying information such as your program or class number.

2 Click the File tab and then click the *Print* option to display the worksheet in the Print backstage area as shown in Figure E1.2.

3 The right side of the backstage area displays the first page of the worksheet as it will look when printed with the current print options. The pages indicator at the bottom left of the preview shows that you are viewing page 1 of 2 pages. Click the Next Page button ▶ at the right of the indicator to display page 2.

Figure E1.2 Print Backstage Area

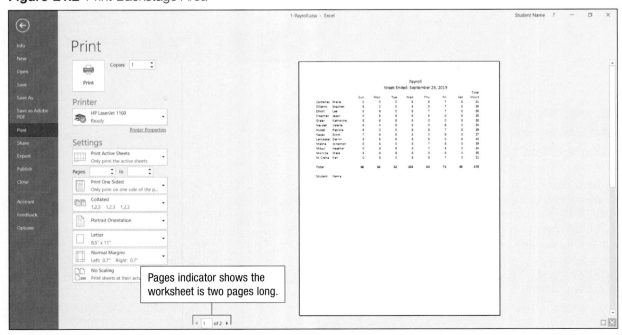

Pages indicator shows the worksheet is two pages long.

In Brief

Preview Worksheet
1. Click File tab.
2. Click *Print*.

Change to Landscape Orientation
1. Click File tab.
2. Click *Print*.
3. Click orientation gallery.
4. Click *Landscape Orientation*.

4 The second page of the printout appears, showing the columns that could not fit on page 1.

5 Click the orientation gallery (currently displays *Portrait Orientation*) in the *Settings* category of the Print backstage area.

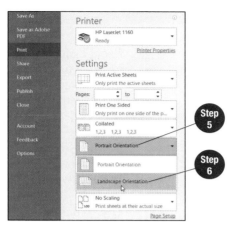

> One method to reduce the printout to one page is to change the orientation of the paper from portrait to landscape. In portrait orientation, the content is printed on paper that is taller than it is wide. In landscape orientation, the data is rotated to print on paper that is wider than it is tall.

6 Click *Landscape Orientation* at the drop-down list.

> The preview updates to show the worksheet in landscape orientation. Notice that all of the columns now fit on one page.

7 Click the Print button.

> The Print backstage area closes and the worksheet prints on the default printer. The default settings in the Print backstage area are to print one copy of all pages in the active worksheet. You will learn how to further adjust page layout and print settings in a later section.

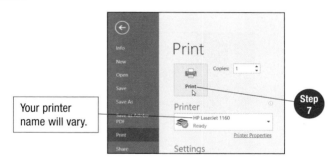

Your printer name will vary.

8 At the worksheet, scroll right, if necessary, until you see the vertical dashed line at the right of the *Gross Pay* column.

> The dashed vertical line is a page break. Page breaks appear after you have previewed or printed a worksheet. A worksheet that spans many rows will display a horizontal dashed line below the last row that can fit on the page. The dashed lines do not print.

9 Save and then close **1-Payroll.xlsx**.

Check Your Work Compare your work with the model answer to ensure that you have completed the activity correctly.

In Addition

Printing Gridlines and Row and Column Headings

By default, the gridlines that create the cells in a worksheet and the row numbers and column letters that label the cells do not print. The Sheet Options group on the Page Layout tab contains check boxes for gridlines and headings. The *View* check boxes for gridlines and headings contain check marks. At these settings, gridlines and row and column headings display on the screen but do not print. To print gridlines and headings, insert check marks in the *Print* check boxes. Complex worksheets may be easier to read with the gridlines printed.

Activity 1.11 Creating a Workbook from a Template

Excel includes worksheets that are formatted and have text and formulas for specific uses such as creating budgets, sales reports, inventories, timecards, and financial statements. These preformatted worksheets are called templates. Templates can be customized and saved with a new name to reflect individual company data. Templates are available at the New backstage area and can be downloaded from Office.com.

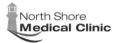
North Shore
Medical Clinic

What You Will Do Darrin Lancaster has asked you to complete an invoice for a recent exam. You decide to use a template to do this since the template has formulas already entered.

Tutorial
Using Templates

1. Click the File tab and then click the *New* option.

2. At the New backstage area, search for invoice templates by clicking in the search text box (displays the text *Search for online templates*), typing invoice that calculates total, and then pressing the Enter key.

3. Double-click the invoice template shown below. (If this template is not available, display the ExcelMedS1 folder on your storage medium and then double-click **TotalsInvoice.xltx**.)

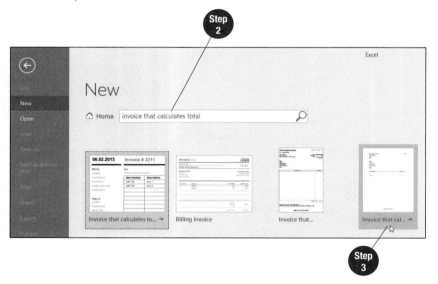

4. Review the template, observing the type of information required and the way data is arranged on the page. Save the workbook in the ExcelMedS1 folder with the name **1-NSMCInvoice**.

5. Click in cell A2 (displays the text *Your Company Name*), type North Shore Medical Clinic, and then press the Enter key.

6. Type 7450 Meridian Street, Suite 150 and then press the Enter key.

7. Type Portland, OR 97202 and then press the Enter key.

8. Type (503) 555-2330 and then press the Enter key.

In Brief

Create Workbook from Template
1. Click File tab.
2. Click *New*.
3. Click in search text box.
4. Type search text.
5. Press Enter.
6. Click template.
7. Click Create button.

⑨ Type dlancaster@ppi-edu.net and then press the Enter key four times.

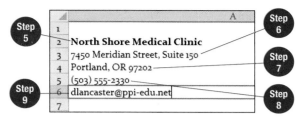

⑩ With cell A10 the active cell (displays the text *Name*), type AJ Estman and then press the Enter key.

⑪ Press the Delete key to remove the text in cell A11 and then press the Enter key.

⑫ Type 430 Island Drive and then press the Enter key.

⑬ Type Portland, OR 97204 and then press the Enter key.

⑭ Type (503) 555-1578 and then press the Enter key.

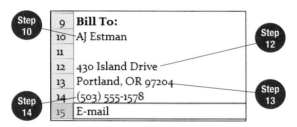

⑮ Press the Delete key to remove the text in cell A15.

⑯ Enter the following data in the specified cells:
A19:   Annual Physical Exam
B19:   143.81
A20:   Lab Analysis: Blood, Urine
B20:   109.45

Notice how the total amount is automatically calculated in cell B21, because the template included a formula.

17				
18	DESCRIPTION	▾	AMOUNT	▾
19	Annual Physical Exam		$	143.81
20	Lab Analysis: Blood, Urine		$	109.45
21	Total		$	253.26
22				

Step 16

⑰ Save, print and then close **1-NSMCInvoice.xlsx**.

Check Your Work Compare your work with the model answer to ensure that you have completed the activity correctly.

In Addition

Pinning a Template

If you use a template on a regular basis, consider pinning the template to the New backstage area. To do this, hover your mouse over the template and then click the gray left-pointing stick pin (*Pin to list*) that displays to the right of the template name. To unpin the template, click the down-pointing stick pin (*Unpin from list*).

Features Summary

Feature	Ribbon Tab, Group	Button, Option	File Tab Option	Keyboard Shortcut
Accounting format	Home, Number	$ ·		
align right	Home, Alignment			
close a workbook			*Close*	Ctrl + F4
copy	Home, Clipboard			Ctrl + C
fill down	Home, Editing	, *Down*		Ctrl + D
fill left	Home, Editing	, *Left*		
fill right	Home, Editing	, *Right*		Ctrl + R
fill up	Home, Editing	, *Up*		
Go To	Home, Editing	, *Go To*		Ctrl + G
Help				F1
insert line break				Alt + Enter
merge and center	Home, Alignment			
new workbook			*New*	Ctrl + N
Open backstage area			*Open*	Ctrl + O
Open dialog box			*Open, Browse*	Ctrl + F12
paste	Home, Clipboard			Ctrl + V
Print backstage area			*Print*	Ctrl + P or Ctrl + F2
save			*Save*	Ctrl + S
save with a new name			*Save As*	F12
show formulas	Formulas, Formula Auditing			Ctrl + `
sort	Home, Editing			
SUM function	Home, Editing	Σ		Alt + =

Workbook — Section study tools and assessment activities are available in the Workbook pages of the ebook. These resources are designed to help you further develop and demonstrate mastery of the skills learned in this section.

Excel

Editing and Formatting Worksheets

Data Files Before beginning section work, copy the ExcelMedS2 folder to your storage medium and then make ExcelMedS2 the active folder.

Skills

- Insert, move, and resize images
- Edit the content of cells
- Clear cells and cell formatting
- Use proofing tools
- Insert and delete columns and rows
- Move and copy cells
- Use the Paste Options button to link cells
- Adjust column widths and row heights
- Change the font, size, style, and color of cell contents
- Apply numeric formats and adjust the number of decimal places
- Use Undo
- Change cell alignment and indentation
- Insert and edit comments
- Add borders
- Use Format Painter
- Apply cell styles
- Apply a theme
- Find and replace cell entries and formats
- Freeze and unfreeze panes
- Change the zoom percentage
- Create formulas with absolute addresses

Precheck Check your current skills to help focus your study of the skills taught in this section.

Activities Overview

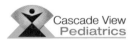
Edit and format a revenue summary report.

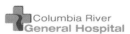
Edit and format a laboratory requisitions billing report, edit and format research data for a medical conference presentation, research and create a workbook on healthcare costs, create a staffing worksheet for the neurology department, and create a radiology requisition form.

Model Answers Preview the model answers for an overview of the activities you will complete in each section.

Activity 2.1   Inserting, Moving, and Resizing Images

Microsoft Office includes a gallery of media images you can insert in a worksheet, such as clip art, photographs, and illustrations. Use the Online Pictures button on the Insert tab to search for and insert images from online sources. Once an image has been inserted, it can be moved, resized, or deleted. Format an image with options at the Picture Tools Format tab. A company logo or other digital image can also be inserted into a worksheet using the Pictures button in the Illustrations group on the Insert tab.

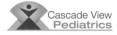

What You Will Do   Sydney Larsen, office manager of Cascade View Pediatrics, has started a January revenue summary report for Dr. Joseph Yarborough. Sydney would like you to enhance the report's appearance before she submits it. You decide to add two images to the worksheet.

Tutorial
Inserting an Image

Tutorial
Modifying Images

1. Open **CVPRevYarborough.xlsx**. *Note: This worksheet contains intentional spelling errors that will be corrected in the next activity.*

2. Save the workbook in the ExcelMedS2 folder with the name **2-CVPRevYarborough**.

3. Make cell A38 the active cell.

4. Click the Insert tab and then click the Online Pictures button 🖼 in the Illustrations group.

   This displays the Insert Pictures window with a search box.

5. Click in the search box, type stethoscope, and then press the Enter key.

6. Click the image shown below and then click the Insert button at the bottom of the window. If this image is not available, close the Insert Pictures window and then click the Pictures button 🖼 on the Insert tab. At the Insert Picture dialog box, navigate to the ExcelMedS2 folder and then double-click *stethoscope.png*.

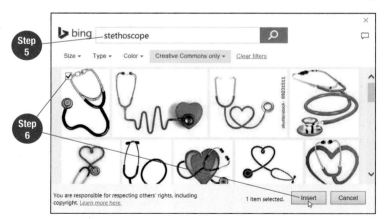

7. Position the mouse pointer on the white sizing handle in the bottom right corner of the image, click and hold down the left mouse button, and then drag down and to the right until the image fits within rows 38 to 43.

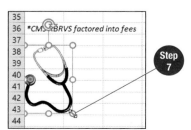

8 Move the mouse pointer over the image until the move icon (four-headed arrow) appears attached to the pointer, click and hold down the left mouse button, drag the image to the right until it is aligned in the center of column E as shown below, and then release the mouse button.

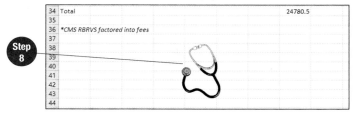

9 Make cell A1 the active cell, click the Insert tab, and then click the Pictures button in the Illustrations group.

10 At the Insert Picture dialog box, navigate to the ExcelMedS2 folder on your storage medium and then double-click **CVPLogo.jpg**.

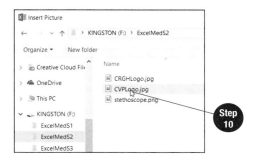

11 Click in the *Shape Height* measurement box in the Size group on the Picture Tools Format tab, type 0.8, and then press the Enter key.

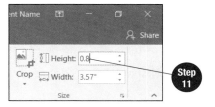

12 Click in any cell to deselect the logo image.

13 Save **2-CVPRevYarborough.xlsx**.

Check Your Work Compare your work with the model answer to ensure that you have completed the activity correctly.

In Addition

Using the Picture Tools Format Tab

When an image inserted from a file is selected, the Picture Tools Format tab becomes available. Customize the image using picture tools or picture styles. For example, use the Crop button to cut an unwanted area from the image, or set a specific height or width measurement for the image with options in the Size group.

Buttons in the Arrange group allow you to group multiple images together, as well as control the alignment, rotation, and order of the image(s) within the worksheet. Use buttons in the Adjust group to control the brightness, contrast, and color of the image(s).

Editing Data; Clearing Cells; Using Proofing Tools

Data in Excel can be edited after it is entered. Edit a cell by double-clicking in the cell and then using the keyboard to make changes. Also, you can click in a cell to make it active and then edit its contents in the Formula bar. Clearing a cell can involve removing the cell contents, formatting, or both. The Spelling feature is a useful tool to assist with correcting typing errors within a worksheet. After completing a spelling check, you will still need to proofread the worksheet since the spelling checker will not highlight all errors and cannot check the accuracy of the formulas or values. Other proofing tools include a Smart Lookup feature to learn more about specific text using online resources, a Thesaurus to find a word with a similar meaning to a selected word, and a Translate tool to translate a selected word into a different language.

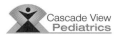
Cascade View
Pediatrics

What You Will Do Sydney's report for Dr. Yarborough contains some typographical errors. It also needs updating after Sydney reviewed the day sheets from the medical accounting program. Sydney has asked you to correct the errors and finish the report.

Tutorial
Editing Data

Tutorial
Clearing Cell Contents and Formatting

Tutorial
Checking Spelling

1 With **2-CVPRevYarborough.xlsx** open, double-click in cell E15.

When you double-click in a cell, the insertion point appears inside it and the word *Edit* appears in the Status bar. The position of the insertion point within the cell varies depending on the location of the cell pointer when Edit mode is activated.

2 Press the Right Arrow or Left Arrow key as needed to move the insertion point between the *4* and *5* and then press the Delete key.

3 Type *3* and then press the Enter key.

4 Make cell E30 the active cell.

5 Position the pointer after *22* in the Formula bar and then click the left mouse button.

The cell pointer changes to an I-beam pointer ⌶ when it hovers over the Formula bar.

Step 3

14	Minor assesment			
15	Annual health exam		60.00	43	80
16	Hospital physicals			
17	Sick notes		15.00	29	48

6 Press the Backspace key to delete *2*, type *4*, and then click the Enter button on the Formula bar.

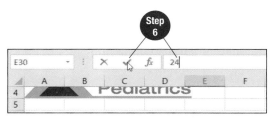
Step 6

7 Make cell A16 the active cell and then press the Delete key.

Pressing the Delete key or the Backspace key clears only the contents of the cell; formatting applied to the cell remains in effect.

8 Select the range F7:F8. Click the Clear button in the Editing group on the Home tab and then click *Clear All* at the drop-down list.

Clicking *Clear All* removes everything from a cell, including formatting and comments.

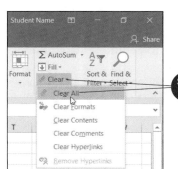
Step 8

In Brief

Edit Data
1. Double-click in cell.
2. Make edits with keyboard.
3. Press Enter.
OR
1. Make cell active.
2. Make edits in Formula bar.
3. Click Enter button.

Clear Cell
1. Make cell active.
2. Click Clear button.
3. Select option at drop-down list.

Check Spelling
1. Click Review tab.
2. Click Spelling button.
3. Click Ignore Once, Ignore All, Change, Change All, or Add to Dictionary as required.
4. Click OK.

Use Thesaurus
1. Make cell active.
2. Click Review tab.
3. Click Thesaurus button.
4. Point to replacement word.
5. Click arrow on replacement word.
6. Click *Insert*.

9 Press Ctrl + Home to make cell A1 the active cell.

10 Click the Review tab and then click the Spelling button in the Proofing group.

> The spelling check begins at the active cell. Words within the worksheet that are not found in the dictionary are highlighted as potential errors. Use buttons in the Spelling dialog box to skip the word (Ignore Once or Ignore All), replace the word with the highlighted word in the *Suggestions* list box (Change or Change All), or add the word to the dictionary if it is spelled correctly (Add to Dictionary).

11 Click the Change button in the Spelling dialog box to instruct Excel to replace *assesment* with *assessment*.

> Excel stops at the next row and flags the same spelling error. A quick glance down the worksheet reveals this word is frequently misspelled throughout the worksheet.

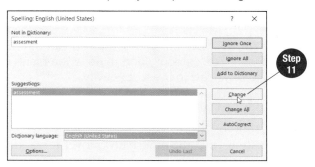

12 Click the Change All button in the Spelling dialog box to replace all occurrences of *assesment* with *assessment*.

13 Click the Change All button to replace *fomr* with *form*. If the spelling checker stops at *RBRVS* in cell A36, click the Ignore Once button.

14 Click OK at the message informing you that the spelling check is complete.

15 Make cell A29 the active cell.

16 Click the Thesaurus button in the Proofing group on the Review tab.

> When you click the Thesaurus button, the Thesaurus task pane displays at the right side of the screen. Use the Thesaurus task pane to replace a word in the worksheet with another word of similar meaning.

17 Point to the word *Replication* in the list box in the Thesaurus task pane, click the down arrow that appears, and then click *Insert* at the drop-down list.

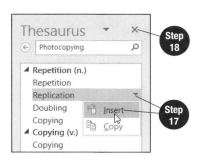

> The word *Photocopying* is replaced with *Replication* in cell A29.

18 Click the Close button in the upper right corner of the Thesaurus task pane.

19 Save **2-CVPRevYarborough.xlsx**.

> **Check Your Work** — Compare your work with the model answer to ensure that you have completed the activity correctly.

Insert rows or columns in a worksheet using options from the Insert button drop-down list in the Cells group on the Home tab or from the context-sensitive shortcut menu that displays when you right-click a selected area. Inserted rows are placed above the active cell or selected rows and existing rows are shifted down. Columns are inserted left of the active cell or selected columns and existing columns are shifted right. Delete rows or columns using options from the Delete button drop-down list or from the context-sensitive shortcut menu that displays when you right-click a selected area. When rows or columns are deleted, data is automatically shifted up or to the left to fill the space and relative references in formulas are updated.

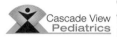
Cascade View Pediatrics

What You Will Do   To improve the layout of the report, you decide to insert blank rows before each fee category and remove the blank row that was created when you deleted *Hospital physicals* in the last activity.

Tutorial
Inserting Columns and Rows

Tutorial
Deleting Columns and Rows

1 With **2-CVPRevYarborough.xlsx** open, position the cell pointer (displays as a right-pointing black arrow) over row indicator 18, click and hold down the left mouse button, drag the mouse down over row indicator 19, and then release the mouse button.

> This selects rows 18 and 19.

2 Click the Home tab, click the Insert button arrow in the Cells group, and then click *Insert Sheet Rows* at the drop-down list.

> Two blank rows are inserted above row 18. All rows below the inserted rows are shifted down.

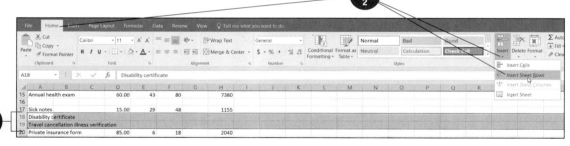

3 Click in cell A18, type Hearing assessment, and then press the Enter key.

4 Type Speech assessment in cell A19 and then press the Enter key.

5 Type the data for hearing and speech assessment as follows:

D18: 26.50	E18: 4	F18: 2
D19: 31.50	E19: 7	F19: 5

6 Enter formulas to calculate the totals for hearing and speech assessment as follows:

H18: =(e18+f18)*d18
H19: =(e19+f19)*d19

Steps 3-6

16					
17	Sick notes	15.00	29	48	1155
18	Hearing assessment	26.50	4	2	159
19	Speech assessment	31.50	7	5	378
20	Disability certificate				
21	Travel cancellation illness verification				

In Brief

Insert Rows or Columns
1. Select required number of rows or columns.
2. Click Insert button arrow.
3. Click *Insert Sheet Rows* or *Insert Sheet Columns*.

Delete Rows or Columns
1. Select rows or columns to be deleted.
2. Click Delete button arrow.
3. Click *Delete Sheet Rows* or *Delete Sheet Columns*.

7 Click row indicator 16 to select the entire row.

8 Click the Delete button arrow 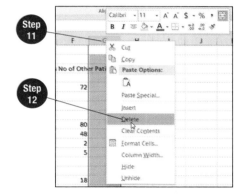 in the Cells group and then click *Delete Sheet Rows* at the drop-down list.

> The contents of row 16 are removed from the worksheet.

9 Select row 11. Hold down the Ctrl key, select rows 24 and 29, and then release the mouse button and the Ctrl key.

> Holding down the Ctrl key allows you to select multiple rows or columns that are not adjacent.

10 Position the cell pointer within any of the three selected rows, right-click to display the shortcut menu and Mini toolbar, and then click *Insert* at the shortcut menu.

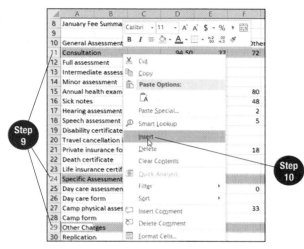

11 Right-click column indicator G.

> Right-clicking the column indicator selects the column and displays the shortcut menu and Mini toolbar at the same time.

12 At the shortcut menu, click *Delete*.

> The contents of the columns to the right of the deleted column are shifted left to fill in the space.

13 Click in any cell in the worksheet to deselect the column.

14 Save **2-CVPRevYarborough.xlsx**.

Check Your Work Compare your work with the model answer to ensure that you have completed the activity correctly.

In Addition

Inserting and Deleting Cells

In this activity, you selected entire rows and columns before inserting or deleting. This practice is the common method when you need to add to or delete data from a worksheet. Another method, used less frequently, is to insert new blank cells or delete a range of cells within the worksheet area. To insert new blank cells, select the number of cells you need to add near the location the cells will be added and then click the Insert button in the Cells group on the Home tab, or click the Insert button arrow and then click *Insert Cells* at the drop-down list

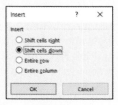

to open the Insert dialog box (shown below). Using the dialog box, you can choose to shift existing cells right or down. Click the Delete button in the Cells group to delete a selected range of cells and shift up the cells below the deleted range. Click the Delete button arrow and then click *Delete Cells* to open the Delete dialog box with options similar to those at the Insert dialog box.

Activity 2.4   Moving, Copying, and Linking Cells

You learned how to use copy and paste to copy formulas in the payroll worksheet for North Shore Medical Clinic. You can also use cut and paste to move the contents of a cell or range of cells to another location in the worksheet. The selected cells being cut or copied are called the source. The cell or range of cells that is receiving the source data is called the destination. If data already exists in the destination cells, Excel replaces the contents. Cells cut or copied to the Clipboard can be pasted more than once in the active workbook, in another workbook, or in another Office application. Link data between cells using the Paste Options gallery or by inserting a simple formula.

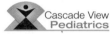
Cascade View
Pediatrics

Tutorial
Moving Cells

Tutorial
Copying and Pasting Cells

Tutorial
Linking Data

What You Will Do   Continue to work on the report by moving, copying, and linking cell contents.

1 With **2-CVPRevYarborough.xlsx** open, make cell A40 the active cell.

2 Click the Cut button [✄] in the Clipboard group on the Home tab.

> A moving marquee surrounds the source after you click the Cut button or Copy button, indicating that the cell contents have been placed in the Clipboard.

3 Make cell A9 the active cell and then click the Paste button in the Clipboard group. (Do not click the Paste button arrow, because this displays a drop-down gallery of options.)

> The text is moved from cell A40 to cell A9. In the next step, you will move the contents of a cell using a method called drag and drop.

4 Make cell A10 the active cell.

5 Point to any one of the four borders surrounding the selected cell.

> When you point to a border, the pointer changes from the thick white cross to a white arrow with the move icon (four-headed arrow) attached to it.

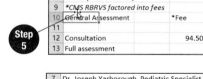

6 Click and hold down the left mouse button, drag the cell down one row to cell A11, and then release the mouse button.

> A green border will appear as you drag, indicating the placement of the range when you release the mouse. The destination range displays in a ScreenTip below the green border.

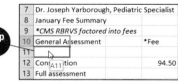

7 Make cell D34 the active cell.

> Dr. Yarborough charges the same fee for telephone prescription renewals and sick notes, so Sydney wants you to link the sick notes fee to the telephone prescription renewal fee. That way, if the fee changes, you will only need to type the new fee in one of the two cells, but they will both be updated.

8 Click the Copy button in the Clipboard group.

In Brief

Move or Copy Cells
1. Select source cells.
2. Click Cut button or Copy button.
3. Select starting destination cell.
4. Click Paste button.

Copy and Link Cells
1. Select source cells.
2. Click Copy button.
3. Select destination cell.
4. Click Paste button arrow.
5. Click Paste Link button.

9 Make cell D17 the active cell, click the Paste button arrow in the Clipboard group, and then click the Paste Link button in the *Other Paste Options* section of the Paste button drop-down gallery.

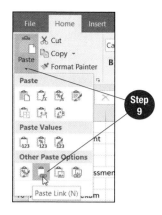

The existing data in cell D17 is replaced with the value copied from cell D34 and the source and destination cells are now linked. Linking the cells means that any change made to the source cell (D34) will automatically be applied to the destination cell (D17). A Paste Options button appears next to the destination cell (D17). Click the button to access the Paste Options drop-down gallery if you want to choose another paste option. Refer to the In Addition section at the bottom of this page for more information on the Paste Options drop-down gallery.

10 Press the Esc key to remove the moving marquee from cell D34.

11 Make cell D34 the active cell, edit the value to read *16.50*, and then press the Enter key.

Notice that the value in cell D17 automatically changes to *16.50*.

12 Select the range E27:G27.

13 Point to any one of the four borders surrounding the selected range until the pointer displays as a white arrow with the move icon attached to it, hold down the Ctrl key, and then drag the mouse to the range E28:G28. Release the mouse button and then release the Ctrl key.

Holding down the Ctrl key while dragging copies cells.

14 Make cell D28 the active cell, type *30.00*, and then press the Enter key.

15 Save **2-CVPRevYarborough.xlsx**.

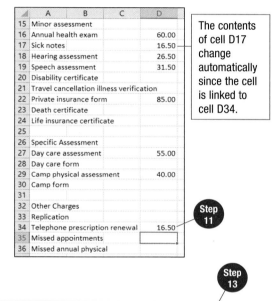

The contents of cell D17 change automatically since the cell is linked to cell D34.

> **Check Your Work** Compare your work with the model answer to ensure that you have completed the activity correctly.

In Addition

Using the Paste Options Gallery

The Paste Options gallery (shown at the right) appears when you click the Paste button arrow in the Clipboard group, when you click the Paste Options button that appears after an entry has been pasted into a cell, or in the shortcut menu that displays when you right-click in a cell. The gallery is divided into three sections: *Paste, Paste Values*, and *Other Paste Options*. Within each section, buttons are included for various paste options. Hover the mouse over a button to view a ScreenTip that describes the button's purpose and to see a preview of the paste option applied to the cell in the worksheet. The Paste Options gallery is context sensitive, meaning the buttons that appear are dependent on the type of content that has been copied and the location in which the content is being (or has been) pasted.

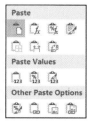

By default, columns are the same width and rows are the same height with columns set by default to a width of 8.11 characters and rows to a height of 14.40 points. Column width and row height can be adjusted manually or automatically. Multiple methods are available for manually adjusting the column width or row height, such as using the Format button in the Cells group on the Home tab, or clicking and dragging column or row heading boundaries. As you learned in Section 1, you can AutoFit a column or row by double-clicking a heading boundary. Excel automatically adjusts the heights of rows to accommodate the size of the text within the cells. Manually increasing the row height adds more space between rows, which can be used to improve readability or as a design technique to draw attention to a series of cells.

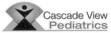

What You Will Do   To improve the readability of the report, you will adjust the widths of columns in which the entire heading is not currently visible and increase the height of the row containing the column headings.

Tutorial
Adjusting Column
Width and Row Height

1 With **2-CVPRevYarborough.xlsx** open, make any cell active in column E.

2 Click the Format button 🔲 in the Cells group on the Home tab and then click *Column Width* at the drop-down list.

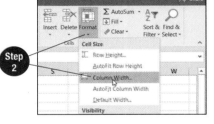

3 At the Column Width dialog box, type 20 and then click OK or press the Enter key.

> In the next step, you will use the mouse to adjust the width of column F.

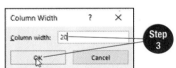

4 Position the mouse pointer on the column heading boundary line between columns F and G until the pointer changes to a vertical line with a left-and-right-pointing arrow ➕.

5 Click and hold down the left mouse button, drag the boundary line to the right until *Width: 17.00 (160 pixels)* displays in the ScreenTip, and then release the mouse button. ***Note: The pixel amount in parentheses will vary depending on your monitor's settings. Use the 17.00 character measurement in this activity.***

> As you drag the boundary line to the right or left, a line appears in the column in the worksheet area, indicating the new width. If, after decreasing a column's width, cells that previously had values in them display as a series of pound symbols (######), the column is now too narrow. Excel displays pound symbols instead of displaying only a part of a numeric value so that you do not confuse the partially displayed value with the actual full value. Widen the column to redisplay the numbers.

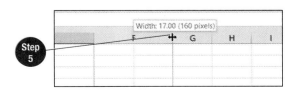

In Brief

Increase or Decrease Column Width
1. Select column(s).
2. Click Format button.
3. Click *Column Width*.
4. Type width.
5. Click OK.

Increase or Decrease Row Height
1. Select row(s).
2. Click Format button.
3. Click *Row Height*.
4. Type height.
5. Click OK.

Adjust Column Width or Row Height Using Mouse
Drag boundary to right of column or below row, or double-click boundary to AutoFit.

6 Make cell A21 active, click the Format button in the Cells group, and then click *AutoFit Column Width* at the drop-down list.

> The *AutoFit Column Width* option adjusts the width of the column to accommodate the content in the active cell. You can also double-click a column's boundary line to AutoFit the width to accommodate the longest entry.

7 Use the Column Width dialog box or drag the column boundary to increase the width of column D to *10 (97 pixels)*.

> After reviewing the worksheet, you decide the two columns with dollar values should be the same width. In the next steps, you will learn how to change the width of multiple columns in one operation.

8 Click column indicator D, hold down the Ctrl key, and then click column indicator G.

9 Position the mouse pointer on either one of the two columns' right boundary lines until the pointer changes to a vertical line with a left-and-right-pointing arrow.

> Any changes made to the width of one column boundary will affect all of the selected columns.

10 Drag the boundary line to the right until *Width: 15.00 (142 pixels)* displays in the ScreenTip and then release the mouse button.

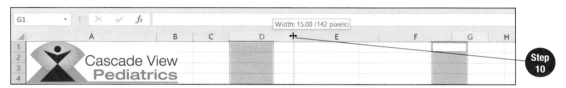

11 Click in any cell to deselect the columns.

> Do not be concerned that the columns appear too wide—you will improve the layout as you work through the next several activities.

12 Position the mouse pointer on the boundary line between rows 10 and 11 until the pointer changes to a horizontal line with an up-and-down-pointing arrow ✛.

13 Drag the boundary line down until *Height: 21.00 (35 pixels)* displays in the ScreenTip and then release the mouse button.

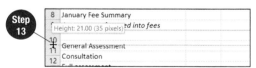

14 Save **2-CVPRevYarborough.xlsx**.

Check Your Work Compare your work with the model answer to ensure that you have completed the activity correctly.

In Addition

Using the Row Height Dialog Box

Just as you adjusted column width at the Column Width dialog box, you can increase or decrease the height of a row with the Row Height dialog box, shown at the right. Click in any cell within the row, click the Format button in the Cells group on the Home tab, and then click *Row* *Height* at the drop-down list. Type the desired height and then press the Enter key or click OK.

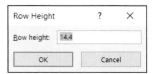

The font is the typeface used to display and print data. The default font in Excel is Calibri, but many other fonts are available. The size of the font is measured in units called points. A point is approximately $\frac{1}{72}$ of an inch measured vertically. The default font size in Excel is 11 points. The larger the point size, the larger the type. Each font's style can be changed to **bold**, *italic*, or ***bold italic***. Change the font color of text to improve worksheet appearance or emphasize certain text, such as changing the font color of negative numbers to red.

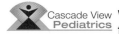
Cascade View
Pediatrics

What You Will Do   To add to the visual appeal of the revenue report, you will change the font and font size and apply formatting such as bold and color.

Tutorial
Applying Font Formatting

Tutorial
Adding Fill Color to Cells

1   With **2-CVPRevYarborough.xlsx** open, make cell A6 the active cell.

2   Click the *Font* option box arrow in the Font group on the Home tab, scroll down the list of fonts in the drop-down gallery, and then point to *Book Antiqua*.

Notice that Excel applies the font to the active cell so that you can preview the result. This feature is called live preview.

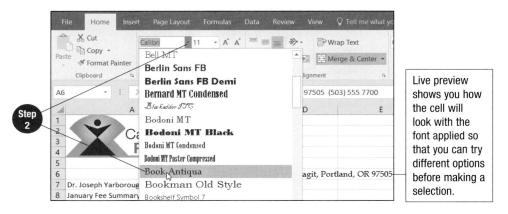

Live preview shows you how the cell will look with the font applied so that you can try different options before making a selection.

3   Click *Book Antiqua* to apply the font to cell A6.

4   With cell A6 still the active cell, click the *Font Size* option box arrow in the Font group and then click *14* at the drop-down list.

The row height is automatically increased to accommodate the larger font size.

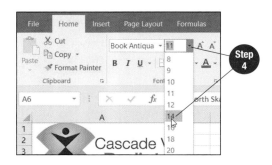

In Brief

Change Font
1. Select cells.
2. Click *Font* option box arrow.
3. Click font option.

Change Font Size
1. Select cells.
2. Click *Font Size* option box arrow.
3. Click size option.

Change Font Color
1. Select cells.
2. Click Font Color button arrow.
3. Click color option.

Change Font Style
1. Select cells.
2. Click attribute button.

5 With cell A6 still selected, click the Bold button **B** in the Font group.

6 With cell A6 still selected, click the Font Color button arrow **A** in the Font group and then click *Orange, Accent 2, Darker 25%* (sixth column, fifth row in the *Theme Colors* section).

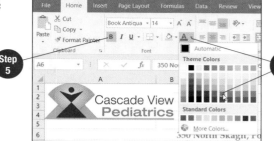
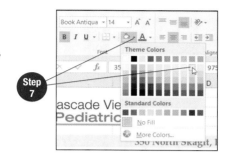

7 With cell A6 still selected, click the Fill Color button arrow in the Font group and then click *Blue, Accent 5, Lighter 80%* (ninth column, second row in the *Theme Colors* section).

> Fill is the color of the background in the cell. Changing the fill color is sometimes referred to as applying shading to a cell.

8 Select the range A7:I7 and then click the Merge & Center button in the Alignment group.

9 With cell A7 the active cell, change the font size to 12 points and then change the font color to Blue, Accent 5, Darker 25% (ninth column, fifth row in the *Theme Colors* section).

10 Select the range A8:I8 and apply the same formatting you applied in Steps 8 and 9.

> Since Blue, Accent 5, Darker 25% is the color you most recently selected from the Font Color button drop-down gallery, you can apply it to cells A8:I8 simply by clicking the Font Color button. You do not need to display the drop-down gallery.

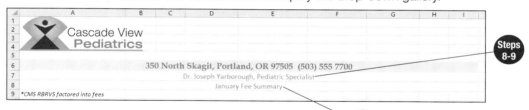

11 Click in any cell to deselect cell A8.

12 Save **2-CVPRevYarborough.xlsx**.

Check Your Work Compare your work with the model answer to ensure that you have completed the activity correctly.

In Addition

Using the Format Cells Dialog Box

You can use the Format Cells dialog box with the Font tab selected (shown at the right) to change the font type, font size, font style, and color of text. Additional Underline style options such as *Single*, *Double*, *Single Accounting*, and *Double Accounting* are available, as well as the special effects options *Strikethrough*, *Superscript*, and *Subscript*. Select the cells you want to change and then click the Font group dialog box launcher to display the Format Cells dialog box with the Font tab selected.

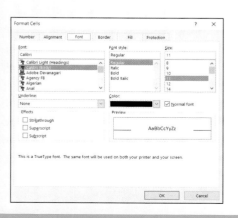

Activity 2.7

Formatting Numeric Cells; Adjusting Decimal Places; Using Undo

Excel provides specialized formatting options for numeric values. The Accounting format adds a dollar symbol ($), a comma in the thousands place, two digits after the decimal point, and displays negative values in brackets. Other numeric formats include Comma, Percentage, and Currency. By default, cells are initially set to the General format, which has no specific numeric style. The number of digits that display after the decimal point in a selected range of cells can be increased or decreased using the Increase Decimal and Decrease Decimal buttons in the Number group on the Home tab. Accountants follow a formatting standard where the top and bottom row containing monetary values display with the dollar symbol and the rest of the values do not include the dollar symbol. Use the Undo button on the Quick Access Toolbar to reverse the last action. Excel stores up to 100 actions that can be undone or redone, and you can repeat actions as many times as you need. Some actions (such as Save) cannot be reversed with Undo.

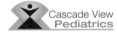 **Cascade View Pediatrics**

What You Will Do   Continue improving the visual appearance of the revenue summary report by applying format options to the numeric cells.

Tutorial
Applying Number Formatting

Tutorial
Using Undo and Redo

1 With **2-CVPRevYarborough.xlsx** open, make cell D12 the active cell.

2 Hold down the Ctrl key and then click in cell G12.

3 Click the Accounting Number Format button in the Number group on the Home tab.

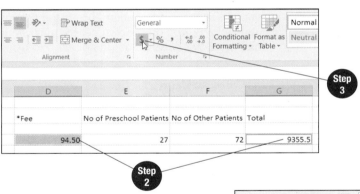

4 Click in any cell to deselect the cells.

5 Select the range G16:G34.

6 Click the Comma Style button in the Number group.

> The Comma Style button formats cells the same as the Accounting Number Format button with the exception of the dollar (or alternative currency) symbol.

7 Click in any cell to deselect the cells and review the numeric values in the worksheet. Only one numeric cell remains that could be improved by applying a format option: cell G38.

8 Make cell G38 the active cell.

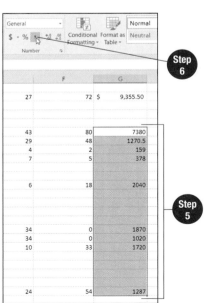

9 Click the Accounting Number Format button in the Number group.

10 Select the range E12:F34 and then click the Increase Decimal button in the Number group two times.

> One digit past the decimal point is added to the cells in the selected range each time you click the Increase Decimal button.

11 With the range E12:F34 still selected, click the Decrease Decimal button in the Number group.

> One digit past the decimal point is removed from the cells in the selected range each time you click the Decrease Decimal button.

12 Click the Undo button on the Quick Access Toolbar.

> Excel adds back one digit past the decimal point in the range E12:F34.

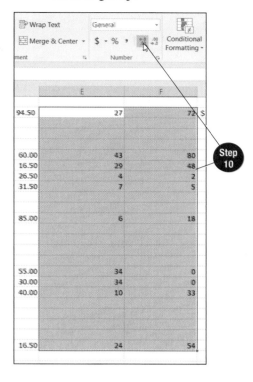

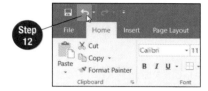

13 Click the Undo button two times to return the cells to their original state and then click in any cell to deselect the range.

14 Save **2-CVPRevYarborough.xlsx**.

Check Your Work Compare your work with the model answer to ensure that you have completed the activity correctly.

In Addition

Accessing Additional Number Format Options

Click the *Number Format* option box arrow in the Number group on the Home tab to display a drop-down list (shown at the right) with additional numeric format options including date, time, fraction, and scientific options. Click the *More Number Formats* option at the bottom of the list to display the Format Cells dialog box with the Number tab selected. Using this dialog box, you can access further customization options for a format, such as displaying negative values in red or creating your own custom format code.

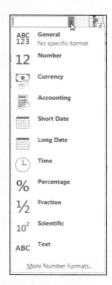

Data in a cell can be left-aligned, right-aligned, or centered within the column. Cells that have Merge & Center applied can be formatted to align the text in the merged cell at the left or right. Use the Increase Indent and Decrease Indent buttons to indent text from the left edge of the cell approximately one character width each time the button is clicked. Using buttons along the top row in the Alignment group on the Home tab, you can change vertical alignment, rotate text, or wrap text within a cell. A *comment* is a pop-up box containing text that can be attached to a cell and that displays when the cell pointer is positioned over a cell with an attached comment. A diagonal red triangle in the upper right corner of the cell alerts the reader that a comment exists. Insert a comment in a cell with the New Comment button in the Comments group on the Review tab.

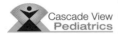
Cascade View Pediatrics

What You Will Do   Continue improving the appearance of the revenue summary report by editing cells, removing columns, adjusting column widths, aligning cells, and indenting labels. You will also add two comments asking Sydney to verify values before the report is submitted to Dr. Yarborough.

Tutorial
Applying Alignment Formatting

Tutorial
Inserting, Editing, and Printing Comments

1 With **2-CVPRevYarborough.xlsx** open, select cell E10 and then edit the contents to read *Preschool Patients*. Select cell F10 and then edit the contents to read *Other Patients*.

2 Select the range E10:F10, click the Format button in the Cells group on the Home tab, and then click *AutoFit Column Width* at the drop-down list.

3 Delete columns B and C from the worksheet. Refer to Activity 2.3 if you need assistance with this step.

4 Delete columns F and G from the worksheet.

Although no data existed in any cells within columns F and G, this step corrected the extended merge and centering applied to rows 6–8.

5 Select the range B10:E10.

6 Click the Center button 🬂 in the Alignment group on the Home tab.

Other buttons in the Alignment group include the Align Left button 🬂, which aligns entries at the left edge of the cell, and the Align Right button 🬂, which aligns entries at the right edge of the cell.

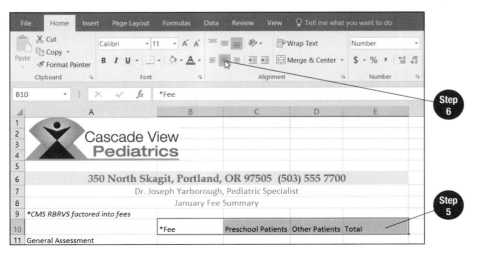

7 Select the range A12:A24.

8 Click the Increase Indent button ⊞ in the Alignment group.

Each time you the click the Increase Indent button, the contents of the selected cells are indented by approximately one character width. If you click the Increase Indent button too many times, click the Decrease Indent button ⊞ to return the text to the previous indent position.

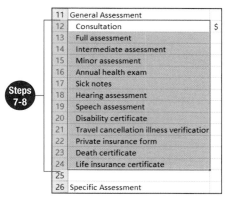

Steps 7-8

11	General Assessment	
12	Consultation	$
13	Full assessment	
14	Intermediate assessment	
15	Minor assessment	
16	Annual health exam	
17	Sick notes	
18	Hearing assessment	
19	Speech assessment	
20	Disability certificate	
21	Travel cancellation illness verification	
22	Private insurance form	
23	Death certificate	
24	Life insurance certificate	
25		
26	Specific Assessment	

9 Select the range A27:A30 and then click the Increase Indent button.

10 Select the range A33:A36 and then click the Increase Indent button.

11 Select the range B10:E10. Hold down the Ctrl key and then click cells A11, A26, A32, and A38.

Use the Ctrl key to select multiple ranges or cells to which you want to apply a formatting option.

Step 11

	A	B	C	D	E
10		*Fee	Preschool Patients	Other Patients	Total
11	General Assessment				
12	Consultation	$ 94.50	27	72	$ 9,355.50
13	Full assessment				
14	Intermediate assessment				
15	Minor assessment				
16	Annual health exam	60.00	43	80	7,380.00
17	Sick notes	16.50	29	48	1,270.50
18	Hearing assessment	26.50	4	2	159.00
19	Speech assessment	31.50	7	5	378.00
20	Disability certificate				
21	Travel cancellation illness verification				
22	Private insurance form	85.00	6	18	2,040.00
23	Death certificate				
24	Life insurance certificate				
25					
26	Specific Assessment				
27	Day care assessment	55.00	34	0	1,870.00
28	Day care form	30.00	34	0	1,020.00
29	Camp physical assessment	40.00	10	33	1,720.00
30	Camp form				
31					
32	Other Charges				
33	Replication				
34	Telephone prescription renewal	16.50	24	54	1,287.00
35	Missed appointments				
36	Missed annual physical				
37					
38	Total				$ 26,480.00

Sheet1   ⊕

12 Click the Bold button in the Font group.

13 Click in any cell to deselect the cells.

14 Select the range B10:E10.

In Activity 2.5, you increased the height of row 10 to 21.00 points. The Alignment group contains buttons that allow you to control the alignment of the text between the top and bottom borders of the row. In the next step, you will center the text vertically within the cells.

15 Click the Middle Align button ≡ in the Alignment group.

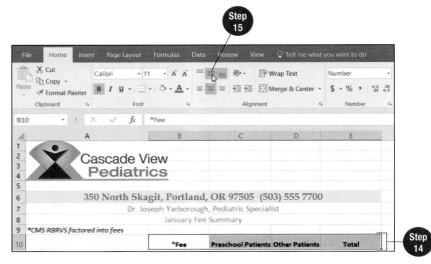

16 Deselect the range.

17 Make cell C30 the active cell.

You want to insert a comment to Sydney Larsen asking her to confirm that there were no charges for camp forms in January.

18 Click the Review tab and then click the New Comment button in the Comments group.

A comment box displays anchored to the active cell with the user's name inserted in bold text at the top of the box. In worksheets accessed by multiple people, the name helps the reader identify who made the comment.

19 Type Sydney, please confirm no camp forms were issued in January. Thanks.

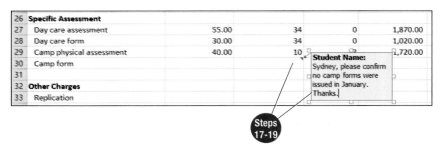

20 Click in any cell outside the comment box.

The comment box closes and a diagonal red triangle appears in the upper right corner of cell C30, indicating that a comment exists for the cell.

21 Right-click cell B28 and then click *Insert Comment* at the shortcut menu.

22 Type Check fee. This is the same rate as last year.

23 Click in any cell outside the comment box.

24 Hover the cell pointer over cell B28.

Hovering the cell pointer over a cell that contains a comment causes the comment box to pop up.

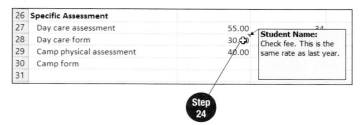

Step 24

25 Right-click cell B28 and then click *Edit Comment* at the shortcut menu.

26 Add the following sentence to the end of the existing comment text:

Should this be the same fee as Dr. Severin's?

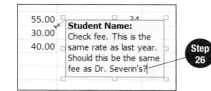

Step 26

27 Click in any cell outside the comment box.

28 Make cell A9 the active cell and then click the Next button 🔲 in the Comments group on the Review tab.

Excel displays the comment box in cell B28.

29 Click the Next button in the Comments group.

Excel displays the comment box in cell C30.

30 Click the Next button and then click Cancel at the message indicating that Excel has reached the end of the workbook. This instructs Excel not to continue the review at the beginning of the workbook.

The Comments group also contains a Previous button 🔲 that can be used to view the comment box prior to the active comment.

31 Click in any cell to close the comment associated with cell C30.

32 Save **2-CVPRevYarborough.xlsx**.

Check Your Work Compare your work with the model answer to ensure that you have completed the activity correctly.

In Addition

Printing Comments

By default, comments do not print with a worksheet. To print a worksheet with the comment boxes, you need to specify a *Comments* option at the Page Setup dialog box. Click the Page Layout tab, click the Page Setup dialog box launcher in the Page Setup group, click the Sheet tab, and then click the *Comments* option box arrow in the *Print* section (shown at the right). You can choose to print the comment text at the end of the sheet or as displayed on the sheet.

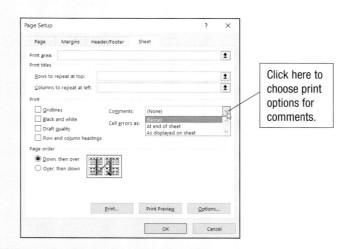

Click here to choose print options for comments.

Activity 2.9   Adding Borders; Using Format Painter

Borders in various styles and colors can be applied to display and print in selected cells within a worksheet. Borders can be added to the top, left, bottom, or right edge of a cell. Use borders to underscore headings or totals or to emphasize cells containing important data. Format Painter copies formatting from a selected cell to another cell. Use this feature to apply multiple format options from one cell to another cell.

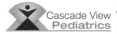
Cascade View Pediatrics

What You Will Do   As you get closer to completing the report, you will spend time improving the appearance of the worksheet by adding borders and shading.

Tutorial
Adding Borders to Cells

Tutorial
Using Format Painter and the Repeat Command

Tutorial
Applying Formatting Using the Format Cells Dialog Box

1 With **2-CVPRevYarborough.xlsx** open, select the range A10:E10.

2 Click the Bottom Border button arrow in the Font group on the Home tab.

A drop-down list of border style options displays.

3 Click *Top and Bottom Border* at the drop-down list.

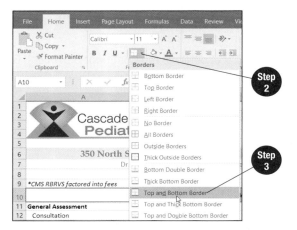

4 Click in any cell to deselect the range and view the border.

5 Make cell A11 the active cell, click the Top and Bottom Border button arrow (previously the Bottom Border button), and then click *Outside Borders* at the drop-down list.

6 Make cell A26 the active cell and then click the Outside Borders button (not the button arrow).

Since the Borders button updates to the most recently selected border style, you can apply the *Outside Borders* option to the active cell without displaying the drop-down list.

7 Make cell A32 the active cell, click the Outside Borders button, and then deselect the cell.

8 Make cell E38 the active cell, click the Outside Borders button arrow, and then click *Top and Double Bottom Border* at the drop-down list.

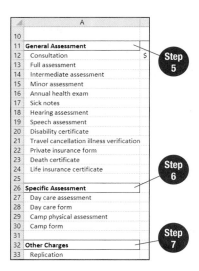

In Brief

Add Borders
1. Select cells.
2. Click Borders button arrow.
3. Click border style.
4. Deselect cells.

Copy Formats
1. Make active cell containing formats.
2. Click (copy once) or double-click (copy more than once) Format Painter button.
3. Click destination cell(s).
4. If necessary, click Format Painter button to turn off feature.

9 Select the range A17:E17, click the Fill Color button arrow, and then click the *More Colors* option.

10 At the Colors dialog box with the Standard tab selected, click the yellow color option shown at the right and then click OK.

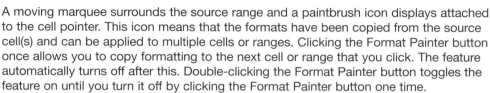

11 With the range A17:E17 still selected, double-click the Format Painter button [icon] in the Clipboard group.

A moving marquee surrounds the source range and a paintbrush icon displays attached to the cell pointer. This icon means that the formats have been copied from the source cell(s) and can be applied to multiple cells or ranges. Clicking the Format Painter button once allows you to copy formatting to the next cell or range that you click. The feature automatically turns off after this. Double-clicking the Format Painter button toggles the feature on until you turn it off by clicking the Format Painter button one time.

12 Select the range A22:E22. Notice that the shading is copied to the range and the paintbrush icon remains attached to the cell pointer.

13 Select the range A34:E34.

14 Click the Format Painter button to turn off the feature.

16	Annual health exam	60.00	43	80	7,380.00
17	Sick notes	16.50	29	48	1,270.50
18	Hearing assessment	26.50	4	2	159.00
19	Speech assessment	31.50	7	5	378.00
20	Disability certificate				
21	Travel cancellation illness verification				
22	Private insurance form	85.00	6	18	2,040.00
23	Death certificate				
24	Life insurance certificate				
25					
26	**Specific Assessment**				
27	Day care assessment	55.00	34	0	1,870.00
28	Day care form	30.00	34	0	1,020.00
29	Camp physical assessment	40.00	10	33	1,720.00
30	Camp form				
31					
32	**Other Charges**				
33	Replication				
34	Telephone prescription renewal	16.50	24	54	1,287.00
35	Missed appointments				

15 Click in any cell to deselect the range.

16 Save **2-CVPRevYarborough.xlsx**.

Check Your Work Compare your work with the model answer to ensure that you have completed the activity correctly.

In Addition

Creating a Custom Border

If none of the borders in the drop-down list suit your needs, you can create a custom border. Click the *More Borders* option at the bottom of the Borders button drop-down list to display the Format Cells dialog box with the Border tab selected, as shown below. At this dialog box, you can change to a different line style by clicking another line option in the *Style* list box and/or change the line color by clicking the *Color* option box arrow and then choosing the desired color at the drop-down gallery. Next, specify the outside border and/or inside border you want by clicking one of the buttons in the *Presets* section, clicking one or more of the Border buttons along the perimeter of the preview box, or clicking inside the preview box at the edge of the cell along which you want the border to appear. When you are finished creating the border, click OK.

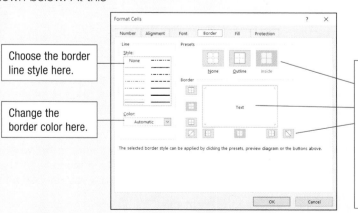

Choose the border line style here.

Change the border color here.

Specify where the border should appear by clicking a button in the *Presets* section, a border button, or inside the preview box along the edge at which you want the border to appear.

Activity 2.10 Applying Cell Styles; Applying and Modifying Themes

Cell styles contain a group of predefined formatting options saved under one name. Styles are an efficient method for consistently applying formats and creating a professional, consistent worksheet appearance. Excel includes several predefined cell styles that you can apply or modify, or you can choose to create your own cell style. A theme is a set of formatting choices that includes a set of colors, a set of heading and body fonts, and a set of lines and fill effects. Excel provides a variety of themes you can use to format a worksheet.

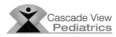
Cascade View Pediatrics

What You Will Do To further finalize the revenue summary report, you will apply cell styles and a theme.

> **Tutorial**
> Applying Cell Styles
>
> **Tutorial**
> Applying and Modifying Themes

1 With **2-CVPRevYarborough.xlsx** open, select the range A7:A8.

> You decide to change the formatting of this range to a predefined cell style.

2 Click the More Cell Styles button ⬇ (may also display as the Cell Styles button 🖾) in the Styles group on the Home tab.

> A drop-down gallery appears with the predefined cell styles grouped into five sections: *Good, Bad and Neutral*; *Data and Model*; *Titles and Headings*; *Themed Cell Styles*; and *Number Format*.

3 Move the mouse over several of the cell style options at the drop-down gallery to display a live preview of the styles applied to the two title rows.

4 Click the *Heading 4* style in the *Titles and Headings* section.

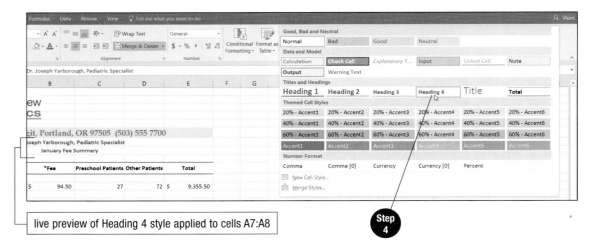

live preview of Heading 4 style applied to cells A7:A8

Step 4

5 Make cell A11 the active cell, click the More Cell Styles button in the Styles group, and then click the *Accent5* style in the *Themed Cell Styles* section.

6 Apply the Accent5 style to cells A26 and A32.

7 Deselect the cell(s).

> In the next steps, you will apply a theme to the worksheet. Changing the theme will cause the fonts, colors, and effects in the cells to change. As with styles, you will be able to live preview of the changes before you choose a theme.

8 Click the Page Layout tab.

9 Click the Themes button in the Themes group.

10 Move the mouse over several of the themes in the drop-down gallery and observe the changes that take place in the worksheet.

> Applying a theme affects the entire worksheet. You do not select a cell or range of cells before you apply a theme.

11 Click *Organic* at the drop-down gallery.

12 Click the Colors button in the Themes group and then click *Slipstream* at the drop-down gallery.

13 Click the Fonts button in the Themes group and then click *Corbel*.

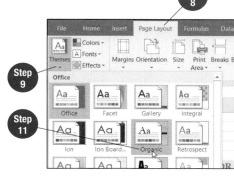

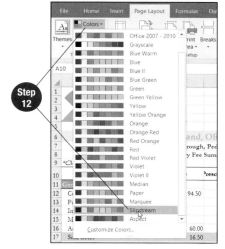

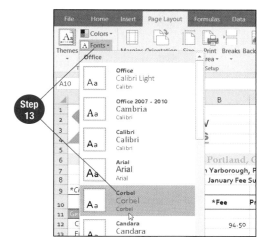

14 Automatically adjust the width of columns A, C, and D to fit the longest entries.

> The theme and theme colors applied in previous steps increased the font size of text, so the columns need to be adjusted to display all of the text.

15 Save **2-CVPRevYarborough.xlsx**.

Check Your Work ▶ Compare your work with the model answer to ensure that you have completed the activity correctly.

In Addition

Creating a New Cell Style

You can create your own cell style using the *New Cell Style* option at the bottom of the Cell Styles drop-down gallery. First, select a cell in the current worksheet and apply all of the formatting to the cell that you want to save in the style. Second, with the cell to which you have applied the desired formats active, click the More Cell Styles button (or Cell Styles button) in the Styles group on the Home tab and then click *New Cell Style* at the drop-down gallery. At the Style dialog box, shown at the right, type a name for the style in the *Style name* text box and then click OK. The new style will appear at

the top of the Cell Styles drop-down gallery in a new section titled *Custom*. Custom styles are saved in the workbook in which they are created. You will not see the new style when you open a new workbook; however, you can copy styles from one workbook to another.

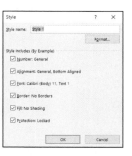

Activity 2.11 Using Find and Replace

Use the Find feature to search for specific labels or values that you want to verify or edit. The Find feature will move to each cell containing the text you specify. The Replace feature will search for a label, value, or format and replace it with another label, value, or format you specify. Use Find and Replace to ensure that all occurrences of the specified label or value are located and, if necessary, edited.

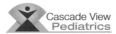

What You Will Do   To double-check your work on the revenue summary report, you decide to search the worksheet to make sure you included all of the forms. Sydney Larsen has also reviewed the report and requested that you change all occurrences of *assessment* to *evaluation*.

Tutorial
Finding Data

Tutorial
Replacing Data

Tutorial
Replacing Formatting

1 With **2-CVPRevYarborough.xlsx** open, press Ctrl + Home to make cell A1 the active cell.

2 Click the Home tab.

3 Click the Find & Select button 🔍 in the Editing group and then click *Find* at the drop-down list.

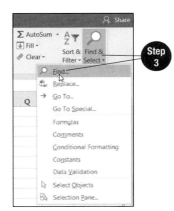

4 Type form in the *Find what* text box and then click the Find Next button.

> Cell A22, which contains the first occurrence of the word *form*, becomes active.

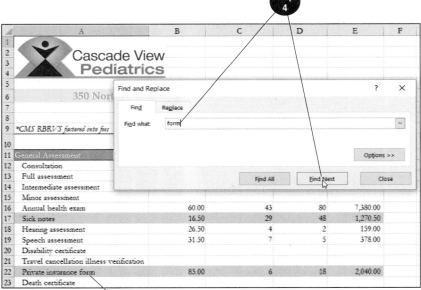

> The Find feature moves to the next occurrence of the text each time you click the Find Next button.

5 Click the Find Next button.

> The cell containing *Day care form* (cell A28) becomes active.

6 Click the Find Next button.

> The cell containing *Camp form* (cell A30) becomes active.

In Brief

Find Label or Value
1. Click Find & Select button.
2. Click *Find*.
3. Type label or value in *Find what* text box.
4. Click Find Next button.

Replace Label or Value
1. Click Find & Select button.
2. Click *Replace*.
3. Type label or value in *Find what* text box.
4. Type replacement label or value in *Replace with* text box.
5. Click Replace or Replace All button.

7 Click the Find Next button.

> Excel returns to the first occurrence of *form*, located in cell A22. Although in this small worksheet you could easily have reviewed the form entries by scanning column A, in a large worksheet with many rows and columns, using the Find feature is an efficient way to locate specific text. Using the Find feature also ensures that you do not miss any instances of the text or formatting for which you are searching.

8 Click the Close button to close the Find and Replace dialog box.

9 Click the Find & Select button in the Editing group and then click *Replace* at the drop-down list.

10 Select *form* in the *Find what* text box and then type assessment.

11 Press the Tab key to move the insertion point to the *Replace with* text box and then type evaluation.

12 Click the Replace All button.

> Excel searches through the entire worksheet and automatically changes all occurrences of *assessment* to *evaluation*.

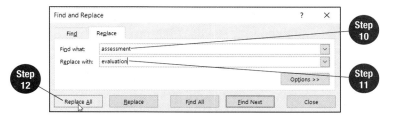

13 Click OK at the message informing you that Excel has completed the search and made nine replacements.

14 Click the Close button to close the Find and Replace dialog box.

15 Click the Page Layout tab, click the *Width* option box arrow (currently displays *Automatic*) in the Scale to Fit group and then click *1 page* at the drop-down list

16 Save and then print **2-CVPRevYarborough.xlsx**.

Check Your Work Compare your work with the model answer to ensure that you have completed the activity correctly.

In Addition

Replacing Formats

You can use the Replace feature to find formatting and replace it with other formatting or remove it. For example, you could find all occurrences of bold and blue font color and replace them with bold and green font color. At the Find and Replace dialog box with the Replace tab selected, click the Options button to expand the dialog box and display Format buttons to the right of the *Find what* and *Replace with* text boxes (shown at the right). Use these buttons to specify the desired formatting options. The Preview boxes (which initially display *No Format Set*) will display the formatting that Excel will find and replace.

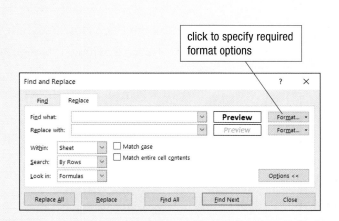

click to specify required format options

When you scroll horizontally or vertically to view other parts of a worksheet, some column or row headings may scroll off the screen, making relating to text or values difficult. Freezing panes causes certain rows and columns, such as those containing headings or labels, to remain fixed when scrolling. Magnify or reduce the worksheet display by dragging the Zoom slider bar button, clicking the Zoom In or Zoom Out buttons, or specifying a zoom percentage at the Zoom dialog box. Changing the zoom does not affect printing since worksheets automatically print at 100% unless scaling options are changed.

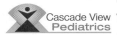
Cascade View Pediatrics

What You Will Do   You will freeze row headings in the report to make sure data is easily understood even when scrolling. You will also experiment with various zoom settings to make more cells visible within the current window.

Tutorial
Freezing and
Unfreezing Panes

Tutorial
Changing the Zoom

1 With **2-CVPRevYarborough.xlsx** open, make cell A11 the active cell.

2 Click the View tab.

3 Click the Freeze Panes button 🔲 in the Window group.

4 Click *Freeze Panes* at the drop-down list.

> The position of the active cell before you freeze panes is important since all rows above and all columns left of the active cell will be frozen. Notice you made cell A11 the active cell, so rows 1-10 are now frozen. A horizontal black line appears, indicating which rows remain fixed when scrolling, as shown in Figure E2.1.

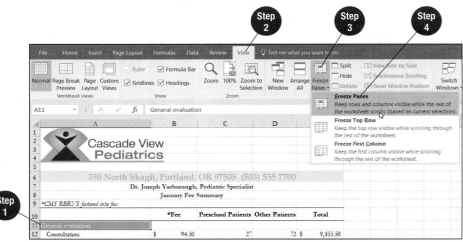

5 Press the Page Down key a few times to scroll down the worksheet.

> Notice that rows 1 through 10 do not scroll off the screen.

6 Press Ctrl + Home. Excel returns to cell A11 instead of cell A1 since cell A1 is frozen.

7 Click the Freeze Panes button in the Window group and then click *Unfreeze Panes* at the drop-down list.

> The *Freeze Panes* option changes to *Unfreeze Panes* when rows or columns have been frozen.

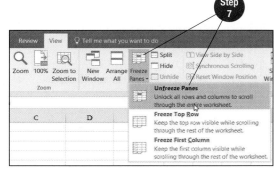

Freeze Panes
1. Make cell active below and right of rows or columns to be frozen.
2. Click View tab.
3. Click Freeze Panes button.
4. Click *Freeze Panes*.

Change Zoom Setting
Drag Zoom slider bar.
OR
Click Zoom In or Zoom Out buttons.
OR
Click zoom percentage value and choose magnification option at Zoom dialog box.

Figure E2.1 Worksheet with Rows 1–10 Frozen

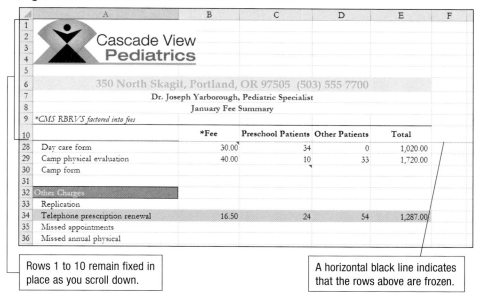

Rows 1 to 10 remain fixed in place as you scroll down.

A horizontal black line indicates that the rows above are frozen.

8 Click and drag the button on the Zoom slider bar at the right side of the Status bar (above the time and date on the Taskbar) and watch the cells grow and shrink as you drag right and left.

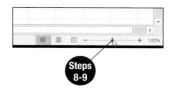

Steps 8-9

9 Drag the Zoom slider button to the halfway mark on the slider bar to redisplay the worksheet at 100%.

10 Click *100%* at the right side of the slider bar to open the Zoom dialog box.

11 Click the *75%* option and then click OK.

12 Click the Zoom In button (plus symbol) at the right side of the Zoom slider bar.

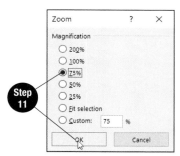

Step 11

13 Continue to click the Zoom In button until the zoom percentage returns to 100%.

When the worksheet is set to 100% magnification, clicking the Zoom In or Zoom Out buttons at either side of the slider bar magnifies or shrinks the display of the worksheet by 10%.

14 Save **2-CVPRevYarborough.xlsx**.

Check Your Work Compare your work with the model answer to ensure that you have completed the activity correctly.

In Addition

Using Buttons in the Zoom Group

The View tab contains a Zoom group with three buttons to change zoom settings, as shown at the right. Click the Zoom button to display the Zoom dialog box. This is the same dialog box that you displayed in Step 10. Click the 100% button to return the zoom to 100%.

Select a range of cells and then click the Zoom to Selection button to scale the zoom setting so that the selected range fills the worksheet area.

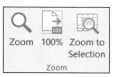

Creating Formulas with Absolute Addressing

In previous activities, when you copied and pasted formulas in worksheets, the cell addresses in the destination cells changed automatically relative to the destination row or column. The formulas in these worksheets used relative addressing. Sometimes you need a cell address to remain fixed when it is copied to another location in the worksheet. To do this, the formulas must include absolute addressing for those cell addresses that you do not want changed. Make a cell address absolute by typing a dollar symbol ($) in front of the column letter or row number that you do not want to change. You can also use the F4 function key to toggle through variations of the address as relative, absolute, or mixed, in which either the row is absolute and the column is relative or vice versa.

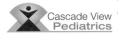

Cascade View Pediatrics

What You Will Do   Dr. Yarborough would like to increase his monthly revenue by approximately $1,500. He has asked you to add columns to the report to determine the percentage by which he needs to increase his fees to achieve this goal.

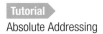

Tutorial
Absolute Addressing

1 With **2-CVPRevYarborough.xlsx** open, make cell F10 the active cell and then type New Fee.

2 Make cell G10 the active cell and then type New Total.

3 Make cell F9 the active cell, type 5%, and then press the Enter key.

> Placing the percent increase in its own cell will allow you to easily try out different percentages until you find the one that will achieve the $1,500 increase in revenue. In the next steps, you will create and copy formulas that will calculate revenue based on a 5% increase in fees.

4 Make cell F12 the active cell, type =(b12*f9, press F4, type)+b12, and then press the Enter key.

> You will be copying this formula to the remaining rows, so you need to make sure that the reference to cell F9 stays the same when the formula is duplicated. Pressing F4 causes Excel to insert dollar symbols in front of the row letter and column number immediately left of the insertion point—f9 becomes $F$9, an absolute address.

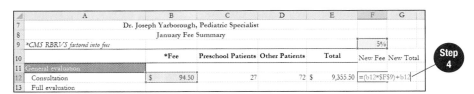

5 Make cell G12 the active cell, type =(c12+d12)*f12, and then press the Enter key.

> The formula to calculate the total revenue does not require an absolute reference. When copying this formula, you want the row numbers to change relative to the destination cells.

Make Cell Address Absolute
With insertion point positioned just after cell address or with cell address selected in Formula bar, press F4.
OR
Type dollar symbol immediately preceding column letter and/or row number.

6 Make cell F16 the active cell, type =(b16*f9)+b16, and then press the Enter key.

> You can type the dollar symbols into the formula rather than pressing F4 to insert them.

B	C	D	E	F	G
eph Yarborough, Pediatric Specialist					
January Fee Summary					
				5%	
*Fee	Preschool Patients	Other Patients	Total	New Fee	New Total
$ 94.50	27	72 $	9,355.50	$ 99.23	$9,823.28
60.00	43	80	7,380.00	=(b16*f9)+b16	
16.50	29	48	1,270.50		

Step 6

7 Make cell F16 the active cell and then click the Copy button in the Clipboard group on the Home tab.

8 Select the range F17:F19, hold down the Ctrl key, and then select cells F22, F27:F29, and F34.

9 Click the Paste button in the Clipboard group.

10 Press the Esc key to remove the moving marquee from cell F12.

11 Click cell F17 and then look at the Formula bar to see the formula that was pasted into the cell: =(B17*$F$9)+B17.

> Notice that the cell address containing the percent value (F9) did not change, while the cell address that contains the original fee for sick notes (B17) changed relative to the destination (row 17).

12 Click a few other cells in column F to view the formula. Notice that in each cell, the address for cell F9 remains the same while the cell address for column B always changes relative to the destination row.

13 Copy the formula in cell G12 and paste it into cells G16:G19, G22, G27:G29, and G34 by completing steps similar to those in Steps 8 through 11.

14 Copy the formula in cell E38, paste it into cell G38, and then AutoFit the width of column G.

15 Make cell A40 the active cell, type Increase in January Revenue:, make cell G40 the active cell, type =g38-e38, and then press the Enter key.

> The increased revenue, $1,324.00, does not meet the $1,500.00 goal.

16 Make cell F9 the active cell and edit the value to read 6%.

17 Look at the updated value in cell G40. Notice that the increased revenue of $1,588.80 now meets the goal set by Dr. Yarborough.

18 Use Format Painter to copy the formatting from cell E10 to the range F10:G10 and then turn on the display of formulas.

19 Save, print, and then close **2-CVPRevYarborough.xlsx**.

Check Your Work Compare your work with the model answer to ensure that you have completed the activity correctly.

In Addition

Learning More about Mixed Addressing

You can instruct Excel to fix only the row number or the column letter of a cell that is copied and pasted to another location. This table shows more ways that a cell address can use absolute referencing. Pressing F4 repeatedly causes Excel to scroll through each of these variations for the selected cell address.

Example	Action
=$A$12*.01	Neither the column nor the row will change.
=$A12*.01	The column will remain fixed at column A, but the row will change.
=A$12*.01	The column will change, but the row remains fixed at row 12.
=A12*.01	Both the column and row will change.

Features Summary

Feature	Ribbon Tab, Group	Button, Option	Keyboard Shortcut
align left	Home, Alignment		
align right	Home, Alignment		
bold	Home, Font	B	Ctrl + B
borders	Home, Font		Ctrl + Shift + &
cell styles	Home, Styles		
center	Home, Alignment		
clear cell	Home, Editing		
Comma format	Home, Number	,	
copy	Home, Clipboard		Ctrl + C
cut	Home, Clipboard		Ctrl + X
decrease decimal	Home, Number		
decrease indent	Home, Alignment		
delete cell, column, or row	Home, Cells		
fill color	Home, Font		
Find	Home, Editing	, *Find*	Ctrl + F
font type	Home, Font		Ctrl + 1
font color	Home, Font	A	Ctrl + 1
font size	Home, Font		Ctrl + 1
Format Painter	Home, Clipboard		
freeze panes	View, Window		
image from file	Insert, Illustrations		
increase decimal	Home, Number		
increase indent	Home, Alignment		
insert cell, column, or row	Home, Cells		
italic	Home, Font	I	Ctrl + I
middle-align	Home, Alignment		
online image	Insert, Illustrations		

Feature	Ribbon Tab, Group	Button, Option	Keyboard Shortcut
paste	Home, Clipboard		Ctrl + V
repeat			Ctrl + Y
Replace	Home, Editing	, *Replace*	Ctrl + H
Spelling	Review, Proofing		F7
theme	Page Layout, Themes		
theme colors	Page Layout, Themes		
theme fonts	Page Layout, Themes		
Thesaurus	Review, Proofing		Shift + F7
undo an action			Ctrl + Z
zoom	View, Zoom		

Workbook Section study tools and assessment activities are available in the Workbook pages of the ebook. These resources are designed to help you further develop and demonstrate mastery of the skills learned in this section.

Excel

Using Functions, Adding Visual Elements, Printing, and Working with Tables

Data Files Before beginning section work, copy the ExcelMedS3 folder to your storage medium and then make ExcelMedS3 the active folder.

Skills

- Create AVERAGE, COUNT, MAX, and MIN formulas to perform statistical analysis
- Create NOW and TODAY formulas
- Create and use range names
- Use an IF function to return a result based on a logical test
- Create, edit, and format a column chart and a pie chart

- Insert and format shapes and text boxes
- Change page layout options for printing, including margins, horizontal and vertical centering, and scaling
- Insert headers and footers in Page Layout view
- Format data as a table
- Sort and filter a table

Precheck Check your current skills to help focus your study of the skills taught in this section.

Activities Overview

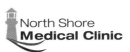

Calculate statistics and set print options for the standard exam room supplies report, compare discounts from two medical supply vendors and add graphics to the report, calculate dates in the dermatology patient tracking worksheet, and create charts summarizing dermatology diagnoses by age group of patient.

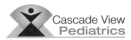

Revise the January fee summary report to calculate fee increases; calculate statistical functions, add dates, calculate expense variance, add a logo, sort, and set print options for a quarterly expense report; and create a chart, draw objects, and format a table in a rent and maintenance cost report.

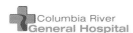

Finish a weekly adult cardiac bypass surgery report; calculate average standard costs for cardiac surgery patient stays; create charts and change print options for a quarterly expense report; format, filter and sort the cardiac nurse casual call list; filter and sort the nursing professional development list; and create and format a patient cost report and a chart on U.S. cancer statistics.

Model Answers Preview the model answers for an overview of the activities you will complete in each section.

189

Activity 3.1   Using Statistical Functions

Until now, you have only used the SUM function when you click the AutoSum button in the Editing group on the Home tab. Excel includes numerous other built-in formulas that are grouped into function categories. The Statistical category contains several functions that can be used to perform statistical analysis on data, such as calculating medians, variances, frequencies, and so on. The structure of a function formula begins with the equals sign (=), followed by the name of the function and then the argument within parentheses. Argument is the term given to the values to be included in the calculation. The structure of the argument is dependent on the function being used and can include a single range of cells, multiple ranges, single cell references, or a combination thereof.

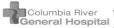Columbia River
General Hospital

What You Will Do   Lee Elliott, office manager of North Shore Medical Clinic, would like you to compile statistics on the cost of supplies for eight exam rooms.

Tutorial
Using Statistical
Functions

1   Open **NSMCSupplies.xlsx** and then save it with the name **3-NSMCSupplies**.

2   Make cell F4 the active cell and then freeze the panes. Refer to Section 2, Activity 2.12, if you need assistance with this step.

3   Type the following labels in the cells indicated:
> A65:   Average exam room standard cost:
> A66:   Maximum exam room standard cost:
> A67:   Minimum exam room standard cost:
> A68:   Count of exam room items:

4   Make cell B65 the active cell.

> In the next steps, you will insert the AVERAGE function to determine the arithmetic mean of the totals in the cells in row 63. If an empty cell or a cell containing text is included in the argument, Excel ignores the cell when determining the result. If, however, the cell contains a zero value, it is included in the average calculation.

5   Click the Home tab and then click the AutoSum button arrow in the Editing group.

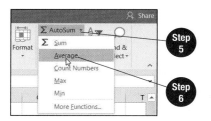

6   Click *Average* at the drop-down list.

> Excel inserts the formula *=AVERAGE()* in the active cell with the insertion point positioned between the parentheses. Since no values exist immediately above or to the left of the active cell, Excel does not offer a suggested range. In the next step, you will drag to select the range in the formula.

7   Position the cell pointer over cell F63, click and hold down the left mouse button, drag right to cell M63, and then release the left mouse button. The range F63:M63 is inserted as the function argument.

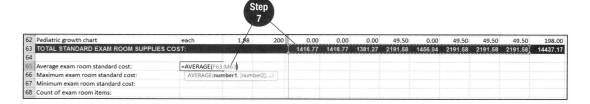

8 Press the Enter key or click the Enter button on the Formula bar.

Excel returns the result *1804.64625* in cell B65.

9 If it is not already active, make cell B66 the active cell.

10 Click the AutoSum button arrow and then click *Max* at the drop-down list.

The MAX function returns the largest value in the argument.

11 Type f63:m63 and then press the Enter key.

Excel returns the result *2191.58* in cell B66. Typing the range into the formula is sometimes faster if you are sure of the starting and ending cell references.

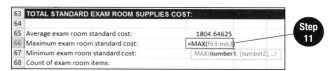

12 With cell B67 the active cell, type the function =min(f63:m63) and then press the Enter key.

The MIN function returns the smallest value in the argument, *1381.27*. You can type the entire function directly into the cell if you know the name of the function you want to use and the structure of the argument.

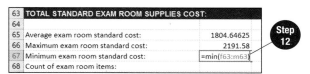

13 With cell B68 the active cell, type the function =count(d4:d62) and then press the Enter key.

COUNT returns the number of cells that contain numbers or numbers that have been formatted as text and dates. Empty cells, text labels, and error values in the range are ignored.

14 Apply the Comma format to the range B65:B67.

15 Click in any cell to deselect the range B65:B67.

16 Save and then close **3-NSMCSupplies.xlsx**.

Check Your Work Compare your work with the model answer to ensure that you have completed the activity correctly.

In Addition

Exploring Other Statistical Functions

Click *More Functions* at the AutoSum button drop-down list to display the Insert Function dialog box. This dialog box will allow you to access Excel's complete list of functions. The following is a sampling of other statistical functions and their descriptions:

Function Name	Description
=COUNTA	counts the number of cells in a range (including those that contain labels); ignores empty cells
=COUNTBLANK	counts the number of empty cells in a range
=MEDIAN	returns the number in the middle of a range

Writing Formulas with Date and Time Functions

Excel provides the TODAY and NOW date and time functions that insert the current date or date and time into a worksheet. The advantage to using the functions rather than just typing the date and time is that the date and time are automatically updated when you open the worksheet. When you type a date in a cell, Excel stores the date as a serial number. Serial numbers in Excel begin with the number 1 (which represents January 1, 1900) and increase sequentially. Because dates are stored as numbers, they can be used in formulas. A date will appear in a cell based on how it is entered. Specify the appearance of dates in a worksheet with options at the Format Cells dialog box with the Number tab selected.

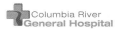
Columbia River
General Hospital

What You Will Do   You will finish the weekly adult cardiac bypass surgery report for Columbia River General Hospital by entering dates and formulas to track patient movement from surgery to the follow-up visit at the surgeon's office 30 days later.

Tutorial
Using Date and Time Functions

1   Open **CRGHCardiacSurgWk45.xlsx** and then save it with the name **3-CRGHCardiacSurgWk45**.

2   Make cell I4 the active cell, type =now(), and then press the Enter key.

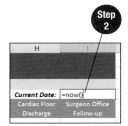
Step 2

> The current date and time are inserted in cell I4. In the next steps, you will delete the date and time and then use the TODAY function to see the difference between the two date functions. Instead of typing a function (as you did in this step), you can insert a date and time function with the Date & Time button on the Formulas tab.

3   Make cell I4 the active cell and then press the Delete key to delete the date and time.

4   With cell I4 the active cell, click the Formulas tab, click the Date and Time button in the Formulas group, and then click *TODAY* at the drop-down list.

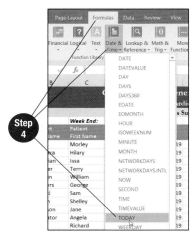
Step 4

5   At the Function Arguments dialog box, click OK.

> The current date is inserted in the cell with the time displayed as *0:00*. Normally, the time does not display with the TODAY function; however, since the NOW function was used first, Excel retained the time format for the cell. In the next steps, you will format the cell to display only the month, day, and year.

6   With cell I4 the active cell, click the Home tab, click the *Number Format* option box arrow in the Number group, and then click *Short Date* at the drop-down list.

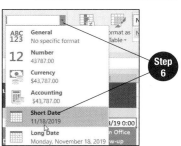
Step 6

> This removes the time from the cell and displays the month, day, and year numerically.

7   Make cell B4 the active cell, click the Formulas tab, click the Date & Time button in the Function Library group, and then click *DATE* at the drop-down list.

> The Function Arguments dialog displays with a text box for each section of the function argument.

8 Type 2019 in the *Year* text box.

9 Press Tab to move the insertion point to the *Month* text box and then type 11.

10 Press Tab to move the insertion point to the *Day* text box, type 10, and then click OK.

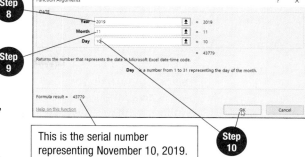

> This is the serial number representing November 10, 2019.

> The Function Arguments dialog box displays the serial number for November 10, 2019, as *43779*. This is the value Excel stores in the cell. Notice that the formula in the Formula bar is *=DATE(2019,11,10)*.

11 Make cell D4 the active cell, type =b4+6, and then press the Enter key.

> Excel displays the result *11/16/2019* in the cell (6 days from the week start date).

12 Make cell G6 the active cell, type =f6+1, and then press the Enter key.

> During this report week, each patient moved through the system at normal speed, which is one day in the CSRU (Cardiac Surgery Recovery Unit).

13 Make cell H6 the active cell, type =g6+4, and then press the Enter key.

> Bypass patients each spent four days on the cardiac floor after CSRU.

14 Make cell I6 the active cell, type =e6+30, and then press the Enter key.

> Bypass patients attend a follow-up visit 30 days after their surgery date.

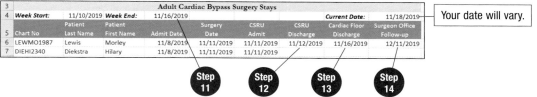

> Your date will vary.

15 Select the range G6:I6 and then use the fill handle to copy the formulas to the remaining rows (G7:I24).

16 Select the range I6:I24.

> In the next steps, you will format the date entries for the surgeon's follow-up visit to display the day of the week.

17 Click the *Number Format* option box arrow in the Number group on the Home tab.

18 Click *Long Date* at the drop-down list.

19 AutoFit the width of column I.

> You now need to change the dates of follow-up visits that fall on a Saturday or Sunday, since the surgeon's office is closed weekends.

20 Make cell I15 the active cell, type =date(2019,12,16), and then press the Enter key.

21 Copy cell I15 to each cell that resulted in a Saturday follow-up visit.

22 Make cell I19 the active cell, type =date(2019,12,17), and then press the Enter key.

23 Copy the contents of cell I19 to each cell that resulted in a Sunday follow-up visit.

24 Save, print, and then close **3-CRGHCardiacSurgWk45.xlsx**.

Check Your Work Compare your work with the model answer to ensure that you have completed the activity correctly.

Activity 3.3 Creating and Using Range Names

Assigning a name to a cell or a range of cells allows you to reference the cell(s) using a descriptive label rather than the cell address or range address when creating formulas, printing, or when navigating a large worksheet. Referencing by name makes a formula easier to understand. For example, a formula such as =*Sales-Expenses* is readily understood. A formula such as =*D3-D13* requires the reader to look at the labels next to the values in the formula cells in order to grasp the formula's purpose. A range name can be a combination of letters, numbers, underscore characters, and periods up to 255 characters. The first character in a range name must be a letter, an underscore, or a backslash (\). Spaces are not valid in a range name. To create a range name, select the desired cells and then type the name in the Name box at the left of the Formula bar.

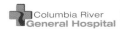
Columbia River General Hospital

What You Will Do   The November cardiac surgery cost report for Dr. Novak has been started. You have been asked to complete the *Standard Cost* column. You decide to begin by naming the cells to help you build the correct formula.

Tutorial

Naming and Using a Range

1 Open **CRGHNovakCardiacCosts.xlsx** and then save it with the name **3-CRGHNovakCardiacCosts**.

> To begin, you want to name the cells in column D *Days*. The first step in naming a range is to select the cell or group of cells with which the name will be associated.

2 Select the range D6:D20.

3 With the range D6:D20 selected, point to the white box at the left side of the Formula bar (currently displays *D6*). Notice the ScreenTip that displays *Name Box*.

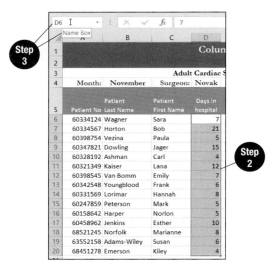

> The white box at the left side of the Formula bar is called the Name box. The Name box displays the address of the active cell. If the active cell has been named, the name appears in the Name box instead. To assign a new name to a cell or selected range, click in the Name box and then type the name.

4 Click in the Name box, type Days, and then press the Enter key.

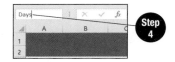

> The range name now appears in the Name box. In the next steps, you will assign a range name to individual cells that will be needed to calculate the standard cost.

5 Make cell G6 the active cell.

6 Click in the Name box, type ShortCost, and then press the Enter key.

7 Make cell H6 the active cell, click in the Name box, type LongCost, and then press the Enter key.

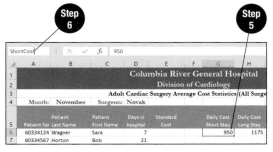

In Brief

Name a Range
1. Select cell(s).
2. Click in Name box.
3. Type range name.
4. Press Enter.

8 Make cell I6 the active cell, click in the Name box, type OvhShort, and then press the Enter key.

9 Make cell J6 the active cell, click in the Name box, type OvhLong, and then press the Enter key.

10 Click the arrow at the right of the Name box.

A drop-down list of range names in the current workbook appears. To move the active cell to a named cell or range, click the name at the drop-down list.

11 Click *Days* at the drop-down list.

The range D6:D20 is selected.

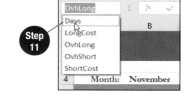

Step 11

12 Make cell B24 the active cell, type Average Days in Hospital:, and then press the Enter key.

13 Make cell D24 the active cell, type =average(days), and then press the Enter key.

Range names are not case sensitive when you use them in a formula. When you type the range name *days* in the formula, notice that Excel color-codes cells D6:D20 to show you the cells that are being referenced in the formula.

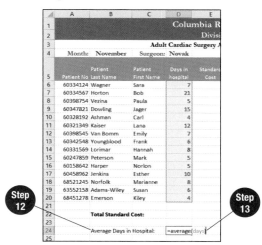

14 Format cell D24 to display zero decimal places.

15 Save **3-CRGHNovakCardiacCosts.xlsx**.

Check Your Work — Compare your work with the model answer to ensure that you have completed the activity correctly.

In Addition

Managing Range Names

To edit or delete a range name, display the Name Manager dialog box, shown at the right. To do this, click the Formulas tab and then click the Name Manager button in the Defined Names group. The Name Manager dialog box displays the range names in the active workbook and provides buttons to edit or delete names.

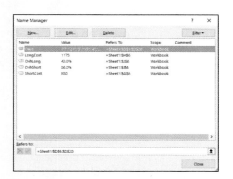

Activity 3.4 Using the Logical IF Function

The IF function, also called a logical test, returns one of two values in a cell based on a true-or-false answer to a question. The format of an IF function is *=IF(logical_test,value_if_true,value_if_false)*. For example, assume a medical supplies salesperson earns a 3% commission if his or her sales are greater than or equal to $100,000, or a 2% commission for sales less than $100,000. Assume the sales value resides in cell B4. The logical test in this example would be *B4>=100000*. Excel can only return a true-or-false answer when this test is performed. The commission will be calculated with either *B4*3%* (*value_if_true*) or *B4*2%* (*value_if_false*). In this example, the IF function formula would be *=IF(B4>=100000,B4*3%,B4*2%)*.

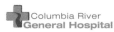 **Columbia River General Hospital**

What You Will Do   Continuing your work on the November cardiac surgery cost report, you now need to calculate standard costs for patient stays. Standard costs are based on a daily cost rate and an overhead charge, both of which are dependent on the duration of the patient's stay.

Tutorial
Using Logical IF Functions

1 With **3-CRGHNovakCardiacCosts.xlsx** open, make cell E6 the active cell.

2 Click the Formulas tab.

3 Click the Logical button [?] in the Function Library group and then click *IF* at the drop-down list.

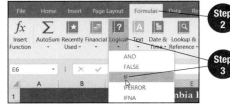

The Function Arguments dialog box for the IF statement displays. Notice the three arguments: *Logical_test, Value_if_true,* and *Value_if_false*. To begin, you want Excel to test whether the value in the Days range is less than or equal to 7. This test determines whether Excel calculates the standard cost at $950 per day and the overhead charge at 36% or $1175 per day with an overhead charge of 43%. You will use range names to make the IF statement easier to create and understand.

4 With the insertion point positioned in the *Logical_test* text box, type days<=7 and then press the Tab key.

Watch the entries that appear at the right of each argument text box as you build the formula. Excel updates these entries to show you how the formula is working as you build each argument. Notice that next to the *Logical_test* text box you now see the TRUE and FALSE results Excel is calculating for each entry in the Days range.

5 With the insertion point positioned in the *Value_if_true* text box, type (days*shortcost)+(days*shortcost*ovhshort) and then press the Tab key.

If the Days value in cell D6 is less than or equal to 7, Excel calculates the standard cost as the days in hospital (D6) times 950 (G6) plus the days in hospital (D6) times 950 (G6) times a 36% overhead charge (I6). Another advantage to using range names is that by default, range names use absolute references. Since the formula will be copied to rows 7–20, absolute references are required for those cells that reference the daily cost and the percentages.

6 With the insertion point positioned in the *Value_if_false* text box, type (days*longcost)+(days*longcost*ovhlong).

If the value in cell D6 is greater than 7, the formula calculates the standard cost as the days in hospital (D6) times 1175 (H6) plus the days in hospital (D6) times 1175 (H6) times a 43% overhead charge (J6). Notice that in the lower left corner of the dialog box, Excel shows the result that will be placed in the active cell (*Formula result = $9,044.00*). The value in cell D6 is 7, so the standard cost is calculated as (7*950)+(7*950*36%).

7 Click OK.

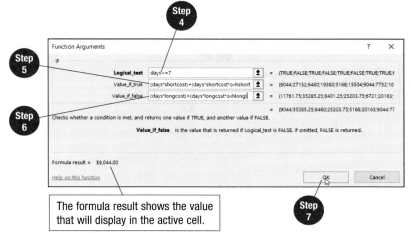

Step 4

Step 5

Step 6

Step 7

The formula result shows the value that will display in the active cell.

8 Drag the fill handle in cell E6 down to row 20 and then click in any cell to deselect the range.

9 Make cell E22 the active cell, click the AutoSum button in the Function Library group, and then press the Enter key to calculate the total standard cost for all of Dr. Novak's November surgeries.

10 Apply the Accounting format to cells E6 and E22 and then apply the Comma format to the range E7:E20.

11 Click cell E6 and review the formula in the Formula bar: *=IF(Days<=7, (Days*ShortCost)+(Days*ShortCost*OvhShort),(Days*LongCost)+(Days*LongCost *OvhLong))*.

The formula may be easier to comprehend if you include the range names when reading it to yourself.

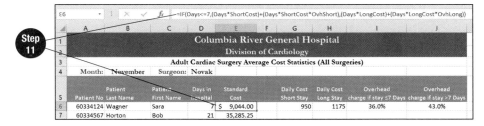

Step 11

12 Save and then close **3-CRGHNovakCardiacCosts.xlsx**.

Check Your Work — Compare your work with the model answer to ensure that you have completed the activity correctly.

In Addition

Exploring the Benefits of the Function Arguments Dialog Box

One advantage to creating an IF function using the Function Arguments dialog box is that the formula automatically appears in the correct syntax. You do not have to worry about typing commas between arguments or the opening and closing brackets; these elements are automatically added to the formula. Another advantage is that the range names in the completed formula are also automatically displayed in the case used when the range name was created. For example, in this activity you typed *days*shortcost*, but the final formula displayed this entry as *Days*ShortCost*.

Activity 3.5   Creating a Column Chart

Numerical values are often more easily understood when presented visually in a chart. Excel includes several chart types, such as column, line, pie, bar, area, and scatter, and others you can use to graphically portray data. The chart can be placed in the same worksheet as the data or it can be inserted into its own sheet. To create a chart, first select the cells containing the data you want to graph and then choose the chart type. Excel graphs the data in a separate object which can be moved, resized, and formatted.

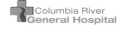
Columbia River
General Hospital

What You Will Do   Hanna Moreland, manager of the Supplies Department at Columbia River General Hospital, has asked you to create a chart to compare operating expenses in each quarter.

> Tutorial
> Creating Charts

> Tutorial
> Changing Chart Design

1 Open **CRGHSuppliesDeptExp.xlsx** and then save it with the name **3-CRGHSuppliesDeptExp**.

2 Select the range A3:E9.

> The first step in creating a chart is to select the range of cells containing the data you want to graph. The range that you are using includes the row labels in column A. Labels are included to provide the frame of reference for each bar, column, or other chart series. If you select multiple ranges, ensure that the data in each range includes a consistent number of cells.

3 Click the Insert tab.

4 Click the Insert Column Chart button [icon] in the Charts group.

5 Click the *3-D Clustered Column* option at the drop-down list (first column, first row in the *3-D Column* section).

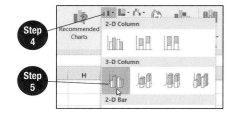

> Excel graphs the data in a 3-D column chart and places the chart inside an object box in the center of the worksheet (see Figure E3.1).

Figure E3.1 3-D Column Chart in an Object Box

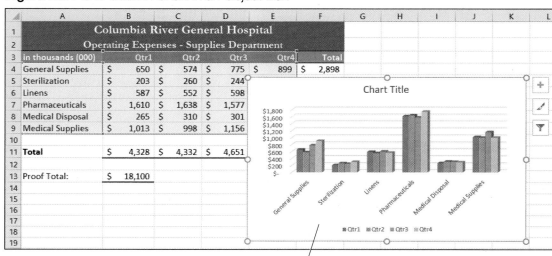

> The 3-D column chart is placed in an object box that can be moved, resized, and formatted as needed.

Create Column Chart
1. Select cells.
2. Click Insert tab.
3. Click Insert Column or Bar Chart button.
4. Click chart type.
5. Move and/or resize chart.
6. Apply design options.

6 Click the Move Chart button 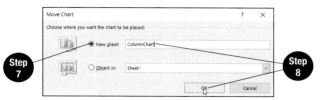 in the Location group on the Chart Tools Design tab.

7 At the Move Chart dialog box, click the *New sheet* option.

8 With *Chart1* selected in the *New sheet* text box, type ColumnChart and then click OK.

> The chart object is moved to a new sheet in the workbook with a tab labeled *ColumnChart*. The chart is automatically scaled to fill the entire page in landscape orientation.

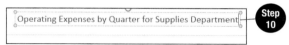

9 Click the Quick Layout button 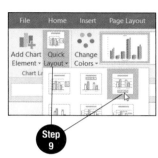 in the Chart Layouts group and then click the layout style in the third column, first row of the drop-down gallery.

> This layout adds a title to the top center of the chart and moves the legend to the bottom center.

10 Click *Chart Title* to select the title object, click at the beginning of the text to position the insertion point inside the chart title box, delete *Chart Title*, and then type Operating Expenses by Quarter for Supplies Department.

Operating Expenses by Quarter for Supplies Department

11 Click inside the chart area to deselect the title text.

12 Click the More Chart Styles button in the Chart Styles group on the Chart Tools Design tab.

13 Click the *Style 10* option in the drop-down gallery (second column, second row).

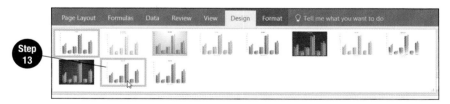

14 Save **3-CRGHSuppliesDeptExp.xlsx**.

> **Check Your Work** Compare your work with the model answer to ensure that you have completed the activity correctly.

In Addition

Creating a Recommended Chart

If you are not sure what type of chart will best illustrate your data, consider letting Excel recommend a chart. To do this, select the data, click the Insert tab, and then click the Recommended Charts button in the Charts group. This displays the data in a chart in the Insert Chart dialog box. Customize the recommended chart with options in the left panel of the dialog box. Click OK to insert the recommended chart in the worksheet. You can also insert a recommended chart in the worksheet with the keyboard shortcut Alt + F1.

Activity 3.6   Creating a Pie Chart

Pie charts illustrate each data point's size in proportion to the total of all items in the data source range. Each slice in a pie chart is a percentage of the whole pie. You can choose to display the percent values, the actual values used to generate the chart, or both values as data labels inside or outside the pie slices. Use a pie chart when you have only one data series to graph and there are no negative or zero values within the data range.

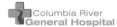
Columbia River
General Hospital

What You Will Do   Hanna Moreland is pleased with the column chart you created for the quarterly operating expenses. Hanna would like you to create another chart that shows each expense as a proportion of the total expenses.

Tutorial
Formatting with Chart Buttons

1 With **3-CRGHSuppliesDeptExp.xlsx** open, click the tab labeled *Sheet1* near the bottom left corner of the window and above the Status bar.

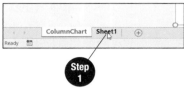

2 Click in any cell to deselect the range that was used to generate the column chart in the previous activity.

3 Select the range A3:A9, hold down the Ctrl key, and then select the range F3:F9.

4 Click the Insert tab.

5 Click the Insert Pie or Doughnut Chart button in the Charts group.

6 Click the *3-D Pie* option in the *3-D Pie* section of the drop-down gallery.

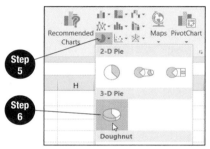

7 Point to the border of the chart object until the mouse pointer displays with the four-headed-arrow move icon, click and hold down the left mouse button, and then drag the chart, positioning it approximately centered below columns A–F with the top edge in row 16.

8 With the chart selected, click the Chart Elements button that displays at the right side of the chart.

> When a chart is selected, three buttons display outside the top right corner of the chart. With these buttons, you can insert or remove chart elements, apply chart styles, and edit what data points and names display in the chart.

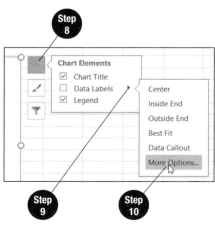

9 Point to the *Data Labels* option at the drop-down list and then click the triangle at the right side of the option.

10 Click *More Options* at the side menu.

> This displays the Format Data Labels task pane at the right side of the screen.

Create Pie Chart
1. Select cells.
2. Click Insert tab.
3. Click Insert Pie or Doughnut Chart button.
4. Click option.
5. Move and/or resize chart.
6. Apply design options.

11 At the Format Data Labels task pane, click the *Percentage* check box below the *Label Contains* heading in the *Label Options* section to insert a check mark and then click the *Value* check box to remove the check mark.

12 Scroll down the Format Data Labels task pane (if necessary), click the expand arrow at the left of *Number*, click the *Category* option box arrow, and then click *Percentage* at the drop-down list.

13 Select the number in the *Decimal places* text box and then type 1.

14 Close the Format Data Labels task pane.

15 Click the Chart Styles button 🖋 that displays at the right side of the chart.

16 Click the *Style 3* option at the side menu (third option).

17 Click the Chart Elements button, click the triangle at the right side of the *Data Labels* option, and then click *Outside End* at the side menu.

> Notice that the data labels move from inside the pie slices to the outer edges of the pie.

18 Change the chart title (currently displays as *Total*) to *Total Operating Expenses*.

> Refer to Activity 3.5, Step 10, if you need assistance with this step.

19 Click in the worksheet area outside the chart to deselect the chart.

20 Save **3-CRGHSuppliesDeptExp.xlsx**.

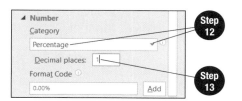

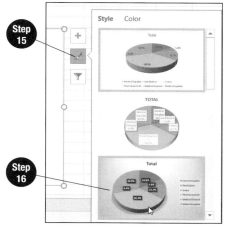

Check Your Work | Compare your work with the model answer to ensure that you have completed the activity correctly.

In Addition

Adding Sparklines

The Insert tab contains a Sparklines group. Sparklines are miniature charts that you can add to a cell. These miniature charts illustrate changes from a specific row or column of data. For example, in the worksheet shown below, the sparkline chart was created in cell G4 based on the values in the range B4:E4. Click the Insert tab

and then click the Line, Column, or Win/Loss buttons in the Sparklines group. At the Create Sparklines dialog box, select the data range that contains the values on which you want to base the chart, select the cell in which to draw the chart, and then click OK.

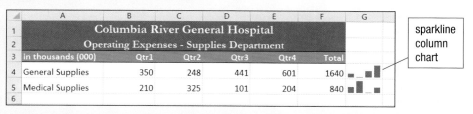

To make changes to an existing chart, click inside the chart or chart element to display a border around the chart object. Click the border to move the chart or click one of the eight sizing handles to resize it. When the chart is selected, the Chart Tools Design and Chart Tools Format tabs become available. Use these tabs to add, delete, or modify the chart or chart elements as needed.

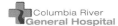
Columbia River
General Hospital

What You Will Do   You will modify the charts created for the Operating Expenses worksheet by formatting the legend, applying bold formatting to the data labels, changing the font in the chart title, and changing the chart type for the column chart.

Tutorial
Changing Chart
Formatting

1 With **3-CRGHSuppliesDeptExp.xlsx** open, click anywhere inside the pie chart to select the chart object.

> Once a chart is selected, two additional tabs become available—the Chart Tools Design tab and the Chart Tools Format tab.

2 Click inside the pie chart legend.

> Eight sizing handles appear around the legend, indicating that the object is selected. You can use these handles to resize the legend or you can drag the legend to a new location.

3 Click the Chart Tools Format tab.

4 Click the Shape Outline button arrow in the Shape Styles group and then click the *Light Blue* option in the drop-down gallery (seventh option from the left in the *Standard Colors* section).

> A thin light blue border appears around the legend.

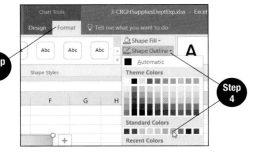

5 Click the chart title, select the text, and then use the *Font* and *Font Size* option boxes on the Mini toolbar to change the title font to 16-point Verdana.

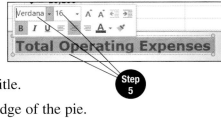

6 Click inside the chart area to deselect the chart title.

7 Click any one of the percent values around the edge of the pie.

> This selects all six data labels.

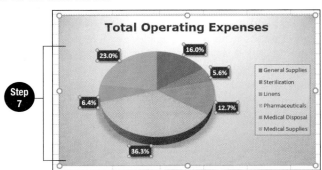

8 Click the Home tab and then click the Bold button in the Font group to turn off bold formatting.

Modify Chart
1. Click to select chart or chart element.
2. Use buttons and options on Chart Tools Design tab or Chart Tools Format tab to modify chart.

9 Click the ColumnChart tab near the bottom left corner of the window and then click inside the column chart to select the chart.

10 If necessary, click the Chart Tools Design tab. Click the Change Chart Type button in the Type group.

11 At the Change Chart Type dialog box, click *Bar* in the left panel and then click the *3-D Clustered Bar* option (fourth option from the left at the top of the right panel).

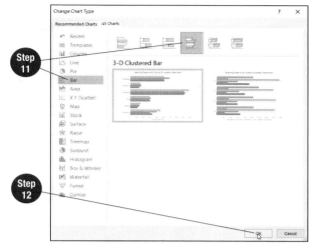

12 Click OK.

13 Click the More Chart Styles button in the Chart Styles group and then click the *Style 5* option at the drop-down gallery.

14 Print the bar chart.

15 Click the Sheet1 tab and then make cell A1 the active cell.

16 Display the Print backstage area.

17 Click the margins gallery in the *Settings* category (currently displays *Normal Margins*), click *Wide* at the drop-down list, and then click the Print button.

18 Save **3-CRGHSuppliesDeptExp.xlsx**.

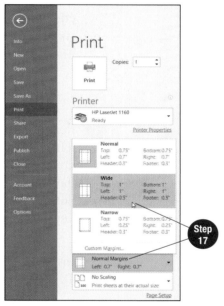

> **Check Your Work** Compare your work with the model answer to ensure that you have completed the activity correctly.

In Addition

Editing Chart Elements

Another way to edit a chart is to right-click a chart element to display the shortcut menu. For example, right-clicking the axis labels in the bar chart displays the shortcut menu shown at the right. The bottom section of the shortcut menu changes depending on the element you click.

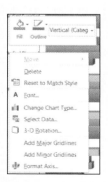

Activity 3.8   Inserting Shapes and Text Boxes

The Shapes button on the Insert tab includes buttons with which you can draw lines, rectangles and other, basic shapes, block arrows, equation shapes, flowchart symbols, stars, banners, and callouts. Draw shapes or insert text boxes to add emphasis or create space for explanatory notes in a worksheet. Text can also be added to enclosed shapes.

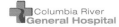
Columbia River General Hospital

What You Will Do   An upcoming price increase from the hospital's medical waste disposal contractor is higher than expected. Hanna Moreland wants you to use a shape and a text box to add an explanatory note to the operating expenses worksheet.

Tutorial
Inserting a Shape

Tutorial
Formatting a Shape

Tutorial
Inserting and Modifying Text Boxes

1   With **3-CRGHSuppliesDeptExp.xlsx** open and the Sheet1 tab active, click the Insert tab.

2   Click the Shapes button in the Illustrations group and then click the line with an arrow shape (second option in the *Lines* section).

> When a shape has been selected from the Shapes button drop-down list, the mouse pointer changes to crosshairs.

3   Position the crosshairs near the bottom left boundary of cell D12, click and drag up toward the value *310* in cell C8, and then release the mouse button. If you are not happy with the arrow, press the Delete key and then try again.

4   Click the Text Box button in the Insert Shapes group on the Drawing Tools Format tab.

> When the Text Box tool has been selected, the mouse pointer changes to a down-pointing arrow.

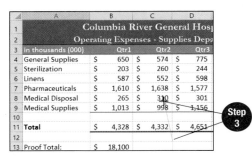

5   Position the mouse pointer at the top left boundary of cell D13, click and drag the mouse pointer down and to the right to draw a text box of the approximate size shown in the image below, and then release the the mouse button.

> The insertion point is positioned inside the box when you release the mouse button, indicating that you can begin typing text.

6   Type Qtr2 next year will be 8% higher! inside the text box.

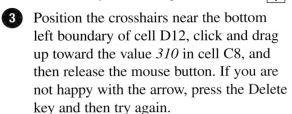

Draw Shape
1. Click Insert tab.
2. Click Shapes button.
3. Click shape option.
4. Click in worksheet or drag to create shape.
5. Move, resize, or format shape.

Draw Text Box
1. Click Insert tab.
2. Click Text Box button.
3. Click in worksheet or drag to create text box.
4. Type text.
5. Click outside text box object.
6. Move, resize, or format text box.

7 Click outside the text box to deselect the object. If necessary, use the sizing handles on the text box to resize it so that all of the text fits on one line.

8 Click the arrow shape to select it, press and hold down the Ctrl key, and then click the text box. Both drawn objects are now selected.

9 If necessary, click the Drawing Tools Format tab.

10 Click the Shape Outline button arrow in the Shape Styles group and then click the *Light Blue* option in the drop-down gallery (seventh option from the left in the *Standard Colors* section).

11 Click the Shape Outline button arrow a second time, point to *Weight*, and then click *1½ pt* at the side menu.

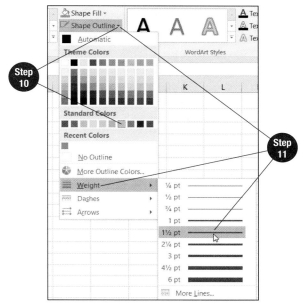

12 Click in any cell to deselect the drawn shapes.

Figure E3.2 shows the text box and arrow after formatting options have been applied.

13 Save **3-CRGHSuppliesDeptExp.xlsx**.

Figure E3.2 Formatted Text Box and Line Arrow Shape

	A	B	C	D	E	F
1	Columbia River General Hospital					
2	Operating Expenses - Supplies Department					
3	in thousands (000)	Qtr1	Qtr2	Qtr3	Qtr4	Total
4	General Supplies	$ 650	$ 574	$ 775	$ 899	$ 2,898
5	Sterilization	$ 203	$ 260	$ 244	$ 298	$ 1,005
6	Linens	$ 587	$ 552	$ 598	$ 564	$ 2,301
7	Pharmaceuticals	$ 1,610	$ 1,638	$ 1,577	$ 1,743	$ 6,568
8	Medical Disposal	$ 265	$ 310	$ 301	$ 288	$ 1,164
9	Medical Supplies	$ 1,013	$ 993	$ 1,156	$ 997	$ 4,164
10						
11	Total	$ 4,328	$ 4,332	$ 4,651	$ 4,789	$ 18,100
12						
13	Proof Total:	$ 18,100		Qtr2 next year will be 8% higher!		
14						

Check Your Work Compare your work with the model answer to ensure that you have completed the activity correctly.

The Page Layout tab contains buttons to modify the page setup and scaling options for printing purposes. You can also change printing options while previewing the worksheet at the Print backstage area. The margins on a worksheet are the blank spaces at the top, bottom, left, and right edges of the page and the beginning of the printed text. The default margins are 0.75-inch top and bottom and 0.7-inch left and right. Smaller worksheets can be centered horizontally and/or vertically on the page to improve the printed appearance. For larger worksheets, you can scale down the size of printed text to force the printout to a maximum number of pages.

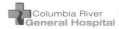
Columbia River General Hospital

What You Will Do   You will modify page layout options at the Print backstage area before printing the two worksheets you have been working on in this section.

Tutorial
Changing Page Layout Options

1 With **3-CRGHSuppliesDeptExp.xlsx** open, display the Print backstage area.

Notice the worksheet is not evenly balanced between the left and right margins. In the next steps you will change the margins to improve the page layout.

2 Click the margins gallery in the *Settings* category (currently displays *Wide Margins*).

3 Click *Custom Margins* at the drop-down list.

The Page Setup dialog box displays with the Margins tab active.

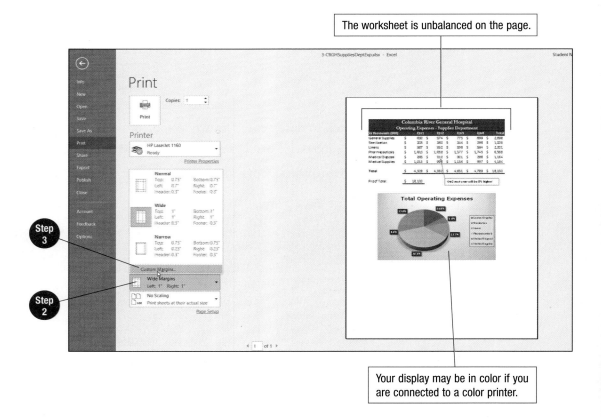

The worksheet is unbalanced on the page.

Your display may be in color if you are connected to a color printer.

In Brief

Change Margins
1. Click Page Layout tab.
2. Click Margins button.
3. Click *Custom Margins*.
4. Change margin options.
5. Click OK.
OR
1. Click File tab.
2. Click *Print*.
3. Click margins gallery.
4. Click *Custom Margins*.
5. Change margin options.
6. Click OK.

4 Select the current entry in the *Top* measurement box and then type 2.2. Select the current entry in the *Left* measurement box, type 1.25, and then click OK.

> The preview pane at the Print backstage area shows the worksheet with the new margins applied. The page layout is improved for printing.

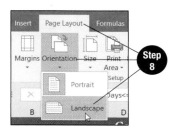

5 Click the Print button.

6 Save and then close **3-CRGHSuppliesDeptExp.xlsx**.

7 Open **3-CRGHNovakCardiacCosts.xlsx**.

8 Click the Page Layout tab, click the Orientation button in the Page Setup group, and then click *Landscape* at the drop-down list.

9 Click the Margins button in the Page Setup group and then click *Custom Margins* at the drop-down list.

> The Page Setup dialog box displays with the Margins tab active. This is another way to display the same Page Setup dialog box you accessed by using the margins gallery at the Print backstage area.

10 In the *Center on page* section, click the *Horizontally* check box to insert a check mark, click the *Vertically* check box to insert a check mark, and then click OK.

> Centering the worksheet horizontally is another method you can use to ensure the worksheet prints balanced between the left and right edges of the page. You can insert check marks in both the *Horizontally* and *Vertically* check boxes to print a worksheet that is centered between both the left and right edges (horizontally), and the top and bottom edges (vertically) of the page.

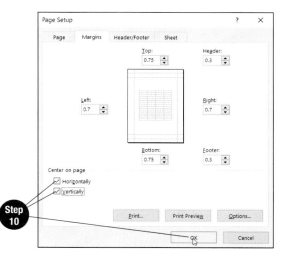

11 Print the worksheet.

12 Save and then close **3-CRGHNovakCardiacCosts.xlsx**.

Check Your Work — Compare your work with the model answer to ensure that you have completed the activity correctly.

In Addition

Printing Column or Row Headings on Multiple Pages

Use the Print Titles button in the Page Setup group on the Page Layout tab to define column or row headings that you want repeated at the top or left edge of each page. Printing column and/or row headings makes the data row and columns in a multipage printout easier to identify.

Using Page Layout View; Inserting Headers and Footers

Page Layout view allows you to view the worksheet along with the print settings. Page Layout view also displays horizontal and vertical rulers to assist with measurements. A header is text that prints at the top of each worksheet and a footer is text that prints at the bottom of each worksheet. Excel includes predefined headers and footers you can select from a drop-down list, or you can create your own custom header or footer text.

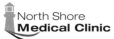
North Shore
Medical Clinic

What You Will Do The operations manager at North Shore Medical Clinic would like a hard copy of the clinic supplies inventory worksheet. Since this is a long worksheet, you decide to add a header and footer to the report to include identifying information. You also decide to add page numbers and experiment with scaling options to fit the printout on two pages.

Tutorial
Inserting Headers and Footers

1 Open **3-NSMCSupplies.xlsx** and then click the Page Layout button at the right side of the Status bar (to the left of the Zoom slider bar).

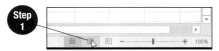

2 At the Microsoft Office Excel message box indicating that freeze panes is not compatible with Page Layout view, click OK to unfreeze the panes and continue.

3 If necessary, use the horizontal and vertical scroll bars to adjust the window so that the worksheet, including the white space for the top margin, is entirely visible.

4 Click the text *Add header* near the top center of the page.

Headers and footers are divided into three boxes. Click in each box to type text or insert header and footer elements. By default, text in the left box is left-aligned, text in the center box is centered, and text in the right box is right-aligned.

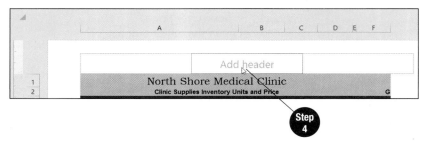

5 Click in the left header box and then type your first and last names.

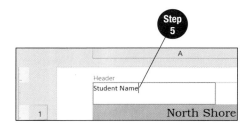

In Brief

Insert Header or Footer
1. Switch to Page Layout view.
2. Click *Add header* or *Add footer*.
3. Insert header and footer elements and/or type text in left, center, or right box.
4. Click in worksheet area to close header or footer section.

6 Click in the right header box, type Date Printed:, and then press the spacebar.

7 Click the Current Date button in the Header & Footer Elements group on the Header & Footer Tools Design tab.

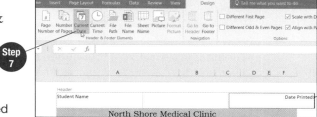

> Excel inserts the code *&[Date]*, which is replaced with the current date when the worksheet is printed.

8 Click the Go to Footer button in the Navigation group on the Header & Footer Tools Design tab.

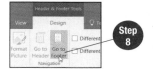

> The right footer box at the bottom of the page is active for editing.

9 Click in the center footer box to select it for editing.

10 Click the File Name button in the Header & Footer Elements group.

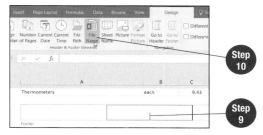

> Excel inserts the code *&[File]*, which is replaced with the workbook file name when the worksheet is printed.

11 Click anywhere in the worksheet area outside the footer to close the footer section.

12 Scroll to the top of the worksheet to view the header. Notice that Excel now displays the current date in place of the *&[Date]* code.

13 Scroll down to the bottom of the worksheet and notice that Excel now displays the file name in place of the *&[File]* code.

14 Click the Page Layout tab.

> By default, the header and footer margins are 0.3 inch. In the next step, you will adjust the header and footer margins to provide more white space at the top and bottom of the page.

15 Click the Margins button in the Page Setup group and then click *Custom Margins* at the drop-down list. At the Page Setup dialog box with the Margins tab active, change the margin settings as follows:

Top:	1	*Header:*	0.5
Bottom:	1	*Footer:*	0.5
Left:	1		

16 Click OK to close the Page Setup dialog box.

17 Review the new margin settings in Page Layout view.

18 Print the worksheet.

19 Click the Normal button located at the right side of the Status bar (to the left of the Zoom slider bar).

20 Save and then close **3-NSMCSupplies.xlsx**.

Check Your Work ▷ Compare your work with the model answer to ensure that you have completed the activity correctly.

Create a table in Excel to manage data independently of other cells in the worksheet or to filter and sort a list. A worksheet can contain more than one range formatted as a table. By default, filter arrows appear in the first row of the table and a border surrounds the table range, with a sizing arrow in the bottom right corner. Excel includes a variety of predefined table styles to apply professional quality formatting features to the table range. The Table Tools Design tab becomes available when a range of cells is defined as a table.

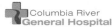

What You Will Do   Luisa Gomez, Cardiac Nurse Manager, often uses a casual relief call list when a full-time nurse calls in sick. Luisa would like the list to be in a format that she can sort and filter based on shift preference and/or experience. You decide to use a table to accomplish this.

Tutorial
Formatting Data as a Table

Tutorial
Adding a Row to a Table

1. Open **CRGHCasualNurses.xlsx** and then save it with the name **3-CRGHCasualNurses**.

2. Select the range A4:J35 and then click the Format as Table button ▨ in the Styles group on the Home tab.

    The first step in defining a table is to specify the range of cells to be included. Do not include cells containing merged titles or other data that should not be included when you sort and filter the rows.

3. Click the blue table style in the drop-down gallery (sixth column, first row in the *Medium* section).

    Excel includes several predefined table styles grouped into *Light*, *Medium*, and *Dark* categories. Use these styles to add color, border, and shading formatting to cells within the table. In addition, you can create your own custom table style and save it with the workbook.

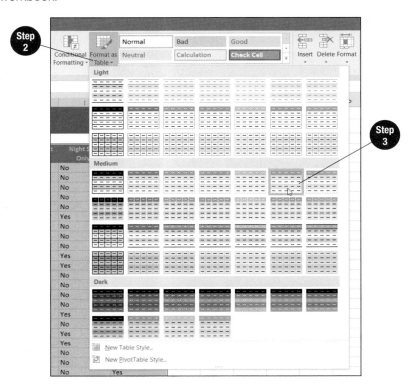

4 At the Format As Table dialog box with
=$A$4:$J$35 selected in the *Where is the data
for your table?* text box, click OK.

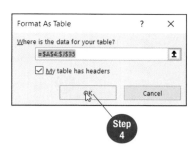

Step
4

> Excel applies the table style formatting to the
> range, displays filter arrows in each cell in the first
> row of the table, adds a border to the table, and
> displays a sizing handle in the bottom right cell.

5 Click in any cell to deselect the range.

6 Right-click the row label for row 36, click *Insert* at the shortcut menu, and then type
the new record in the columns indicated. Press the Enter key after typing the last cell.

Employee Number:	99823
Employee Last Name:	Awad
Employee First Name:	Rania
Hire Date:	=date(2019,1,31)
Telephone:	555-4652
Years Experience:	7
OR Experience:	Yes
Day Shift Only?:	No
Night Shift Only?:	No
Can Work Either Shift:	Yes

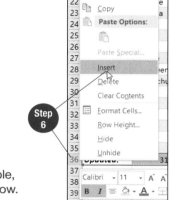

Step
6

> Since you typed data in the row immediately below the table,
> Excel automatically expands the table to include the new row.
> You can also insert a new row at the bottom of a table by
> selecting the last cell in the table and then pressing the Tab key.

7 Make cell J36 the active cell and then press the Tab key.

> A new row is inserted at the bottom of the table.

8 Type the following text in row 37 in the columns indicated. Press the Enter key after
typing the last cell. (Do not press the Tab key, as this action will cause another new
row to be added to the table.)

Employee Number:	99828
Employee Last Name:	Fernandez
Employee First Name:	Natalio
Hire Date:	=date(2019,1,31)
Telephone:	555-7643
Years Experience:	3
OR Experience:	Yes
Day Shift Only?:	No
Night Shift Only?:	Yes
Can Work Either Shift:	Weekends only

35	99754 Valdez	Linda	1/30/2019	555-3498	16	Yes	No	No	Yes	
36	99823 Awad	Rania	1/31/2019	555-4652	7	Yes	No	No	Yes	
37	99828 Fernandez	Natalio	1/31/2019	555-7643	3	Yes	No	Yes	Weekends only	
38	*Updated:*	31-Jan-19								

Steps
6-8

9 Make active any cell within the table.

The contextual Table Tools Design tab is not available unless the active cell is positioned within the table.

10 If necessary, click the Table Tools Design tab. Click the *Banded Rows* check box in the Table Style Options group to remove the check mark.

When a table has banded rows, it means that every other row is formatted differently (for example, odd rows might be shaded in blue while even rows remain white). Banding makes it easier to read text across multiple columns in a list. The style of formatting for the banded rows is dependent on the table style that has been applied. Notice that once you remove the check mark from the check box, all rows are formatted the same.

11 Click the *Banded Columns* check box in the Table Style Options group to insert a check mark.

Notice that every other column is now shaded in blue.

12 Click the *First Column* check box in the Table Style Options group to insert a check mark.

The contents of the cells in the first column now appear in bold. The type of formatting applied by clicking the *First Column* check box depends on the table style.

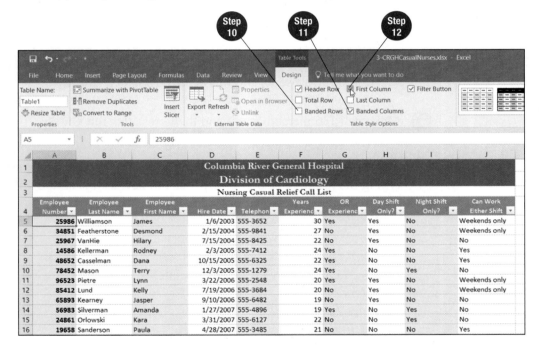

13 Select the range E5:J37, click the Home tab, and then click the Center button in the Alignment group.

14 Select the range A4:J4 and then click the Middle Align button in the Alignment group.

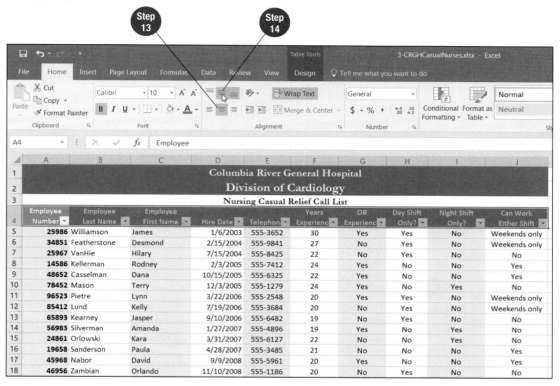

Step 13

Step 14

15 Click in any cell to deselect the range and then save **3-CRGHCasualNurses.xlsx**.

Check Your Work Compare your work to the model answer to ensure that you have completed the activity correctly.

In Addition

Converting a Table to a Normal Range

A range that has been formatted as a table can be converted back to a normal range using the Convert to Range button in the Tools group on the Table Tools Design tab (shown at the right). Convert a table to a range if you no longer need to treat the data range independently from the rest of the worksheet. For example, you may want to format a range as a table simply to apply the color, shading, and border effects that are available through table styles. Converting a table to a normal range preserves this formatting; however, features unique to a table, such as the ability to apply banding, add a total row, and check for duplicates, will no longer be available to the range.

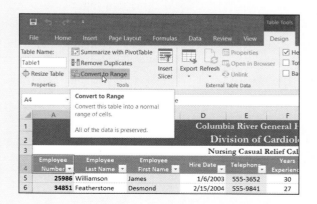

In Section 1, you learned to sort a payroll worksheet alphabetically by last name. Sorting rows in a table by single or multiple criteria involves the same process you used in Section 1. To sort by a single column, click in any cell in the column by which you wish to sort and then use the *Sort A to Z* or the *Sort Z to A* options at the Sort & Filter button drop-down list. To group the rows first by one column and then sort the grouped rows by another column, display the Sort dialog box. You can continue to group and sort by multiple criteria as needed.

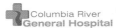
Columbia River General Hospital

What You Will Do   You decide to print the nursing casual relief call list with the data sorted alphabetically by last name. Next, you want to print the list grouped first in descending order by years of experience, second by OR experience, and third by whether the individual can work either shift.

Tutorial
Sorting a Table

1   With **3-CRGHCasualNurses.xlsx** open, click in any cell in column B of the table.

2   Click the Sort & Filter button in the Editing group on the Home tab.

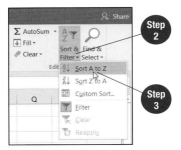

3   Click *Sort A to Z* at the drop-down list.

> The table is sorted in ascending order by last name. Excel displays a black arrow in the filter arrow button to indicate that the table is sorted by the *Employee Last Name* column.

4   Print the worksheet.

5   Click the Sort & Filter button and then click *Custom Sort* at the drop-down list.

6   At the Sort dialog box, click the *Sort by* option box arrow in the *Column* section and then click *Years Experience* at the drop-down list.

7   Click the *Order* option box arrow (currently reads *Smallest to Largest*) and then click *Largest to Smallest* at the drop-down list.

8   Click the Add Level button.

9   Click the *Then by* option box arrow in the *Column* section and then click *OR Experience* at the drop-down list.

10   Click the *Order* option box arrow (currently reads *A to Z*) and then click *Z to A* at the drop-down list.

> If the employee has OR experience, you want them to be listed first within the group of employees with the same number of years of experience. Since cells in this column have only a Yes or No in the cell, sorting in descending order will ensure that those with OR experience are shown first.

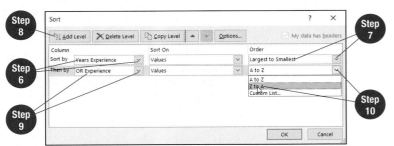

Sort Table by Single Column
1. Click in any row within column by which to sort.
2. Click Sort & Filter button.
3. Click *Sort A to Z* or *Sort Z to A*.

Sort Table by Multiple Columns
1. Click Sort & Filter button.
2. Click *Custom Sort*.
3. Select first column to sort by.
4. Select sort order.
5. Click Add Level.
6. Repeat Steps 3–5 for each sort column.
7. Click OK.

11 Click the Add Level button.

12 In the new row, click the *Then by* option box arrow in the *Column* section and then click *Can Work Either Shift* at the drop-down list.

13 Click the *Order* option box arrow (currently reads *A to Z*) and then click *Z to A* at the drop-down list.

> If the employee can work either shift, *Yes* will appear in the cell in the *Can Work Either Shift* column. Sorting in descending order will ensure that those who have no shift restrictions will be listed first within the groups of employees who have OR experience and the most years of experience.

14 Click OK to apply the sort.

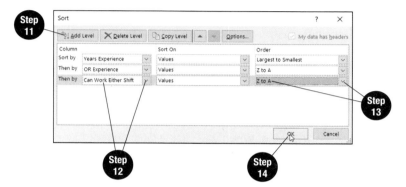

15 Examine the sorted worksheet and compare your results with Figure E3.3.

16 Print the worksheet.

17 Save **3-CRGHCasualNurses.xlsx**.

Figure E3.3 Sorted Partial Table

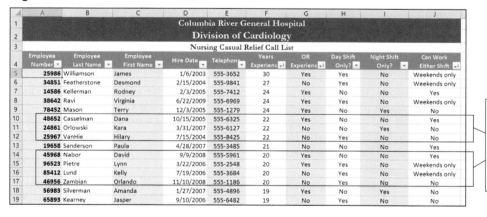

Employee Number	Employee Last Name	Employee First Name	Hire Date	Telephone	Years Experience	OR Experience	Day Shift Only?	Night Shift Only?	Can Work Either Shift
25986	Williamson	James	1/6/2003	555-3652	30	Yes	Yes	No	Weekends only
34851	Featherstone	Desmond	2/15/2004	555-9841	27	No	Yes	No	Weekends only
14586	Kellerman	Rodney	2/3/2005	555-7412	24	Yes	No	No	Yes
38642	Ravi	Virginia	6/22/2009	555-6969	24	Yes	Yes	No	Weekends only
78452	Mason	Terry	12/3/2005	555-1279	24	Yes	No	Yes	No
48652	Casselman	Dana	10/15/2005	555-6325	22	Yes	No	No	Yes
24861	Orlowski	Kara	3/31/2007	555-6127	22	No	No	Yes	No
25967	VanHie	Hilary	7/15/2004	555-8425	22	No	Yes	No	No
19658	Sanderson	Paula	4/28/2007	555-3485	21	No	No	No	Yes
45968	Nabor	David	9/9/2008	555-5961	20	Yes	No	No	Yes
96523	Pietre	Lynn	3/22/2006	555-2548	20	Yes	Yes	No	Weekends only
85412	Lund	Kelly	7/19/2006	555-3684	20	No	Yes	No	Weekends only
46956	Zambian	Orlando	11/10/2008	555-1186	20	No	Yes	No	No
56983	Silverman	Amanda	1/27/2007	555-4896	19	Yes	No	Yes	No
65893	Kearney	Jasper	9/10/2006	555-6482	19	No	Yes	No	No

Columbia River General Hospital
Division of Cardiology
Nursing Casual Relief Call List

> Notice that if employees have the same years of experience and OR experience, those with *Yes* in the *Can Work Either Shift* column are listed before those who have a restriction on the shift they can work.

Check Your Work Compare your work with the model answer to ensure that you have completed the activity correctly.

In Addition

Understanding Sort Order

By default, Excel sorts the data in a column alphanumerically. Alphanumeric sorting arranges rows with entries that begin with symbols first, then numbers, then letters. The *Sort On* option box in the Sort dialog box also provides three additional methods by which you can group rows: *Cell Color*, *Font Color*, or *Cell Icon*.

Activity 3.13   Filtering a Table

A filter is used to display only the table records that meet specified criteria. The records that do not meet the filter criteria are temporarily hidden from view. Using a filter, you can view and/or print a subset of rows within a table. For example, you might want to print a list of employees who have OR experience. Once you have printed the list, removing the filter redisplays all of the rows. In the first row of a table, Excel displays filter arrow buttons that you can use to specify the filter criteria.

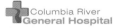
Columbia River
General Hospital

What You Will Do   Luisa Gomez has asked you for two lists: one with employees who can only work the night shift and another with employees with OR experience who can work either shift.

Tutorial
Filtering a Table

1 With **3-CRGHCasualNurses.xlsx** open, click the filter arrow button ▼ next to the column label *Night Shift Only?*

A filter arrow button displays for each column in the table. When you click a filter button, Excel displays a drop-down list with each unique field value that exists within the column. In addition, the options *Sort A to Z, Sort Z to A,* and *Sort by Color* appear at the top of the list.

2 Click the *No* check box to remove the check mark.

Removing a check mark from a check box instructs Excel to hide those rows within the table that match the check box entry. Since the only other entry in the column is *Yes,* the criterion for the filter is to display only those rows within the table that have the text entry *Yes* in column I.

3 Click OK.

Excel hides any records that have a value other than *Yes* in column I, as shown in Figure E3.4. The row numbers of the matching items that were found are displayed in blue and a filter icon appears in the filter arrow button in cell I4 to indicate the column by which the table is filtered. The Status bar also indicates that 9 of 33 records were found. A filtered table can be edited, formatted, charted, or printed.

The filter icon indicates that this column was used to filter the table.

Figure E3.4 Filtered Table

Excel hides rows that do not meet the criterion. Matching row numbers are displayed in blue.

	A	B	C	D	E	F	G	H	I	J
1				Columbia River General Hospital						
2				Division of Cardiology						
3				Nursing Casual Relief Call List						
4	Employee Number	Employee Last Name	Employee First Name	Hire Date	Telephone	Years Experience	OR Experience	Day Shift Only?	Night Shift Only?	Can Work Either Shift
9	78452	Mason	Terry	12/3/2005	555-1279	24	Yes	No	Yes	No
11	24861	Orlowski	Kara	3/31/2007	555-6127	22	No	No	Yes	No
18	56983	Silverman	Amanda	1/27/2007	555-4896	19	Yes	No	Yes	No
23	27846	Fairchild	Tina	8/10/2009	555-7822	11	Yes	No	Yes	No
25	99576	Diaz	Anna	1/13/2018	555-9378	10	Yes	No	Yes	Yes
27	69417	LaPierre	Denis	4/23/2010	555-8643	10	Yes	No	Yes	No
30	34668	Fontana	Mario	7/31/2010	555-7433	10	No	No	Yes	No
31	99027	Kumar	Hashil	6/10/2017	555-2398	8	No	No	Yes	No
37	99828	Fernandez	Natalio	1/31/2019	555-7643	3	Yes	No	Yes	Weekends only
38	Updated:	31-Jan-19								

In Brief

Filter Table
1. Click filter arrow button.
2. Remove check marks from check boxes for items you do not want to view.
3. Click OK.

Remove Filter
1. Click filter arrow button.
2. Click *Clear Filter From "column title."*

4. Print the filtered worksheet.

5. Point to the filter icon in the filter arrow button in cell I4. Notice that the filter criterion displays in a ScreenTip.

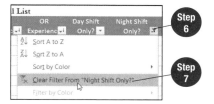

6. Click the filter arrow button in cell I4.

7. Click *Clear Filter From "Night Shift Only?"* at the drop-down list.

   All rows in the table are restored to view.

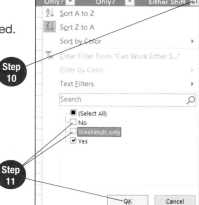

8. Click the filter arrow button in cell G4.

9. Click the *No* check box to remove the check mark and then click OK.

   Only the employees with OR experience are displayed.

10. Click the filter arrow button in cell J4.

11. Click the *No* and *Weekends only* check boxes to remove the check marks and then click OK.

   Only those employees with OR experience who can work either shift are now displayed (see Figure E3.5). Notice that you can continue to filter a table until only those records that meet your criteria are displayed.

12. Print the filtered worksheet.

13. Redisplay all records for both filtered columns.

14. Save and then close **3-CRGHCasualNurses.xlsx**.

Figure E3.5 Filtered Table Using Two Criteria

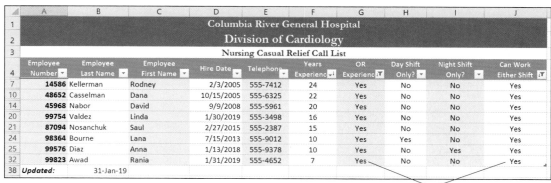

Only those employees with OR experience who can work either shift are shown.

Check Your Work   Compare your work with the model answer to ensure that you have completed the activity correctly.

In Addition

Filtering Data Not Formatted as a Table

Data in a worksheet that has not been formatted as a table can also be filtered using techniques similar to those you learned in this activity. Select the range of cells that you wish to filter, click the Sort & Filter but-ton in the Editing group on the Home tab, and then click *Filter* at the drop-down list. Excel adds filter arrow buttons to each column of the first row of the selected range.

Features Summary

Feature	Ribbon Tab, Group	Button
change chart type	Chart Tools Design, Type	
change margins	Page Layout, Page Setup OR File, *Print*	
create a column chart	Insert, Charts	
create a pie chart	Insert, Charts	
Date & Time functions	Formulas, Function Library	
draw a shape	Insert, Illustrations	
draw a text box	Insert, Text	
filter table	Home, Editing	
format table	Home, Styles	
header or footer	Insert, Text OR Page Layout View	
Logical functions	Formulas, Function Library	
move chart	Chart Tools Design, Location	
Normal view	View, Workbook Views	OR
Page Layout view	View, Workbook Views	OR
scale page width and/or height	Page Layout, Scale to Fit OR File, *Print*	
sort table	Home, Editing	

Workbook   Section study tools and assessment activities are available in the Workbook pages of the ebook. These resources are designed to help you further develop and demonstrate mastery of the skills learned in this section.

Integrating Programs

Word and Excel

Data Files Before beginning section work, copy the IntegratingMed1 folder to your storage medium and then make IntegratingMed1 the active folder.

Skills

- Copy and paste Word data into an Excel worksheet
- Link an Excel worksheet with a Word document
- Update linked data
- View linked data as an icon

- Link an Excel chart with a Word document
- Embed an Excel worksheet into a Word document
- Edit an embedded worksheet

Precheck Check your current skills to help focus your study of the skills taught in this section.

Activities Overview

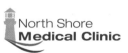
North Shore **Medical Clinic**

Copy and paste quarterly statistics on new patients; calculate depreciation values, edit data, and link an equipment worksheet to a Word document; link and update a chart depicting actual and projected expenditures to an Operations Report in Word; and embed a flu shot clinic form from Excel into a Word document.

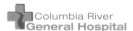
Columbia River **General Hospital**

Copy and paste volunteer information from a worksheet to a Word document; link and update tuition fee billing data and a chart from a worksheet to a Word document; and embed a fact sheet into a hospital foundation document.

Model Answers Preview the model answers for an overview of the activities you will complete in each section.

Copying and Pasting Word Data into an Excel Worksheet

Microsoft Office is a suite that allows for integration, which is the combining of data from two or more programs into one file. Integration can occur by copying and pasting data between programs. The program containing the data to be copied is called the source program and the program where the data is pasted is called the destination program. For example, you can copy data from a Word document into an Excel worksheet. Copy and paste data between programs in the same manner as you would copy and paste data within a program.

North Shore Medical Clinic

What You Will Do   You will copy data on new patients at North Shore Medical Clinic from a Word document into an Excel worksheet and then use Excel to total the number of patients per month and per specialty.

1 Open Word and then open **NSMCNewPatientRpt.docx**.

2 Open Excel and then open **NSMCNewPatients-Qtr1.xlsx**.

3 Save the workbook with the name **1-NSMCNewPatients-Qtr1**.

4 Click the Word button on the taskbar.

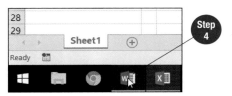

5 Select the last six rows of the table, as shown below.

6 Click the Copy button in the Clipboard group on the Home tab.

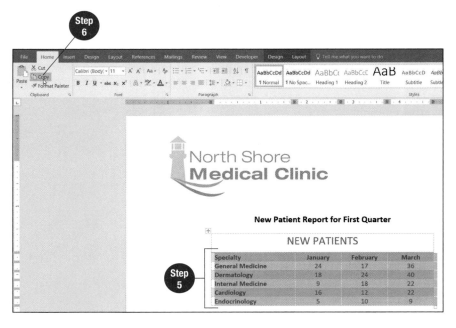

New Patient Report for First Quarter

NEW PATIENTS

Specialty	January	February	March
General Medicine	24	17	36
Dermatology	18	24	40
Internal Medicine	9	18	22
Cardiology	16	12	22
Endocrinology	5	10	9

7 Click the Excel button on the taskbar.

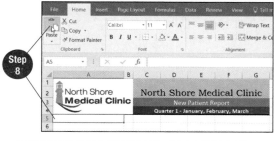

8 Make sure cell A5 is the active cell and then click the Paste button in the Clipboard group.

9 Click the Paste Options button and then click the Match Destination Formatting button.

10 Click in any cell to deselect the range.

11 Select the range B5:D10, click and hold down the left mouse button on one of the borders surrounding the selected cells, and then drag the range to cells C5:E10.

12 Make cell G5 the active cell and then type Total.

13 Make cell G6 the active cell, click the AutoSum button Σ in the Editing group on the Home tab, and then press the Enter key to calculate the total of the range C6:F6.

14 Use the fill handle to copy the formula in cell G6 down to the range G7:G10.

15 Make cell A12 the active cell and then type Total.

16 Make cell C12 the active cell and then use the AutoSum button in the Editing group to calculate the total of the range C6:C11.

17 Use the fill handle to copy the formula in cell C12 to the range D12:G12.

18 Clear the contents of cell F12 to remove the zero.

19 Apply formatting changes as desired to improve the appearance of the worksheet.

20 Save, print, and then close **1-NSMCNewPatients-Qtr1.xlsx**.

21 Click the Word button on the taskbar.

22 Close **NSMCNewPatientRpt.docx**. If prompted to save changes to the document, click Don't Save.

Check Your Work Compare your work with the model answer to ensure that you have completed the activity correctly.

In Addition

Cycling through Open Programs

Switch between open programs by clicking the button on the taskbar representing the desired program. You can also cycle through open programs by pressing Alt + Tab. Pressing Alt + Tab causes a window to display. Continue holding down the Alt key and pressing the Tab key until the desired program icon is selected in the window and then release the Tab key and the Alt key.

In the previous activity, you copied data from a Word document and pasted it into an Excel worksheet. If you continuously update the data in the Word document, you would need to copy and paste the data into the Excel worksheet to keep it updated as well. To keep data updated in all programs, consider copying and linking the data. When data is linked, it exists in the source program but not as separate data in the destination program. The destination program contains only a code that identifies the name and location of the source program and the location of the data in the source file. Since the data is saved only in the source program, changes made to the data in the source program are reflected in the destination program. Office updates linked data automatically whenever you open the destination program or edit the linked data in the destination program.

North Shore Medical Clinic

What You Will Do   You will open a worksheet with equipment purchase information, use a function to calculate straight-line depreciation, and then copy and link the data to a Word document.

1   With Word active, open **NSMCEquipGERm3-SLD.docx**.

2   Save the document with the name **1-NSMCEquipGERm3-SLD**.

3   Make Excel active and then open **NSMCEquipGERm3.xlsx**.

4   Save the workbook with the name **1-NSMCEquipGERm3**.

> In the next steps, you will use Excel's SLN function to calculate the annual depreciation value to be recorded for each equipment item. Straight-line depreciation requires three values: the equipment's original cost, the estimated value of the equipment when taken out of service (salvage), and the expected number of years the clinic will use the item (life).

5   Make cell H6 active and then click the Insert Function button f_x on the Formula bar.

6   Type straight-line depreciation in the *Search for a function* text box and then press the Enter key or click Go.

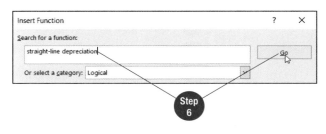

7   If necessary, click to select *SLN* in the *Select a function* list box and then click OK.

8   With the insertion point positioned in the *Cost* text box, type E6 and then press the Tab key.

9   Type F6 in the *Salvage* text box and then press the Tab key.

10   Type G6 in the *Life* text box and then press the Enter key.

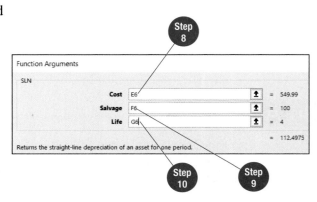

> Excel returns the value *$112.50* in cell H6. In the Formula bar, the function is *=SLN(E6,F6,G6)*.

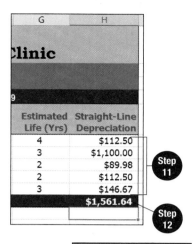

Step 11

Step 12

11 Copy the formula in cell H6 to the range H7:H10.

12 Make cell H11 the active cell and then use the AutoSum button to calculate the total of the range H6:H10.

13 Select the range A5:H11 and then click the Copy button in the Clipboard group on the Home tab.

14 Click the Word button on the taskbar.

15 Press Ctrl + End to move the insertion point to the end of the document.

16 Click the Paste button arrow and then click *Paste Special* at the drop-down list.

17 Click *Microsoft Excel Worksheet Object* in the *As* list box, click the *Paste link* option, and then click OK.

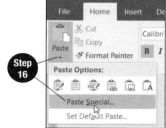

Step 16

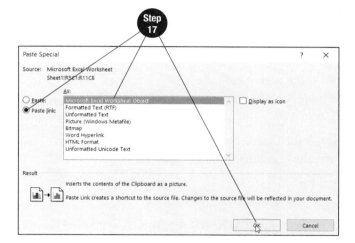

Step 17

18 Save, print, and then close **1-NSMCEquipGERm3-SLD.docx**.

19 Click the Excel button on the taskbar.

20 Press the Esc key to remove the marquee around the range A5:H11 and then click any cell to deselect the range.

21 Save, print, and then close **1-NSMCEquipGERm3.xlsx**.

> **Check Your Work** — Compare your work with the model answer to ensure that you have completed the activity correctly.

In Addition

Linking Data within a Program

Linking does not have to be between two different programs—you can link data between files in the same program. For example, you can create an object in a Word document, such as a table or chart, and then link the object with another Word document (or several Word documents). If you make a change to the object in the original document, the linked object in the other document (or documents) is automatically updated.

The advantage of linking data over copying data is that editing the data in the source program will automatically update the data in the destination program. To edit linked data, open the file in the source program, make the desired edits, and then save the file. The next time you open the file in the destination program, the data will be updated. The display of the linked data in the destination program can be changed to a clickable icon. The icon represents the file and program to which the object is linked. This feature is useful when the source file contains multiple pages, worksheets, or presentation slides.

North Shore Medical Clinic

What You Will Do   Lee Elliott, office manager for North Shore Medical Clinic, has given you revised estimates for salvage value and estimated life for two equipment items in the linked worksheet. You will open the worksheet, update the values, and then view the updated information in Word.

1   With Excel active, open **1-NSMCEquipGERm3.xlsx**.

> The salvage value and estimated life numbers for the AudioScope have been revised to *$75.00* and *3*, respectively.

2   Make cell F6 the active cell and then change the contents to *$75.00*.

3   Make cell G6 the active cell and then change the contents to *3*.

4   Save and close **1-SMCEquipGERm3.xlsx** and then close Excel.

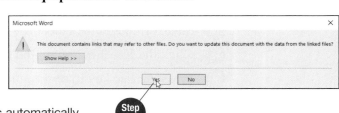

5   With Word active, open **1-NSMCEquipGERm3-SLD.docx**.

6   Click Yes at the message asking if you want to update the document with the data from the linked files.

> The document opens and is automatically updated to reflect the changes you made in *1-NSMCEquipGERm3.xlsx*.

7   Review the Word document. Notice that the estimated salvage and estimated life values for the AudioScope have been updated.

8   Position the mouse pointer over the linked object and then double-click the left mouse button.

> Excel opens and displays *1-NSMCEquipGERm3.xlsx* in the Excel window. The linked range is highlighted. You need to change the salvage value and estimated life for the wall transformer to *$50.00* and *2*, respectively.

9   Make cell F10 active and then change the contents to *$50.00*.

10   Make cell G10 active and then change the contents to *2*.

11   Click the Save button on the Quick Access Toolbar and then close Excel.

In Brief

Update Linked Data
1. Open file in source program.
2. Make edits.
3. Save and close file.
4. Open file in destination program.
5. Click Yes to update links.
6. Save and close file.

Display Linked Object as an Icon
1. Select object.
2. Right-click in object.
3. Point to *Linked Worksheet Object* and then click *Convert*.
4. At Convert dialog box, click *Display as icon* check box.
5. Click OK.

12 Notice that the values in the linked object in Word have been updated.

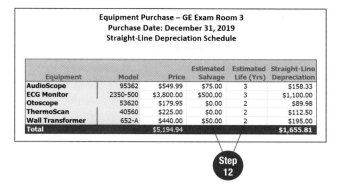

Equipment Purchase – GE Exam Room 3
Purchase Date: December 31, 2019
Straight-Line Depreciation Schedule

Equipment	Model	Price	Estimated Salvage	Estimated Life (Yrs)	Straight-Line Depreciation
AudioScope	95362	$549.99	$75.00	3	$158.33
ECG Monitor	2350-500	$3,800.00	$500.00	3	$1,100.00
Otoscope	53620	$179.95	$0.00	2	$89.98
ThermoScan	40560	$225.00	$0.00	2	$112.50
Wall Transformer	652-A	$440.00	$50.00	2	$195.00
Total		$5,194.94			$1,655.81

Step 12

13 Save and then print **1-NSMCEquipGERm3-SLD.docx**.

14 Display the linked table as an icon. Begin by right-clicking the table, pointing to *Linked Worksheet Object* at the shortcut menu, and then clicking *Convert* at the side menu.

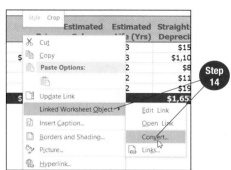

Step 14

15 At the Convert dialog box, click the *Display as icon* check box to insert a check mark and then click OK.

Notice how the table changes to an icon representing the linked document.

16 Print **1-NSMCEquipGERm3-SLD.docx**.

17 Make sure the linked object icon is selected and then redisplay the table. To begin, right-click the icon, point to *Linked Worksheet Object* at the shortcut menu, and then click *Convert* at the side menu.

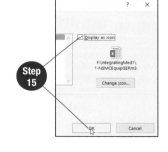

Step 15

18 At the Convert dialog box, click the *Display as icon* check box to remove the check mark and then click OK.

19 Save and then close **1-NSMCEquipGERm3-SLD.docx**.

Check Your Work | Compare your work with the model answer to ensure that you have completed the activity correctly.

In Addition

Breaking a Link

The link between an object in the destination and source programs can be broken. To break a link, right-click the object icon, point to *Linked Worksheet Object*, and then click *Links*. At the Links dialog box, click the Break Link button. At the question asking if you are sure you want to break the link, click Yes.

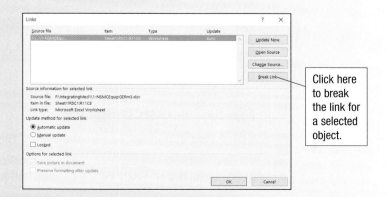

Click here to break the link for a selected object.

While a worksheet does an adequate job of representing data, you can present some data more effectively in a chart. A chart is a visual representation of numeric data and, like a worksheet, can be linked to a document in another program. Link a chart in the same manner as you would link a worksheet.

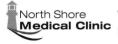

North Shore Medical Clinic

What You Will Do   You will link an Excel chart depicting North Shore Medical Clinic's projected and actual expenditures with the Operations Report document saved in Word. After linking the chart, you will update the data used to generate the chart.

Tutorial

Linking an Object

1. With Word active, open **NSMCOpRpt.docx**.

2. Save the document with the name **1-NSMCOpRpt**.

3. Make Excel active and then open **NSMCQtrlyExp.xlsx**.

4. Save the workbook with the name **1-NSMCQtrlyExp**.

5. Click the chart to select it. (A border displays around the chart.)

    Make sure you do not select an individual chart element when you select the chart. If you see a thin border with sizing handles around a chart element, click outside the chart and select the chart again. Click a white area around the inside perimeter to select the chart without selecting an individual chart element.

6. Click the Copy button in the Clipboard group on the Home tab.

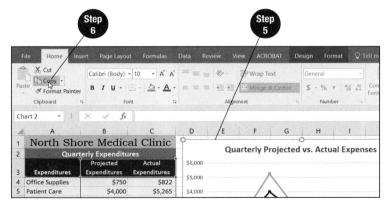

7. Click the Word button on the taskbar.

8. Press Ctrl + End to move the insertion point to the end of the document.

9. Click the Center button in the Paragraph group on the Home tab.

10. Click the Paste button arrow in the Clipboard group and then click *Paste Special*.

11. Click *Microsoft Excel Chart Object* in the *As* list box, click *Paste link*, and then click OK.

12. Save **1-NSMCOpRpt.docx**.

13. Make Excel active and then press the Esc key to remove the border from the chart.

    The actual expenditure value for Diagnostics is incorrect. You will enter the correct value and then examine the change in the chart in both Excel and Word.

14 Make cell C8 the active cell and then change the contents to *$3,400*.

15 Examine the revised chart in Excel.

16 Save and then close **1-NSMCQtrlyExp.xlsx**.

17 Make Word active.

18 Update the chart by clicking the File tab and then clicking *Edit Links to Files* at the bottom right side of the Info backstage area.

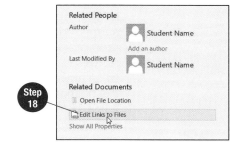

19 At the Links dialog box with the linked object selected in the list box, click the Update Now button.

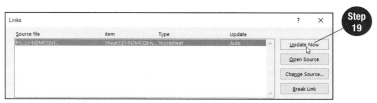

20 Click OK to close the Links dialog box.

21 Click the Back button to return to the document.

22 Change the percent value in the second-to-last sentence in the paragraph above the chart to *16.7%*. The sentence should now read *Overall, the clinic spent 16.7% more on operations than projected.*

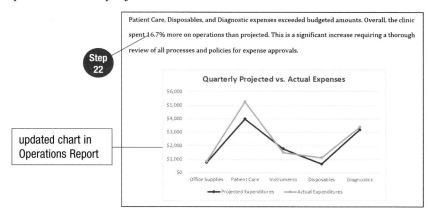

23 Save, print, and then close **1-NSMCOpRpt.docx**.

> **Check Your Work** — Compare your work with the model answer to ensure that you have completed the activity correctly.

In Addition

Customizing a Link

By default, a linked object is updated automatically and can be edited. You can change these defaults with options at the Links dialog box. Display this dialog box by right-clicking the linked object, pointing to *Linked Worksheet Object*, and then clicking *Links*. At the Links dialog box, click the *Manual update* option if you want to control when to update linked data. With the *Manual update* option selected, update linked objects by clicking the Update Now button at the right side of the Links dialog box. If you do not want a linked object updated, click the *Locked* check box in the Links dialog box to insert a check mark.

In addition to copying and linking, another way to integrate data among different files in the same or different programs is by embedding it. While a linked object resides in the source program and is represented by a code in the destination program, an embedded object resides in the source program and in the destination program. When you make a change to an embedded object in the source program, the change is not made to the object in the destination program. Since an embedded object is not automatically updated, unlike a linked object, the only advantage to embedding rather than simply copying and pasting is that you can edit an embedded object in the destination program using the tools of the source program.

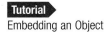
North Shore Medical Clinic

What You Will Do   You will copy and embed a flu shot clinic form created by Heather Mitsui, RMA at North Shore Medical Clinic, from an Excel worksheet into a Word document.

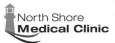
Tutorial
Embedding an Object

1. With Word active, open **NSMCShotClinics.docx**.

2. Save the document with the name **1-NSMCShotClinics**.

3. Make Excel active and then open **NSMCShotForm.xlsx**.

4. Save the workbook with the name **1-NSMCShotForm**.

   Heather Mitsui used Excel to create a flu shot dispensing record form for the upcoming flu shot clinics. You decide to embed Heather's form into a Word document, since the Word document has the clinic's letterhead at the top of the page.

5. Select the range A9:K27 and then click the Copy button in the Clipboard group on the Home tab.

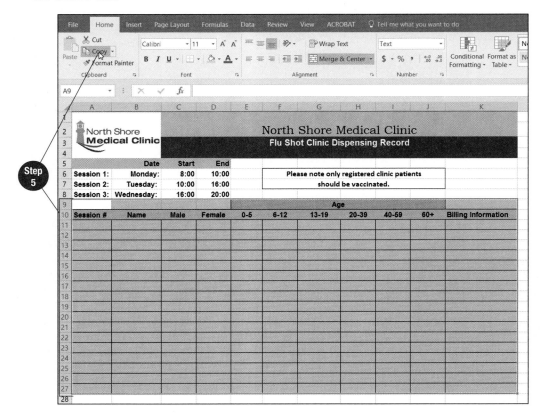

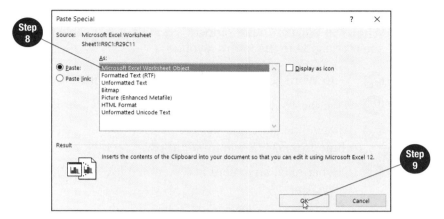

In Brief

Embed Data
1. Open programs and files.
2. Select data in source program.
3. Click Copy button.
4. Click button on taskbar representing destination program.
5. Click Paste button arrow.
6. Click *Paste Special*.
7. Click object in *As* list box.
8. Click OK.

6 Make Word active and then press Ctrl + End to move the insertion point to the end of the document.

7 Click the Paste button arrow in the Clipboard group and then click *Paste Special* at the drop-down list.

8 Click *Microsoft Excel Worksheet Object* in the *As* list box.

   Make sure you do not click the *Paste link* option.

9 Click OK.

10 Display the Print backstage area to see how the form will look when printed.

11 Click the Back button to return to the form.

12 Save, print, and then close **1-NSMCShotClinics.docx**.

13 Make Excel active and then press the Esc key to remove the marquee from the selected range.

14 Click in any cell to deselect the range.

15 Close **1-NSMCShotForm.xlsx** and then close Excel.

Check Your Work Compare your work with the model answer to ensure that you have completed the activity correctly.

In Addition

Inserting an Embedded Object from an Existing File

In this activity, you embedded an Excel worksheet in a Word document using the Copy button and options at the Paste Special dialog box. Another method is available for embedding an object from an existing file. In the destination program document, position the insertion point where you want the object embedded and then click the Object button in the Text group on the Insert tab. At the Object dialog box, click the Create from File tab. At the Object dialog box with the Create from File tab selected, as shown at the right, type the desired file name in the *File name* text box or click the Browse button and then select the file from the appropriate folder. At the Object dialog box, make sure the *Link to file* check box does not contain a check mark and then click OK.

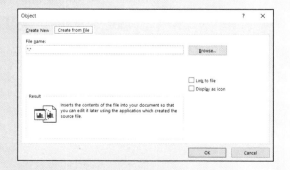

Activity 1.6   Editing an Embedded Worksheet

An embedded object can be edited in the destination program using the tools of the source program. Double-click the embedded object in the file in the destination program and the ribbon from the source program becomes active. For example, if you double-click an Excel worksheet that is embedded in a Word document, the Excel ribbon displays at the top of the Word document window.

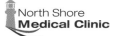

What You Will Do   After embedding the flu shot clinic form into Word, you decide to make some changes to the form's layout.

1. With Word active, open **1-NSMCShotClinics.docx**.

2. Save the document with the name **1-NSMCShotClinics-Edit**.

3. Change the start time for the Session 3 clinic from *04:00 pm* to *06:30 pm*.

4. Double-click anywhere in the embedded worksheet.

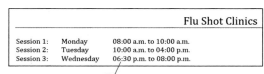

> In a few moments, the worksheet displays surrounded by column and row designations and the Excel ribbon displays at the top of the Word window.

5. Click in any cell within the embedded worksheet to deselect the range.

6. Select columns E through J and then change the column widths to *6.00 (61 pixels)*.

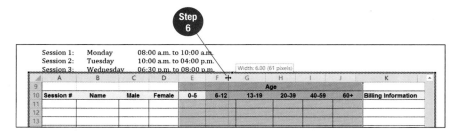

7. Click in any cell to deselect the columns.

8. Select the range A9:D9 and cell K9 and then apply Blue, Accent 5 fill color (ninth column, first row in the *Theme Colors* section).

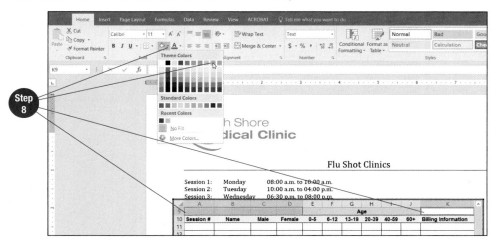

In Brief

Edit Embedded Object
1. In source program, double-click embedded object.
2. Make edits.
3. Click outside object.

9 Insert a new column between columns D and E and then change the width of the new column to *6.00 (61 pixels)*.

10 Type the label *0-1* in cell E10.

11 Change the label in cell F10 from *0-5* to *2-5*.

12 If necessary, drag the middle right sizing handle of the embedded worksheet to the right to make sure columns A through L are visible within the object's border.

13 Merge and center the label *Age* over columns E through K.

14 Select cell E9 (contains the label *Age*) and then apply an outside border.

15 Select the range A9:L9 and then apply an outside border.

16 Make sure the only cells visible within the embedded object border are in the range A9:L27. If any other cells from the source worksheet are visible, use the horizontal and vertical scroll arrows to adjust the window.

Figure I1.1 illustrates a portion of the embedded worksheet with the revised formatting applied in Steps 8 through 15. If this portion of your worksheet does not appear as shown in Figure I1.1, review Steps 8 through 15 to determine if you have missed a step. Also note that you may need to scroll within the worksheet to ensure that columns A through L and rows 1 through 29 are visible within the object's border.

17 Click outside the worksheet to deselect the embedded object.

18 Save, print, and then close **1-NSMCShotClinics-Edit.docx**.

Figure I1.1 Excel Worksheet Embedded in a Word Document

Session 1:	Monday	08:00 a.m. to 10:00 a.m.
Session 2:	Tuesday	10:00 a.m. to 04:00 p.m.
Session 3:	Wednesday	06:30 p.m. to 08:00 p.m.

	A	B	C	D	E	F	G	H	I	J	K	L
9								Age				
10	Session #	Name	Male	Female	0-1	2-5	6-12	13-19	20-39	40-59	60+	Billing Information
11												
12												
13												
14												
15												
16												
17												

Check Your Work Compare your work with the model answer to ensure that you have completed the activity correctly.

In Addition

Troubleshooting Linking and Embedding Problems

If you double-click a linked or embedded object and a message appears telling you that the source file or source program cannot be opened, consider the following troubleshooting options:

- Check to make sure that the source program is installed on your computer. If the source program is not installed, convert the object to the file format of a program that is installed.

- Try closing other programs to free up more memory and make sure you have enough memory to run the source program.
- Check to make sure the source program does not have any dialog boxes open.
- If you are trying to open a linked object, check to make sure no one else is working in the source file.

Unit **3**

Using PowerPoint in the Medical Office

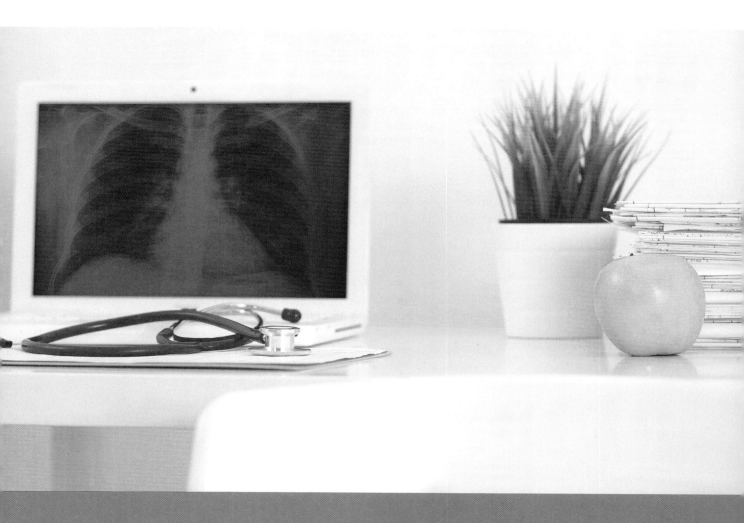

Introducing PowerPoint 2016

Create colorful and powerful presentations using PowerPoint, the full-featured presentation program included in the Microsoft Office suite. With PowerPoint, you can organize and display information and create visual aids. PowerPoint provides a wide variety of editing and formatting features as well as sophisticated visual elements such as images, WordArt, lines, shapes, and diagrams.

In Section 1, you will choose design templates for presentations; insert slides; choose slide layouts; select, move, and size placeholders; use the Tell Me and Help features; check spelling in presentations; run slide shows; and add transitions and transition sounds to presentations. Section 2 focuses on editing slides and slide elements. In that section, you will rearrange, delete, and hide slides; cut, copy, and paste text within and between slides; apply font and font effects; apply formatting such as alignment, spacing, headers, and footers; change slide design themes; insert and format images, WordArt, and SmartArt graphics; and apply animation schemes.

In the two PowerPoint sections, you will prepare medical presentations for two clinics and a hospital as described below.

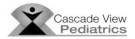

Cascade View Pediatrics is a full-service pediatric clinic that provides comprehensive primary pediatric care to infants, children, and adolescents.

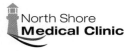

North Shore Medical Clinic is an internal medicine clinic dedicated to providing exceptional care to all patients. The physicians in the clinic specialize in a number of fields including internal medicine, family practice, cardiology, and dermatology.

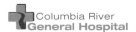

Columbia River General Hospital is an independent, not-for-profit hospital with the mission of providing high-quality, comprehensive care to patients and improving the health of members of the community.

PowerPoint

Preparing a Presentation

Data Files Before beginning section work, copy the PowerPointMedS1 folder to your storage medium and then make PowerPointMedS1 the active folder.

Skills

- Open, save, and close a presentation
- Run a slide show
- Choose a design theme
- Add a new slide to a presentation
- Navigate in a presentation
- Change the slide layout
- Change the presentation view
- Rearrange, delete, and hide slides
- Use the Tell Me and Help features

- Check spelling in a presentation
- Use Thesaurus to display synonyms for words
- Run a slide show and use the pen during a slide show
- Use ink tools
- Add transitions and transition sounds to a presentation
- Print and preview a presentation

Precheck Check your current skills to help focus your study of the skills taught in this section.

Activities Overview

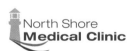
North Shore **Medical Clinic**

Prepare a presentation introducing PowerPoint 2016; prepare, edit, and format a presentation on diabetes; prepare a presentation on cystic fibrosis; and edit and format a presentation containing information on the clinic.

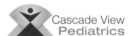
Cascade View Pediatrics

Prepare, edit, and format a presentation containing information on the clinic and prepare, edit, and format a presentation on chickenpox.

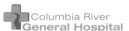
Columbia River **General Hospital**

Prepare, edit, and format a presentation on fibromyalgia and prepare, edit, and format a presentation containing information on the hospital.

Model Answers Preview the model answers for an overview of the activities you will complete in each section.

PowerPoint is a presentation graphics program you can use to organize and present information. With PowerPoint, you can create visual aids for a presentation and then print copies of the aids as well as run the slide show. To open a predesigned PowerPoint template, open the PowerPoint program, click the desired template, and then click the Create button. The presentation screen contains a variety of features for working with a presentation, such as the Title bar, Quick Access Toolbar, ribbon, and Status bar. After creating a presentation, save the presentation so it is available for future use. Save a presentation with options at the Save As backstage area.

North Shore Medical Clinic

What You Will Do You are an employee of North Shore Medical Clinic and Office 2016 has just been installed on your computer. You need to prepare a presentation in the near future, so you decide to open a presentation provided by PowerPoint and experiment with running the slide show.

Tutorial
Opening a Presentation Based on a Template

Tutorial
Exploring the PowerPoint Screen

Tutorial
Running a Slide Show

Tutorial
Saving to a Removable Disk

Tutorial
Closing a Presentation and Closing PowerPoint

1 At the Windows 10 desktop, click the Start button and then click the PowerPoint 2016 tile at the Start menu.

Depending on your system configuration, these steps may vary.

2 At the PowerPoint 2016 opening screen, click the *Welcome to PowerPoint* template.

If this template is not visible, you will need to search for it. To do this, click in the search text box, type Welcome to PowerPoint, and then press the Enter key.

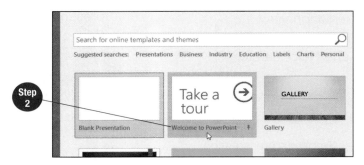

3 Click the Create button.

The Welcome to PowerPoint template opens in the PowerPoint window. What displays in the PowerPoint window will vary depending on what type of presentation you are creating. However, the PowerPoint window contains some consistent elements, such as those identified in Figure P1.1. Refer to Table P1.1 for a description of the window elements.

4 Run the slide show by clicking the Start From Beginning button on the Quick Access Toolbar.

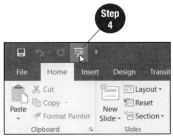

Figure P1.1 PowerPoint Window

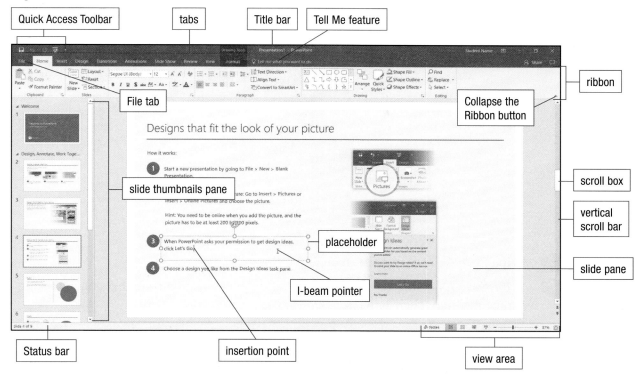

Quick Access Toolbar | tabs | Title bar | Tell Me feature | File tab | Collapse the Ribbon button | ribbon | scroll box | vertical scroll bar | slide pane | slide thumbnails pane | placeholder | I-beam pointer | Status bar | insertion point | view area

Table P1.1 PowerPoint Window Elements

Feature	Description
Collapse the Ribbon button	when clicked, removes ribbon from screen
File tab	when clicked, displays backstage area that contains options for working with and managing presentations
I-beam pointer	used to move the insertion point or to select text
insertion point	indicates location of next character entered at keyboard
placeholder	location on a slide with a dotted border; holds text or objects
Quick Access Toolbar	contains buttons for commonly used commands
ribbon	area containing the tabs with options and buttons divided into groups
scroll box	used to scroll through slides in a presentation; click and hold mouse button on scroll box to view slide number and title
slide pane	displays slide and slide contents
slide thumbnails pane	area on the left side of the screen; displays slide thumbnails
Status bar	displays slide number, view buttons, and Zoom slider bar
tabs	contain commands and buttons organized into groups
Tell Me feature	used to look up features and provide options for using them
Title bar	displays presentation name followed by program name
vertical scroll bar	used to display specific slides
view area	contains buttons for changing presentation view

5 When the first slide fills the screen, read the information and then click the left mouse button. Continue reading the information in each slide and clicking the left mouse button to advance to the next slide. When a black screen displays, click the left mouse button to end the slide show.

6 Save the presentation by clicking the Save button ⊞ on the Quick Access Toolbar.

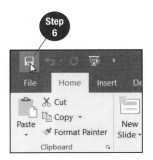

7 At the Save As backstage area, click the *Browse* option.

8 At the Save As dialog box, click the drive in the Navigation pane that contains your storage medium (such as *Removable Disk (F:)*).

Press the F12 function key to display the Save As dialog box without displaying the Save As backstage area.

9 Double-click the *PowerPointMedS1* folder in the Content pane.

10 Click in the *File name* text box, type 1-PowerPoint2016, and then press the Enter key (or click the Save button).

PowerPoint automatically adds the file extension *.pptx* to the end of a presentation name.

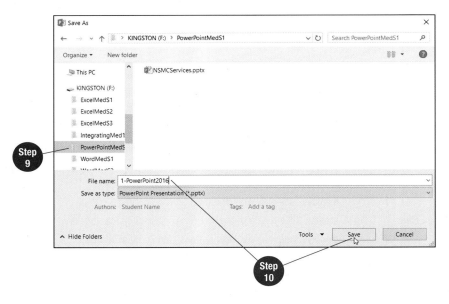

In Brief

Create Presentation from Installed Template
1. Click File tab.
2. Click *New*.
3. Click template.
4. Click Create button.

Save Presentation
1. Click Save button on Quick Access Toolbar.
2. Click *Browse*.
3. Navigate to location.
4. At Save As dialog box, type presentation file name.
5. Press Enter.

Run Slide Show
1. Click Start From Beginning button on Quick Access Toolbar.
2. Click left mouse button to advance slides and to end slide show.

Print Presentation in Outline Layout
1. Click File tab.
2. Click *Print*.
3. Click second gallery in *Settings* category.
4. Click *Outline*.
5. Click Print button.

Close Presentation
1. Click File tab.
2. Click *Close*.

11 At the PowerPoint window, print the presentation information in outline layout by clicking the File tab and then clicking the *Print* option.

> The File tab is in the upper left corner of the screen at the left side of the Home tab. When you click the File tab, the backstage area displays with options for working with and managing presentations.

12 At the Print backstage area, click the second gallery in the *Settings* category (the gallery containing the text *Full Page Slides*) and then click *Outline* in the *Print Layout* section of the drop-down list.

13 Click the Print button. ***Note: If working in a lab, check with your instructor before printing.***

14 Close the presentation by clicking the File tab and then clicking the *Close* option.

> If a message displays asking if you want to save the presentation, click Yes.

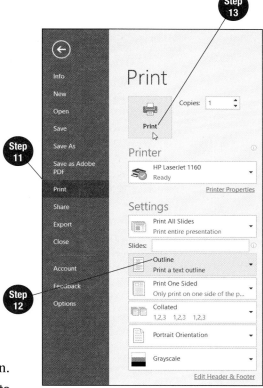

15 Close PowerPoint by clicking the Close button that displays in the upper right corner of the screen.

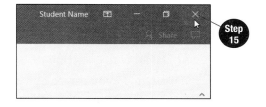

Check Your Work Compare your work with the model answer to ensure that you have completed the activity correctly.

In Addition

Using Tabs

The ribbon displays below the Quick Access Toolbar. PowerPoint features are organized into tabs that display in the ribbon area. The buttons and options on the ribbon area vary depending on the tab selected and the width of the window displayed on the screen. Commands and buttons are organized into groups within a tab. For example, the Home tab, which is the default tab, contains the Clipboard, Slides, Font, Paragraph, Drawing, and Editing groups. When you hover the mouse over a button, a ScreenTip displays with the name of the button, a keyboard shortcut (if any), and a description of the purpose of the button.

Create a PowerPoint presentation using an installed template as you did in the previous activity, or begin with a blank presentation and apply your own formatting or a slide design theme. To display a blank PowerPoint presentation, use the keyboard shortcut Ctrl + N, or click the File tab, click the *New* option, and then click the *Blank Presentation* template in the New backstage area. A PowerPoint presentation screen displays in Normal view with the slide pane in the center and the slide thumbnails pane at the left side of the screen. Insert a new slide in the presentation by clicking the New Slide button in the Slides group on the Home tab or the Insert tab.

North Shore Medical Clinic

What You Will Do   Dr. St. Claire will be presenting information on diabetes at the Greater Portland Healthcare Workers Association meeting. She has asked you to prepare a PowerPoint presentation that she will use during the meeting. You decide to prepare the presentation using a design template provided by PowerPoint.

Tutorial
Opening a Blank Presentation

Tutorial
Applying a Design Theme

Tutorial
Inserting and Deleting Text in a Slide

Tutorial
Inserting a New Slide

1. Open PowerPoint.

2. At the PowerPoint 2016 opening screen, click the *Blank Presentation* template.

3. At the PowerPoint window, click the Design tab.

4. Click the More Themes button ⏷ in the Themes group.

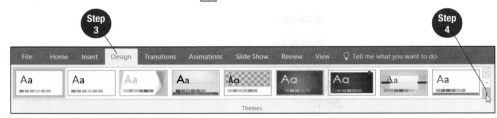

5. Click *Organic* in the *Office* section of the drop-down gallery.

> When you click the More Themes button, a drop-down gallery displays. This gallery contains the live preview feature. When you hover your mouse pointer over one of the design themes, the slide in the slide pane displays with the design theme formatting applied. With the live preview feature, you can preview a design theme before actually applying it to the presentation.

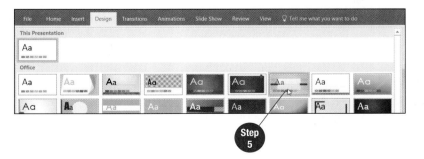

6. Click the fourth thumbnail from the left in the Variants group.

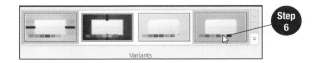

7 Click anywhere in the *Click to add title* placeholder that displays in the slide in the slide pane and then type Understanding Diabetes.

> A placeholder is a location on a slide that is marked with a border and holds text or an object.

8 Click anywhere in the *Click to add subtitle* placeholder that displays in the slide and then type Greater Portland Healthcare Workers Association.

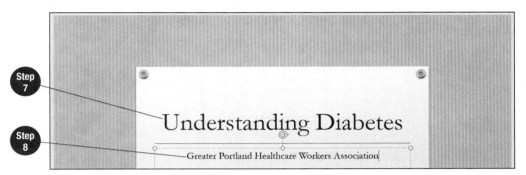

9 Click the Home tab and then click the New Slide button in the Slides group.

> When you click this button, a new slide displays in the slide pane with the Title and Content layout. You will learn more about slide layouts in Activity 1.3.

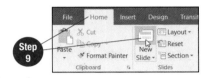

10 Click anywhere in the *Click to add title* placeholder that displays in the slide and then type Statistics of Diabetes.

11 Click anywhere in the *Click to add text* placeholder that displays in the slide and then type Prevalence of diabetes in the United States.

12 Press the Enter key and then type Total number of people diagnosed with diabetes.

13 Press the Enter key and then type Diabetes by age group.

> You can use keys on the keyboard to move the insertion point to various locations within a placeholder in a slide. Refer to Table P1.2 on the next page for a list of insertion point movement commands.

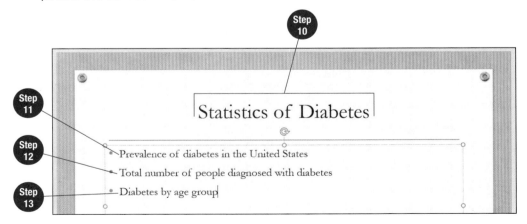

14 Click the New Slide button in the Slides group on the Home tab.

Table P1.2 Insertion Point Movement Commands

To move insertion point	Press
One character left	Left Arrow
One character right	Right Arrow
One line up	Up Arrow
One line down	Down Arrow
One word to the left	Ctrl + Left Arrow
One word to the right	Ctrl + Right Arrow
To end of line of text	End
To beginning of line of text	Home
To beginning of current paragraph in placeholder	Ctrl + Up Arrow
To beginning of previous paragraph in placeholder	Ctrl + Up Arrow two times
To beginning of next paragraph in placeholder	Ctrl + Down Arrow
To beginning of text in placeholder	Ctrl + Home
To end of text in placeholder	Ctrl + End

15 Click anywhere in the *Click to add title* placeholder that displays in the slide and then type Types of Diabetes.

16 Click anywhere in the *Click to add text* placeholder that displays in the slide and then type the bulleted text as shown below. Press the Enter key after each item except the last item.

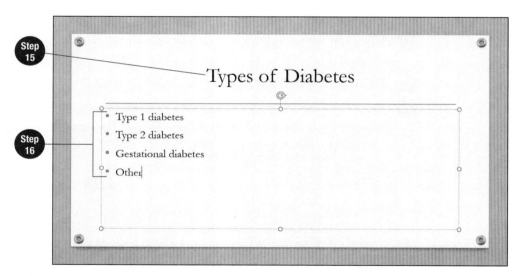

17 Click the New Slide button in the Slides group on the Home tab.

In Brief

Choose Design Theme
1. Click Design tab.
2. Click More Themes button.
3. Click theme at drop-down gallery.

Insert New Slide
1. Click Home tab.
2. Click New Slide button.

18 Click anywhere in the *Click to add title* placeholder that displays in the slide and then type Treatment of Diabetes.

19 Click anywhere in the *Click to add text* placeholder that displays in the slide and then type the bulleted text as shown below. Press the Enter key after each item except the last item.

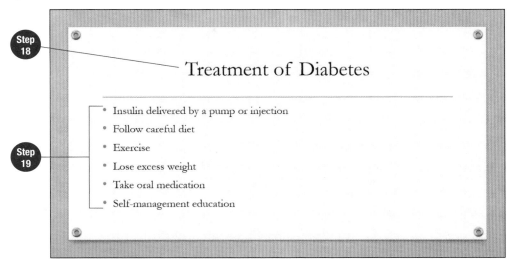

20 Click the Save button on the Quick Access Toolbar.

21 At the Save As backstage area, click the *Browse* option.

22 At the Save As dialog box, click the drive in the Navigation pane that contains your storage medium.

23 Double-click the *PowerPointMedS1* folder in the Content pane.

24 Click in the *File name* text box, type 1-Diabetes, and then press the Enter key (or click the Save button).

25 Close the presentation by clicking the File tab and then clicking the *Close* option.

Check Your Work ▷ Compare your work with the model answer to ensure that you have completed the activity correctly.

In Addition

Planning a Presentation

Consider the following basic guidelines when preparing content for a presentation:

- **Determine the main purpose.** Do not try to cover too many topics. Identifying the main point of the presentation will help you stay focused and convey a clear message to the audience.
- **Determine the output.** To help decide the type of output needed, consider the availability of equipment, the size of the room where you will make the presentation, and the number of people who will be attending the presentation.
- **Show one idea per slide.** Each slide in a presentation should convey only one main idea. Too many ideas on a slide may confuse the audience and cause you to stray from the purpose of the slide.

- **Maintain a consistent design.** A consistent design and color scheme for slides in a presentation will create continuity and cohesiveness. Do not use too much color or too many images or other graphic elements.
- **Keep slides uncluttered and easy to read.** Keep slides simple to make them easy for your audience to understand. Keep words and other items, such as bullets, to a minimum.
- **Determine printing needs.** Will you be providing audience members with handouts? If so, will these handouts consist of a printing of each slide? an outline of the presentation? a printing of each slide with space for taking notes?

Open an existing presentation by displaying the Open backstage area and then clicking the presentation in the *Recent* option list. You can also open a presentation at the Open dialog box. Display the Open dialog box by clicking the File tab and then clicking the *Open* option. At the Open backstage area, click the *Browse* option. Navigate through slides in a presentation with buttons on the vertical scroll bar, by clicking slide thumbnails in Normal view, or by using keys on the keyboard. Insert a new slide with a specific layout by clicking the New Slide button arrow in the Slides group on the Home tab and then clicking the desired layout at the drop-down list. Choose the layout that matches the type of text or object you want to insert in the slide.

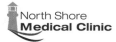
North Shore
Medical Clinic

What You Will Do Dr. St. Claire has asked you to add more information to the diabetes presentation. You will insert a new slide between the third and fourth slides in the presentation and another at the end of the presentation.

Tutorial
Opening from a
Removable Disk

Tutorial
Navigating to Slides

Tutorial
Choosing a Slide
Layout

Tutorial
Saving with the Same
Name

1 Click the File tab and then click the *Open* option.

2 At the Open backstage area, click the *Browse* option.

3 In the Navigation pane of the Open dialog box, click the drive where your storage medium is located (such as *Removable Disk (F:)*).

> You can also display the Open dialog box without displaying the Open backstage area by pressing Ctrl + F12.

4 Double-click the *PowerPointMedS1* folder in the Content pane.

5 Double-click *1-Diabetes.pptx* in the Content pane.

6 With **1-Diabetes.pptx** open, click the Next Slide button near the bottom of the vertical scroll bar.

> Clicking this button displays the next slide, Slide 2, in the presentation. Notice that *Slide 2 of 4* displays at the left side of the Status bar.

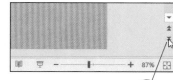

Step 6

7 Click the Previous Slide button ⏫ near the bottom of the vertical scroll bar to display Slide 1.

> When you click the Previous Slide button, Slide 1 displays in the slide pane and *Slide 1 of 4* displays at the left side of the Status bar.

8 Display Slide 3 in the slide pane by clicking the third slide in the slide thumbnails pane (the slide titled *Types of Diabetes*).

9 Insert a new slide between Slides 3 and 4 by clicking the New Slide button in the Slides group on the Home tab.

> When you select a slide in the slide thumbnails pane and then click the New Slide button, the new slide is inserted after the selected slide.

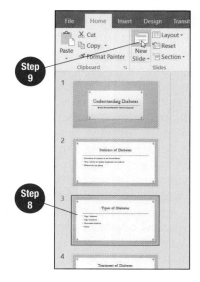

Step 9

Step 8

10 Click in the *Click to add title* placeholder in the slide in the slide pane and then type Symptoms of Diabetes.

In Brief

Open Presentation from Removable Disk
1. Press Ctrl + F12.
2. In the Navigation pane of the Open dialog box, click the drive containing the removable disk.
3. Double-click folder in Content pane.
4. Double-click presentation in Content pane.

11. Click in the *Click to add text* placeholder in the slide and then type the bulleted text as shown at the right. Press the Enter key after each item except the last item.

12. Click below the Slide 1 thumbnail in the slide thumbnails pane.

   When you click below the slide thumbnail, an orange horizontal line displays between Slides 1 and 2.

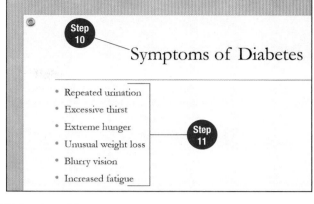

13. Click the New Slide button arrow on the Home tab and then click the *Title Slide* option at the drop-down list.

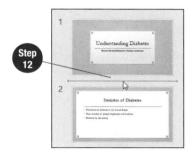
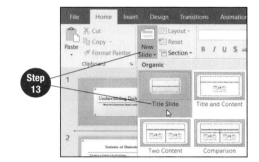

14. Click in the *Click to add title* placeholder and then type What is Diabetes?

15. Click in the *Click to add subtitle* placeholder and then type the text shown at the right.

16. Make Slide 6 active in the slides pane.

17. Click the New Slide button arrow and then click the *Title Only* option at the drop-down list.

18. Click in the *Click to add title* placeholder and then type Discussing Diabetes.

19. Save **1-Diabetes.pptx**.

Check Your Work Compare your work with the model answer to ensure that you have completed the activity correctly.

In Addition

Opening a Presentation from the *Recent* Option List

At the Open backstage area with the *Recent* option selected, a list of the most recently opened presentations displays. The presentations are grouped into categories such as *Today*, *Yesterday*, and possibly *This Week*, *Last Week*, and *Older*. To open a presentation from the *Recent* option list, open PowerPoint to display the opening screen or display the Open backstage area with the *Recent* option selected and then click the desired presentation.

Activity 1.4 Changing Views

PowerPoint provides different viewing options for a presentation. Change the presentation view with buttons in the Presentation Views group on the View tab or in the view area on the Status bar. Normal view is the default view, and you can change the view to Outline view, Slide Sorter view, Notes Page view, or Reading view. Choose the view based on the type of activity you are performing in the presentation. Another method for entering text in a slide is in Outline view. When Outline view is active, the slide thumbnails pane changes to an outline pane for entering text. Insert speaker's notes into a presentation using the notes pane, which can be displayed by clicking the Notes button on the Status bar.

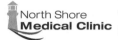
North Shore **Medical Clinic**

What You Will Do   After reviewing the diabetes presentation, Dr. St. Claire has asked you to edit a slide and add a new slide.

Tutorial
Changing Views

Tutorial
Entering Text in the Outline Pane

Tutorial
Changing the Display of a Slide in the Slide Pane

1 With **1-Diabetes.pptx** open, click the View tab and then click the Outline View button in the Presentation Views group.

2 In the third slide, click immediately to the right of the text *Total number of people diagnosed with diabetes*.

3 Press the Enter key and then type Total number of people with undiagnosed diabetes.

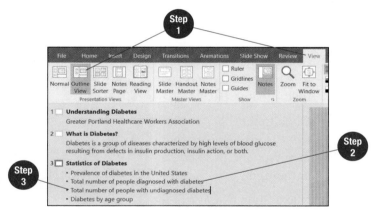

4 Make Slide 4 the active slide, click anywhere in the text *Click to add notes* in the notes pane, and then type Discuss other types of diabetes resulting from surgery, drugs, malnutrition, and infection.

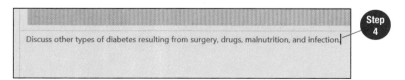

5 Display the slides in Notes Page view by clicking the Notes Page button in the Presentation Views group on the View tab.

> In Notes Page view, an individual slide displays on a page with any added notes displayed below the slide. Notice the note you created about other diabetes displays below the slide in the page.

6 Click the Previous Slide button on the vertical scroll bar until Slide 1 displays.

In Brief

Display in Normal View
1. Click View tab.
2. Click Normal button.
OR
Click Normal button on Status bar.

Display in Outline View
1. Click View tab.
2. Click Outline View button.

Display in Slide Sorter View
1. Click View tab.
2. Click Slide Sorter button.
OR
Click Slide Sorter button on Status bar.

Display in Notes Page View
1. Click View tab.
2. Click Notes Page button.

7. Increase the zoom by clicking the Zoom button in the Zoom group on the View tab, clicking the *100%* option at the Zoom dialog box, and then clicking OK.

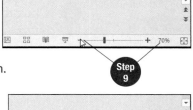

8. You can also change the zoom by using the Zoom slider bar. Position the mouse pointer on the Zoom slider bar button at the right side of the Status bar. Click and hold down the left mouse button, drag to the right until the zoom percentage at the left side of the Zoom slider bar displays as *138%*, and then release the mouse button.

9. Click the Zoom Out button — at the left side of the Zoom slider bar until *70%* displays at the right side of the slider bar.

> Click the Zoom Out button to decrease the zoom and click the Zoom In button + to increase the zoom.

10. View all slides in the presentation as thumbnails by clicking the Slide Sorter button in the view area on the Status bar.

11. View the presentation in Reading view by clicking the Reading View button in the Presentation Views group.

> Use Reading view to show a presentation to someone viewing the presentation on his or her own computer. You can also use Reading view to make it easier to navigate within a presentation. In Reading view, navigation buttons display in the lower right corner of the screen, immediately to the left of the view area on the Status bar.

12. View the presentation in Reading view by clicking the left mouse button until a black screen displays. At the black screen, click the mouse button again.

> This returns the presentation to the previous view—in this case, Slide Sorter view.

13. Return the presentation to Normal view by clicking the Normal button in the Presentation Views group.

14. If necessary, close the notes pane by clicking the Notes button on the Status bar.

15. Save **1-Diabetes.pptx**.

Check Your Work Compare your work with the model answer to ensure that you have completed the activity correctly.

In Addition

Navigating Using the Keyboard

You can also use the keyboard to display slides in a presentation. In Normal view, press the Down Arrow or Page Down key to display the next slide, or press the Up Arrow or Page Up key to display the previous slide in the presentation. Press the Home key to display the first slide in the presentation and press the End key to display the last slide in the presentation. Navigate in Outline view and Slide Sorter view by using the arrow keys on the keyboard. Navigate in Reading view by using the Right Arrow key to move to the next slide and the Left Arrow key to move to the previous slide.

Changing the Slide Layout; Selecting and Moving a Placeholder

So far, you have created slides based on a default slide layout. Change the slide layout by clicking the Layout button in the Slides group on the Home tab and then clicking the desired layout at the drop-down list. Objects in a slide, such as text, charts, tables, or other graphic elements, are generally positioned in placeholders. Click the text or object to select the placeholder, and a dashed border will surround the placeholder. You can move, size, and/or delete a selected placeholder.

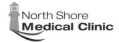

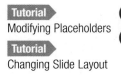

North Shore Medical Clinic

What You Will Do   You have decided to make a few changes to the layout of the slides in the diabetes presentation.

Tutorial
Modifying Placeholders

Tutorial
Changing Slide Layout

1 With **1-Diabetes.pptx** open, make Slide 2 the active slide.

2 Click the Home tab, click the Layout button in the Slides group, and then click the *Title Only* option at the drop-down list.

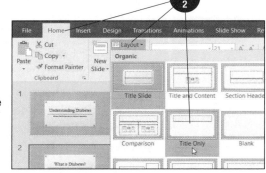

> Position the mouse pointer on an option in the drop-down list and the name of the layout displays in a box. When you click the *Title Only* layout, the text is moved down in the slide and a bullet is inserted before the text describing diabetes.

3 Click in the text describing diabetes to display the placeholder borders.

4 Move the placeholder by positioning the mouse pointer on the border of the placeholder until the mouse pointer displays with a four-headed arrow attached, clicking and holding down the left mouse button, dragging to the left until the text is positioned as shown in Figure P1.2, and then releasing the mouse button.

5 Click in the title *What is Diabetes?* and then move the title. To do this, position the mouse pointer on the border of the placeholder until the mouse pointer displays with a four-headed arrow attached, click and hold down the left mouse button, drag down until the title is positioned as shown in Figure P1.2, and then release the mouse button.

6 Click the Next Slide button on the vertical scroll bar until Slide 4 displays.

7 Click anywhere in the bulleted text to display the placeholder border.

Figure P1.2 Slide 2

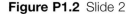

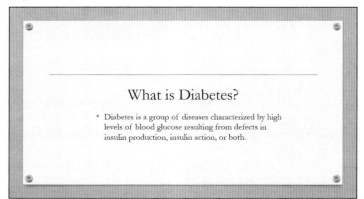

Change Slide Layout
1. Make slide active.
2. Click Home tab.
3. Click Layout button.
4. Click layout option.

Move Placeholder
1. Click in placeholder.
2. Drag border with mouse to new position.

Size Placeholder
1. Click inside placeholder.
2. Drag sizing handles to increase or decrease size.

8 Decrease the size of the placeholder by positioning the mouse pointer on the bottom right sizing handle (displays as a white circle) until the arrow pointer turns into a diagonal double-headed arrow.

9 Click and hold down the left mouse button, drag up and to the left until the placeholder displays as shown below, and then release the mouse button.

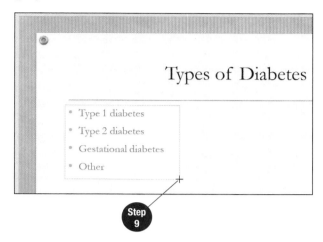

Step 9

10 Move the placeholder by positioning the mouse pointer on the border of the placeholder until the mouse pointer displays with a four-headed arrow attached, clicking and holding down the left mouse button, dragging to the right to the approximate location shown at the right, and then releasing the mouse button.

11 Click outside the placeholder to deselect it.

12 Save **1-Diabetes.pptx**.

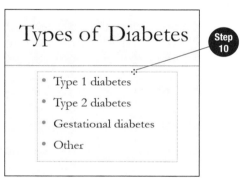

Step 10

Check Your Work Compare your work with the model answer to ensure that you have completed the activity correctly.

In Addition

Using the AutoFit Options Button

If you decrease the size of a placeholder so the existing text does not fit within it, PowerPoint will automatically decrease the size of the text so it fits in the placeholder. If you click anywhere in the text that has been decreased in size, an AutoFit Options button displays at the left side of the placeholder. Click the AutoFit Options button and a list of choices displays for positioning objects in the placeholder, as shown at the right. The *AutoFit Text to Placeholder* option is selected by default and tells PowerPoint to fit text within the boundaries of the placeholder. Click the middle choice, *Stop Fitting Text to This Placeholder*, and PowerPoint will

not automatically fit the text or object within the placeholder. Choose the last option, *Control AutoCorrect Options*, to display the AutoCorrect dialog box with the AutoFormat As You Type tab selected. Additional options may display depending upon the placeholder and the type of data it contains.

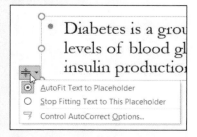

Activity 1.6   Rearranging, Deleting, and Hiding Slides

As you edit a presentation, you may need to rearrange, delete, or hide specific slides. PowerPoint provides various views for creating and managing a presentation. Manage slides in the slide thumbnails pane or in Slide Sorter view. Switch to Slide Sorter view by clicking the Slide Sorter button in the view area on the Status bar or by clicking the View tab and then clicking the Slide Sorter button in the Presentation Views group.

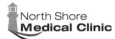
North Shore
Medical Clinic

Tutorial
Rearranging Slides

Tutorial
Deleting Slides

Tutorial
Hiding and Unhiding Slides

What You Will Do   Dr. St. Claire has asked you to make some changes to the presentation, including rearranging the slides, deleting a slide, and hiding a slide.

1   With **1-Diabetes.pptx** open, click Slide 7 in the slide thumbnails pane and then press the Delete key on the keyboard.

> You can also delete a slide by right-clicking the slide in the slide thumbnails pane and then clicking *Delete Slide* at the shortcut menu.

2   Click the Slide Sorter button in the view area on the Status bar.

3   Click Slide 5 to make it active.

> A selected slide displays with an orange border.

4   Position the mouse pointer on Slide 5, click and hold down the left mouse button, drag the slide (the arrow pointer will display with a square attached) to the left of Slide 3, and then release the mouse button.

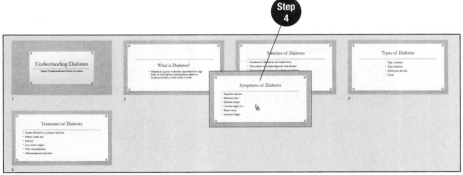

Step 4

5   Click the Normal button in the view area on the Status bar.

6   Position the mouse pointer on the Slide 5 thumbnail in the slide thumbnails pane, click and hold down the left mouse button, drag up until the slide displays immediately below the Slide 2 thumbnail, and then release the mouse button.

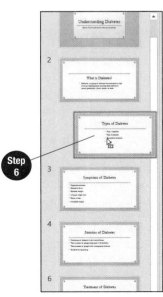

Step 6

Delete Slide
1. Click slide in slide thumbnails pane.
2. Press Delete key.
OR
1. Right-click slide thumbnail.
2. Click *Delete Slide*.

Move Slide
1. Click Slide Sorter button on Status bar.
2. Click slide.
3. Drag slide to new position.
OR
1. Click slide in slide thumbnails pane.
2. Drag slide to new position.

Hide Slide
1. Click slide thumbnail.
2. Click Slide Show tab.
3. Click Hide Slide button.

7 With the Slide 3 thumbnail selected in the slide thumbnails pane (thumbnail displays with an orange border), hide the slide by clicking the Slide Show tab and then clicking the Hide Slide button 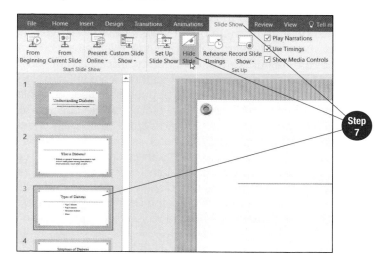 in the Set Up group.

When a slide is hidden, the slide thumbnail displays dimmed and the slide number displays with a diagonal line across it.

8 Run the slide show by clicking the From Beginning button 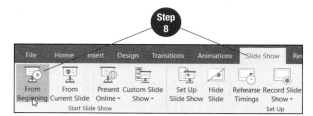 in the Start Slide Show group. Click the left mouse button to advance each slide until a black screen displays. At the black screen, click the left mouse button again.

9 After running the slide show, you decide to redisplay the hidden slide. To do this, make sure the Slide 3 thumbnail is selected in the slide thumbnails pane and then click the Hide Slide button in the Set Up group.

10 Save **1-Diabetes.pptx**.

Check Your Work Compare your work with the model answer to ensure that you have completed the activity correctly.

In Addition

Copying Slides within a Presentation

Copying a slide within a presentation is similar to moving a slide. To copy a slide, position the arrow pointer on the desired slide, press and hold down the Ctrl key, and then click and hold down the left mouse button. Drag to the location where you want the slide copied, release the left mouse button, and then release the Ctrl key. When you drag with the mouse, the mouse pointer displays with a square and a plus symbol attached.

PowerPoint includes the Tell Me feature, which provides information on a function as well as guidance on how to complete it. To use Tell Me, click in the *Tell Me* text box that displays on the ribbon to the right of the View tab and then type the function for which you want help. As you type a search phrase in the *Tell Me* text box, a drop-down list displays with options that are refined as you continue typing. The drop-down list will have options for completing the function, displaying the top three help links most related to the search, or displaying the Help task pane. The Help task pane can also be displayed by pressing the F1 function key on the keyboard. Use PowerPoint's spelling checker to find and correct misspelled words and duplicated words (such as *and and*). The spelling checker compares words in your slides with words in its dictionary. If a match is found, the word is passed over. If no match is found, the spelling checker stops, selects the word, and offers replacements. Use the Thesaurus to find synonyms, antonyms, and related words for a particular word. To use the Thesaurus, click the word for which you want to display synonyms and antonyms, click the Review tab, and then click the Thesaurus button in the Proofing group. This displays the Thesaurus task pane with information about the word in which the insertion point is positioned.

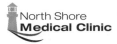
North Shore
Medical Clinic

What You Will Do To enhance the appearance of Slide 1 in the presentation, you will use the Tell Me feature to change the font color of the title. Because several changes have been made to the presentation, you know that checking the spelling of all the slide text is important, but you are not sure how to do it. You will use the Help feature to learn how to complete a spelling check and then use the Thesaurus to replace two words with synonyms.

Tutorial ▶
Using the Tell Me Feature

Tutorial ▶
Using the Help Feature

Tutorial ▶
Checking Spelling

Tutorial ▶
Using the Thesaurus

1 With **1-Diabetes.pptx** open, make Slide 1 the active slide, click in the title *Understanding Diabetes*, and then click the border of the placeholder to select it.

2 Click in the *Tell Me* text box and then type font color.

> The *Tell Me* text box is on the ribbon to the right of the View tab and contains the text *Tell me what you want to do*. When you click in the text box, the last five functions entered will display in a drop-down list.

3 Position the mouse pointer on the arrow at the right of the *Font Color* option in the drop-down list and then click the *Dark Red, Accent 6* option (last column, first row in the *Theme Colors* section) at the side menu that displays.

> The font color of the title changes to a dark red color.

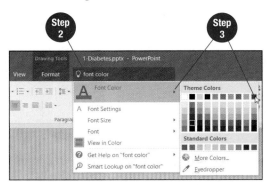

4 Display Slide 6 in the slide pane and then click the New Slide button in the Slides group on the Home tab.

> This inserts a new slide at the end of the presentation.

Figure P1.3 Slide 7

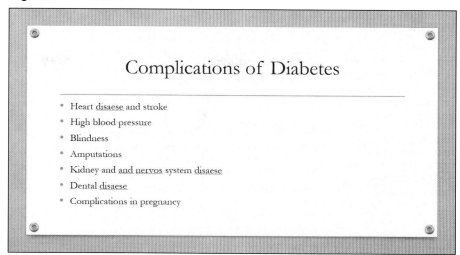

⑤ Click in the *Click to add title* placeholder and then type Complications of Diabetes.

⑥ Click in the *Click to add text* placeholder and then type the text shown in Figure P1.3.

Type the words exactly as shown. You will check the spelling in a later step. If Word's AutoCorrect feature automatically changes the word *disaese* to the correct spelling *disease*, immediately press Ctrl + Z (the Undo command) to return the word to the incorrect spelling.

⑦ Learn how to complete a spelling check. Start by pressing the F1 function key to display the Help task pane.

⑧ At the Help task pane, click in the search text box, type check spelling, and then press the Enter key.

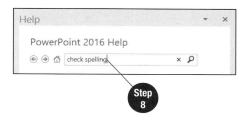

⑨ Click a hyperlink in the Help task pane that will display information on checking spelling.

⑩ Read the information about checking spelling and then click the Close button ☒ in the upper right corner of the Help task pane.

⑪ Complete a spelling check by moving the insertion point to the beginning of the word *Heart*, clicking the Review tab, and then clicking the Spelling button in the Proofing group.

⑫ When the spelling checker selects *disaese* in Slide 7 and displays *disease* in the list box in the Spelling task pane, click the Change All button.

Refer to Table P1.3 for a description of the buttons in the Spelling task pane.

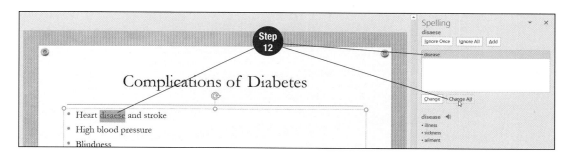

Table P1.3 Buttons in the Spelling Task Pane

Button	Function
Ignore Once	skips that occurrence of the word and leaves currently selected text as written
Ignore All	skips that occurrence of the word and all other occurrences of the word in the presentation
Delete	deletes the currently selected word(s)
Change	replaces the selected word with the selected word in the suggestions list box
Change All	replaces the selected word and all other occurrences of the word in the presentation with the selected word in the suggestions list box
Add	adds the selected word to the main spelling check dictionary

13 When the spelling checker selects *and* in Slide 7, click the Delete button.

14 When the spelling checker selects *nervos* in Slide 7, click *nervous* in the list box in the Spelling task pane and then click the Change button.

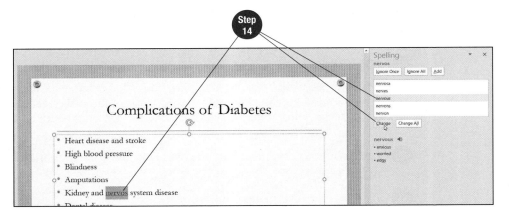

15 At the message telling you that the spelling check is complete, click OK.

16 Display Slide 4 in the slide pane and then click the word *Repeated* in the first bulleted item (*Repeated urination*).

17 Look up synonyms for *Repeated* by clicking the Thesaurus button in the Proofing group on the Review tab.

The Thesaurus task pane displays at the right side of the screen and contains lists of synonyms for *Repeated*. Depending on the word you are looking up, the words in the Thesaurus task pane list box may display followed by *(n.)* for *noun*, *(adj.)* for *adjective*, or *(adv.)* for *adverb*. Antonyms may also display, generally at the end of the list of related synonyms, followed by the word *(Antonym)*.

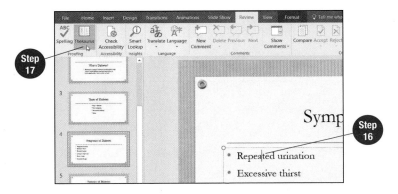

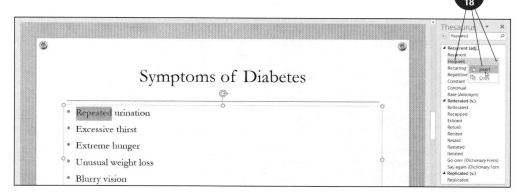

18 Position the mouse pointer on the word *Frequent* in the Thesaurus task pane, click the down arrow at the right of the word, and then click *Insert* at the drop-down list.

This replaces *Repeated* with *Frequent*.

19 Close the Thesaurus task pane by clicking the Close button in the upper right corner of the task pane.

20 Display Slide 7 in the slide pane, right-click the word *Complications* in the last bulleted item, point to *Synonyms* at the shortcut menu, and then click *Difficulties* at the side menu.

The shortcut menu offers another way to display synonyms of words.

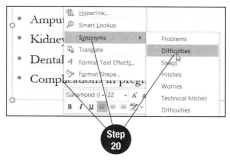

21 Save **1-Diabetes.pptx**.

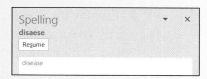

Check Your Work Compare your work with the model answer to ensure that you have completed the activity correctly.

In Addition

Changing Spelling Options

Control spelling options at the PowerPoint Options dialog box with the *Proofing* option selected. Display this dialog box by clicking the File tab and then clicking *Options*. At the PowerPoint Options dialog box, click *Proofing* at the left side of the dialog box. With options in the dialog box, you can tell the spelling checker to ignore certain types of text, create custom dictionaries, and hide the red, wavy lines that indicate spelling errors in the presentation.

Editing While Checking Spelling

When checking the spelling in a presentation, you can temporarily leave the Spelling task pane by clicking in the slide. To resume the spelling check, click the Resume button in the Spelling task pane, as shown below.

You can run a slide show in PowerPoint manually, advance the slides automatically, or set up a slide show to run continuously for demonstration purposes. In addition to the Start From Beginning button on the Quick Access Toolbar, you can run a slide show with the From Beginning button on the Slide Show tab or the Slide Show button on the Status bar. Run the slide show beginning with the currently active slide by clicking the From Current Slide button in the Start Slide Show group or clicking the Slide Show button in the view area. Use the mouse or keyboard to advance through the slides. You can also use buttons on the Slide Show toolbar that displays when you move the mouse pointer while running a slide show. Use the pen tool to emphasize major points or draw the attention of the audience to specific items in a slide during a slide show. To use the pen tool on a slide, run the slide show, and when the desired slide displays, move the mouse to display the Slide Show toolbar. Click the Pen button on the toolbar and then click *Pen*. Use the mouse to underline, circle, or otherwise emphasize specific text in the slide. Options at the Pen button drop-down list also include a laser pointer, highlighter, and eraser. You can also write and highlight on a slide in Normal view with options on the Ink Tools Pens tab. Display this tab by clicking the Start Inking button in the Ink group on the Review tab. This feature is useful when using a pen, stylus, or finger to draw on a tablet.

North Shore
Medical Clinic

What You Will Do   You are now ready to run the diabetes slide show. You will use the mouse to perform various actions while running the slide show and use the pen tool and ink tools to emphasize points in slides.

Tutorial
Running a Slide Show

Tutorial
Changing the Display when Running a Slide Show

Tutorial
Displaying Slide Show Help and Hiding Slides during a Slide Show

Tutorial
Using the Pen Tool during a Slide Show

Tutorial
Using Ink Tools

1   With **1-Diabetes.pptx** open, click the Slide Show tab and then click the From Beginning button in the Start Slide Show group.

> Clicking this button begins the slide show, and Slide 1 fills the entire screen.

2   After viewing Slide 1, click the left mouse button to advance to the next slide.

3   After viewing Slide 2, click the left mouse button to advance to the next slide.

4   At Slide 3, move the mouse pointer until the Slide Show toolbar displays dimmed in the lower left corner of the slide and then click the Previous button (displays as a left arrow) on the toolbar to display the previous slide (Slide 2).

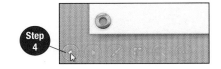

> With buttons on the Slide Show toolbar, you can display the next slide, the previous slide, or another specific slide; use the pen, laser pointer, and highlighter to emphasize text on the slide; display slide thumbnails; and zoom in on elements of a slide. You can also display the Slide Show Help dialog box, shown in Figure P1.4, which describes all the navigation options available while running a slide show. Display this dialog box by clicking the More slide show options button on the Slide Show toolbar and then clicking *Help* at the pop-up list.

5   Click the right arrow button on the Slide Show toolbar to display the next slide (Slide 3).

6   Display the previous slide (Slide 2) by right-clicking anywhere in the slide and then clicking *Previous* at the shortcut menu.

> Right-clicking displays a shortcut menu with a variety of options, including options to display the previous or next slide.

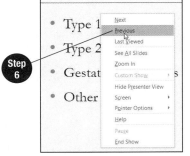

Figure P1.4 Slide Show Help Dialog Box

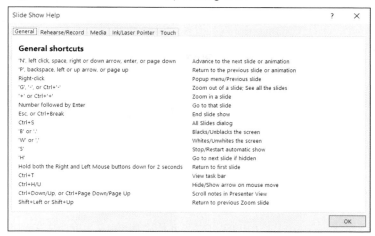

7. Display Slide 5 by pressing the number 5 key and then pressing the Enter key.

   Move to any slide in a presentation by typing the slide number and then pressing the Enter key.

8. Change to a black screen by pressing the letter B on the keyboard.

   When you type the letter B, the slide is removed from the screen and the screen displays black. This might be useful in a situation where you want to discuss something with your audience that is unrelated to the slide.

9. Return to Slide 5 by pressing the letter B on the keyboard.

   Pressing the letter B switches between the slide and a black screen. Press the letter W if you want to switch between the slide and a white screen.

10. Zoom in on the bulleted items in Slide 5 by clicking the Zoom into the slide button (displays as a magnifying glass) on the Slide Show toolbar, hovering the magnification area over the bulleted items, and then clicking the left mouse button.

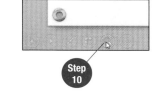

11. Right-click anywhere on the screen to display Slide 5 without magnification.

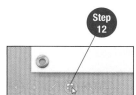

12. Display thumbnails of all the slides in the presentation while viewing the slide show by clicking the See all slides button on the Slide Show toolbar.

13. Click the Slide 3 thumbnail on the screen.

    This displays Slide 3 in the slide show.

14. Click the left mouse button to display Slide 4. Continue clicking the left mouse button until a black screen displays. At the black screen, click the left mouse button again.

    This returns the presentation to Normal view.

15. Click Slide 2 in the slide thumbnails pane.

16. Click the From Current Slide button in the Start Slide Show group on the Slide Show tab.

    Clicking this button starts the slide show from the active slide.

17. Run the slide show by clicking the left mouse button at each slide until Slide 5 is active (contains the title *Statistics of Diabetes*).

18 Move the mouse to display the Slide Show toolbar, click the Pen button, and then click *Laser Pointer* at the pop-up list.

> This turns the mouse pointer into a red, hollow, glowing circle.

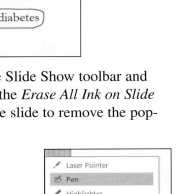

19 Practice moving the laser pointer around the screen.

20 Click the Pen button on the Slide Show toolbar and then click *Pen*.

> This turns the mouse pointer into a small circle.

21 Using the mouse, draw a circle around the text *Total number of people with undiagnosed diabetes*.

22 Using the mouse, draw a line under *Diabetes by age group*.

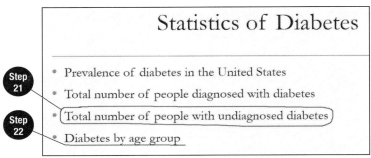

23 Erase the pen markings by clicking the Pen button on the Slide Show toolbar and then clicking *Erase All Ink on Slide* at the pop-up list. If the *Erase All Ink on Slide* option is dimmed so that you cannot access it, click in the slide to remove the pop-up list and then click the Pen button again.

24 Change the color of the ink by clicking the Pen button and then clicking the *Blue* option at the pop-up list (third option from the right).

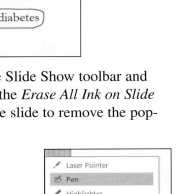

25 Draw a blue line under the words *United States*.

26 Return the mouse pointer back to an arrow by pressing the Esc key.

27 Click the left mouse button to advance to Slide 6.

28 Click the Pen button and then click *Highlighter* at the pop-up list.

> This changes the mouse pointer to a light yellow rectangle.

29 Using the mouse, drag through the words *Insulin delivered by a pump or injection* to highlight them.

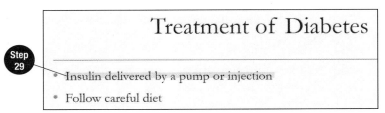

30 Return the mouse pointer back to an arrow by pressing the Esc key.

31 Press the Esc key on the keyboard to end the slide show without viewing the remaining slides. At the message asking if you want to keep your ink annotations, click the Discard button.

32 Make Slide 3 the active slide and then draw a circle around text to display when running a slide show. Begin by clicking the Review tab and then clicking the Start Inking button 🖊 in the Ink group.

> The Ink Tools Pens tab will display with options for writing or highlighting on a slide. This feature is particularly useful for tablets. The mouse pointer will display as a small circle.

33 Click the aqua highlighter option in the seventh column, first row of the Pens gallery.

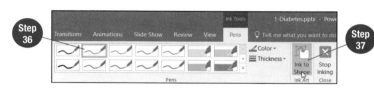

34 Using the mouse, drag through the words *Type 1 diabetes*.

35 Using the mouse, drag through the words *Type 2 diabetes*.

36 Click the red pen option in the second column, first row of the Pens gallery.

37 Click the Ink to Shape button 🗒 in the Ink Art group.

38 Using the mouse, draw a rectangle around the text *Gestational diabetes*.

> Notice that PowerPoint automatically converted the drawn rectangle into a more precise rectangle with a light red fill color. Since the drawn rectangle was converted to a shape, the Ink Tools Pens tab closes and the Drawing Tools Format tab becomes active. If you are not satisfied with the appearance of the rectangle, click the Undo button on the Quick Access Toolbar two times, click the Ink Tools Pens tab, click the Pen button 🖊 in the Write group, and then draw the rectangle again.

39 Click anywhere in the slide to deselect the rectangle.

40 Click the Slide Show button in the view area on the Status bar.

41 Notice that the aqua highlighting and red rectangle display on the slide and then press the Esc key to return the presentation to Normal view.

42 Save **1-Diabetes.pptx**.

Check Your Work ▶ Compare your work with the model answer to ensure that you have completed the activity correctly.

In Addition

Hiding and Displaying the Mouse Pointer

When running a slide show, the mouse pointer is set, by default, to be hidden after three seconds of inactivity. The mouse pointer will appear again when you move the mouse. Change this default setting by clicking the More slide show options button on the Slide Show toolbar, clicking *Arrow Options*, and then clicking *Visible* if you want the mouse pointer to always be visible or *Hidden* if you do not want the mouse to display at all as you run the slide show. The *Automatic* option is the default setting.

You can apply a variety of transitions and transition sounds to a presentation. A transition is how one slide is removed from the screen during a slide show and the next slide is displayed. Interesting transitions, such as fades, dissolves, push, cover, wipes, stripes, and bar can add interest to your presentation. You can also insert a sound that you want to play as one slide is removed from the screen and the next slide is displayed. Add transitions and transition sounds with options on the Transitions tab.

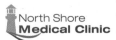
North Shore
Medical Clinic

What You Will Do   Dr. St. Claire has asked you to enhance the presentation by adding transitions and transition sounds to the slides.

Tutorial ▶
Adding Transitions

Tutorial ▶
Adding Sound to Slide Transitions

1   With **1-Diabetes.pptx** open, click the Transitions tab.

2   Click the More Transitions button at the right side of the transition thumbnails in the Transition to This Slide group.

3   Click the *Cube* option in the *Exciting* section of the drop-down list.

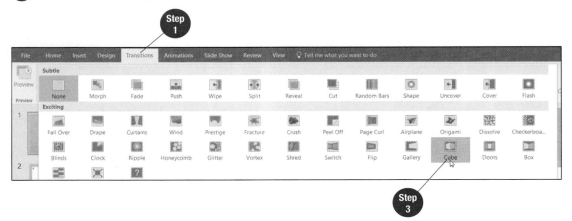

4   Click the Effect Options button [⬜] in the Transition to This Slide group and then click *From Top* at the drop-down list.

The available effect options change depending on the transition selected.

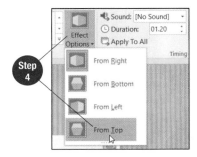

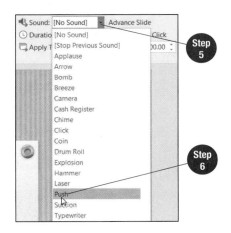

5   Click the *Sound* option box arrow in the Timing group.

6   Click the *Push* option at the drop-down list.

7 Apply three seconds to each slide transition by clicking in the *Duration* measurement box, typing 3, and then pressing the Enter key.

8 Click the Apply To All button 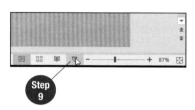 in the Timing group.

Notice that Play Animation star icons display below the slide numbers in the slide thumbnails pane.

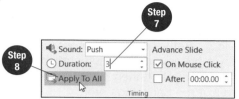

9 Run the slide show by clicking the Slide Show button in the view area on the Status bar.

10 Click the left mouse button to advance each slide.

11 At the black screen that displays after the last slide, click the left mouse button to return the presentation to Normal view.

12 Click the More Transitions button in the Transition to This Slide group.

13 Click the *Wind* option in the *Exciting* section of the drop-down list.

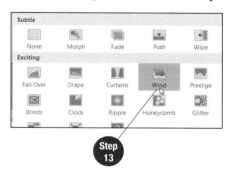

14 Click the *Sound* option box arrow and then click *Wind* at the drop-down list.

15 Click the *Duration* measurement box down arrow until *01.25* displays.

16 Click the Apply To All button in the Timing group.

17 With Slide 1 active, run the slide show.

18 Save **1-Diabetes.pptx**.

In Addition

Running a Slide Show Automatically

Slides in a slide show can be advanced automatically after a specific number of seconds by inserting a check mark in the *After* check box in the Timing group and removing the check mark from the *On Mouse Click* check box. Change the time in the *After* measurement box by clicking the *After* measurement box up or down arrows or by selecting the text in the measurement box and then typing the specific time. If you want the transition time to affect all slides in the presentation, click the Apply To All button. In Slide Sorter view, the transition time displays below each affected slide. Click the Slide Show button to run the slide show. The first slide displays for the specified amount of time and then the next slide automatically displays.

Activity 1.10 Previewing and Printing a Presentation

You can print each slide in a presentation on a separate piece of paper; print each slide at the top of a separate page, leaving the bottom of the page for notes; print up to nine slides or a specific number of slides on a single piece of paper; or print the slide titles and topics in outline form. Before printing a presentation, consider previewing it. Choose print options and display a preview of the presentation in the Print backstage area. Display this view by clicking the File tab and then clicking the *Print* option. Click the Back button or press the Esc key to exit the backstage area.

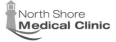
North Shore
Medical Clinic

What You Will Do   Dr. St. Claire needs the slides in the diabetes presentation printed as handouts and as an outline. You will preview and then print the presentation in various formats.

Tutorial
Previewing Slides and
Printing

① With **1-Diabetes.pptx** open, display Slide 1 in the slide pane.

② Click the File tab and then click the *Print* option.

> Slide 1 of the presentation displays at the right side of the screen as it will appear when printed. Use the Next Page button (right-pointing arrow) below and to the left of the preview slide to view the next slide in the presentation, click the Previous Page button (left-pointing arrow) to display the previous slide in the presentation, use the Zoom slider bar to increase or decrease the size of the slide, and click the Zoom to Page button to fit the slide in the viewing area of the Print backstage area. The left side of the Print backstage area displays three categories—*Print*, *Printer*, and *Settings*. Galleries display below each category name. For example, the *Printer* category has one gallery that displays the name of the currently selected printer. The *Settings* category has a number of galleries that describe how the slides will print.

③ Click the Next Page button below and to the left of the preview slide to display the next slide in the presentation.

> This displays Slide 2 in the preview area.

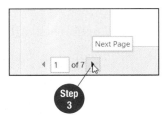

Step
3

④ Click the Zoom In button ➕ that displays at the right side of the Zoom slider bar two times.

> Clicking the Zoom In button increases the size of the slide, and clicking the Zoom Out button decreases the size of the slide.

⑤ Click the Zoom to Page button ⊡ at the right side of the Zoom slider bar.

> Click the Zoom to Page button to fit the entire slide in the viewing area of the Print backstage area.

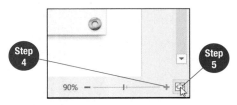

Step
4

Step
5

In Brief

Print Presentation
1. Click File tab.
2. Click *Print*.
3. At Print backstage area, specify printing options.
4. Click Print button.

Preview Presentation
1. Click File tab.
2. Click *Print*.
3. View preview in right side of Print backstage area.

6 You decide to create handouts with all of the slides printed on one page, but first you want to preview how the slides will appear on the page. To do this, click the second gallery in the *Settings* category (contains the text *Full Page Slides*) and then click *4 Slides Horizontal* in the *Handouts* section.

> Notice how four slides display on the preview page.

7 Click the Print button at the top of the Print backstage area.

8 You want to print all slide text on one page so that Dr. St. Claire can use the printout as a reference. To do this, click the File tab and then click the *Print* option.

9 At the Print backstage area, click the second gallery in the *Settings* category (contains the text *4 Slides Horizontal*) and then click *Outline* in the *Print Layout* section.

10 Click the Print button in the *Print* category.

> With the *Outline* option selected, the presentation prints on one page with slide numbers, slide icons, and slide text in outline form.

11 You need a printout of Slide 5. To do this, click the File tab and then click the *Print* option.

12 At the Print backstage area, click the second gallery in the *Settings* category (contains the text *Outline*) and then click *Full Page Slides* in the *Print Layout* section.

13 Click in the *Slides* text box below the first gallery in the *Settings* category, type 5, and then click the Print button.

14 Save **1-Diabetes.pptx**.

15 Close the presentation by clicking the File tab and then clicking the *Close* option.

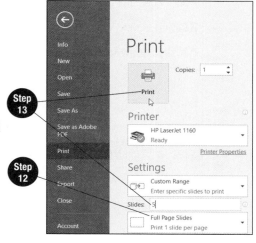

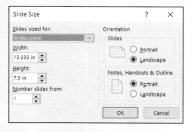

> **Check Your Work** Compare your work with the model answer to ensure that you have completed the activity correctly.

In Addition

Using Options at the Slide Size Dialog Box

You can change orientation at the Slide Size dialog box, shown at the right. Display this dialog box by clicking the Design tab, clicking the Slide Size button in the Customize group, and then clicking *Customize Slide Size* at the drop-down list. With options at this dialog box, you can specify slide size; page width and height; orientation for slides; and orientation for notes, handouts, and outlines.

Features Summary

Feature	Ribbon Tab, Group	Button	File Tab Option	Keyboard Shortcut
apply transitions and sound to all slides	Transitions, Timing			
close a presentation			*Close*	Ctrl + F4
close PowerPoint				
Help				F1
hide slide	Slide Show, Set Up			
ink tools	Review, Ink			
layout	Home, Slides			
new slide	Home, Slides OR Insert, Slides			Ctrl + M
Normal view	View, Presentation Views			
Notes Page view	View, Presentation Views			
Open backstage area			*Open*	Ctrl + O
open blank presentation				Ctrl + N
Outline view	View, Presentation Views			
Print backstage area			*Print*	Ctrl + P
Reading view	View, Presentation Views			
run slide show from current slide	Slide Show, Start Slide Show			Shift + F5
run slide show from Slide 1	Slide Show, Start Slide Show			F5
save			*Save*	Ctrl + S
Save As backstage area			*Save As*	F12
Slide Sorter view	View, Presentation Views			
spelling checker	Review, Proofing			F7
themes	Design, Themes			
Thesaurus	Review, Proofing			Shift + F7
transitions	Transitions, Transition to This Slide			
transition duration	Transitions, Timing			
transition sound	Transitions, Timing			
Zoom dialog box	View, Zoom			

PowerPoint

Editing Slides and Slide Elements

Skills

Data Files — Before beginning section work, copy the PowerPointMedS2 folder to your storage medium and then make PowerPointMedS2 the active folder.

- Increase and decrease the indent of text
- Select, cut, copy, and paste text
- Apply font and font effects
- Find and replace fonts
- Apply formatting with Format Painter
- Change alignment and line and paragraph spacing
- Draw text boxes and shapes

- Insert headers and footers
- Change the design theme, theme colors, and theme fonts
- Insert and format images
- Insert and format WordArt
- Insert and format a SmartArt graphic
- Apply an animation to an object in a slide

Precheck — Check your current skills to help focus your study of the skills taught in this section.

Activities Overview

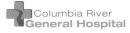

Open an existing presentation containing information on classes offered by the Education Department and then save, edit, and format the presentation; open an existing presentation containing information on the Community Commitment reorganization plan and then save, edit, and format the presentation.

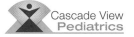

Open an existing presentation on opening a clinic in Vancouver, save the presentation with a new name, and then edit and format the presentation.

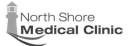

Open an existing presentation containing information on sickle cell anemia and then save, edit, and format the presentation; prepare a presentation on cholesterol.

Model Answers — Preview the model answers for an overview of the activities you will complete in each section.

Text that is formatted as a bulleted list in a slide can have multiple levels. Click the Increase List Level button in the Paragraph group or press the Tab key to demote text to the next level. Click the Decrease List Level button in the Paragraph group on the Home tab or press Shift + Tab to promote text to the previous level. You can also demote text levels (increase the text indent) and/or promote text levels (decrease the text indent) in the slide in Outline view.

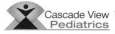 Cascade View Pediatrics

What You Will Do   The doctors at Cascade View Pediatrics are considering expanding by opening a clinic in the Vancouver, Washington, area. Dr. Severin has prepared a presentation with facts about Vancouver and has asked you to edit the presentation by increasing and decreasing the indent of text in slides.

Tutorial
Increasing and Decreasing Indent

1 Open **CVPVancouver.pptx** from the PowerPointMedS2 folder on your storage medium and then save it with the name **2-CVPVancouver**.

2 Display Slide 6 in the slide pane.

3 Looking at the text in Slide 6, you realize that the school names below *University of Portland* should not be indented. To decrease the indent and move them up to the previous list level, start by positioning the insertion point immediately to the left of the *C* in *Clark* and then clicking the Decrease List Level button in the Paragraph group on the Home tab.

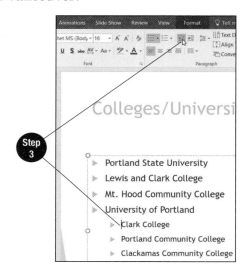

> You can also decrease the indent by pressing Shift + Tab.

4 Position the insertion point immediately to the left of the *P* in *Portland Community College* and then move the text to the previous level by pressing Shift + Tab.

5 Use steps similar to those in either Step 3 or Step 4 to move *Clackamas Community College* to the previous level.

6 Make Slide 2 active. Move the two bulleted items below *Estimated population* down to the next level by clicking immediately left of the *5* in *51%* and then clicking the Increase List Level button in the Paragraph group on the Home tab.

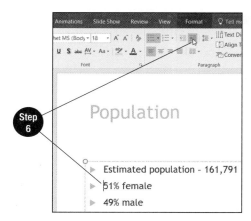

> You can also increase the indent by pressing the Tab key.

7 Position the insertion point immediately to the left of the *4* in *49%* and then press the Tab key.

8 Display Slide 4 in the slide pane.

9 Click the View tab and then click the Outline View button in the Presentation Views group.

10 Looking at Slide 4, you notice that the slide contains too much text. You decide to move some of it to a new slide. To do this, click immediately to the left of the *E* in *Employing* in the outline pane (previously the slide thumbnails pane) and then press Shift + Tab.

Pressing Shift + Tab moves the text to the previous level and creates a new slide with *Employing industries* as the title.

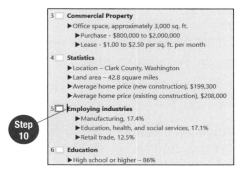

11 Change the title of the slide by typing Employment and then pressing the Enter key.

As you type *Employment*, the text *Employing industries* moves to the right. When you press the Enter key, *Employing industries* moves to the next line and begins a new slide.

12 Move the text *Employing industries* by pressing the Tab key.

The new slide now contains the title *Employment* with *Employing industries* as a bulleted item with three bulleted items below it.

13 Click the Normal button in the Presentation Views group on the View tab.

14 If necessary, click the Notes button on the Status bar to close the notes pane.

15 Save **2-CVPVancouver.pptx**.

Check Your Work Compare your work with the model answer to ensure that you have completed the activity correctly.

In Addition

Rearranging Text in Outline View

You can use the mouse to move text in the outline pane. To do this, position the mouse pointer on the slide icon or bullet at the left side of the text until the arrow pointer turns into a four-headed arrow. Click and hold down the left mouse button, drag the arrow pointer to the desired location (a thin horizontal line displays), and then release the mouse button. If you position the arrow pointer on the bullet and then click and hold down the left mouse button, all text following that bullet is selected. Dragging selected text with the mouse moves the text to a new location in the presentation. You can also copy selected text. To do this, click the slide icon or click the bullet to select the desired text. Position the arrow pointer in the selected text, press and hold down the Ctrl key, and then click and hold down the left mouse button. Drag the arrow pointer (displays with a light gray box and a plus sign attached) to the desired location, release the mouse button, and then release the Ctrl Key.

Selecting, Cutting, Copying, and Pasting Text

Text in a slide can be selected and then deleted from the slide, cut from one location and pasted into another, or copied from one location and pasted into another. Select text using the mouse or the keyboard. Use buttons in the Clipboard group on the Home tab to cut, copy, and paste text.

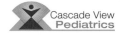

What You Will Do As you review the Vancouver presentation again, you decide to delete, move, and copy specific text items.

Tutorial
Selecting Text

Tutorial
Cutting, Copying, and Pasting Text

1 With **2-CVPVancouver.pptx** open, make sure the presentation displays in Normal view and then display Slide 7 in the slide pane.

2 Click anywhere in the bulleted text.

> Clicking in the bulleted text selects the placeholder containing the text.

3 Position the mouse pointer on the bullet that displays before *University of Portland* until the pointer turns into a four-headed arrow and then click the left mouse button.

> Refer to Table P2.1 for additional information on selecting text.

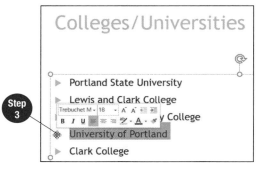

4 Click the Cut button ✂ in the Clipboard group on the Home tab.

5 Position the insertion point immediately to the left of the *L* in *Lewis and Clark College* and then click the Paste button 📋 in the Clipboard group.

6 Position the mouse pointer on the bullet that displays before *George Fox University* until the pointer turns into a four-headed arrow and then click the left mouse button.

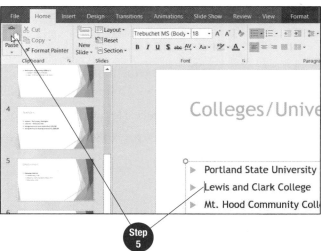

Table P2.1 Selecting Text

To select	Perform this action
entire word	Double-click word.
entire paragraph	Triple-click anywhere in paragraph.
text mouse pointer passes through	Click and drag with mouse.
all text in selected object box	Press Ctrl + A or click Select button in Editing group and then click *Select All*.

Cut and Paste Text
1. Select text.
2. Click Cut button.
3. Position insertion point.
4. Click Paste button.

Copy and Paste Text
1. Select text.
2. Click Copy button.
3. Position insertion point.
4. Click Paste button.

7 Click the Cut button in the Clipboard group.

8 Position the insertion point immediately to the left of the *L* in *Lewis and Clark College* and then click the Paste button in the Clipboard group.

9 Make Slide 6 active, move the insertion point so it is positioned immediately to the right of *7.4%*, and then press the Enter key.

10 Type Area Universities and then press the Enter key.

11 Make Slide 7 active; select *Portland State University*, *University of Portland*, and *George Fox University*; and then click the Copy button in the Clipboard group.

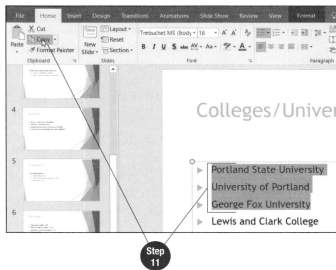

Step 11

When selecting the text, do not include the space after *George Fox University*. If you include the space, which is actually an invisible paragraph symbol, you will get an extra blank line when you paste the text.

12 Make Slide 6 active and then click below the heading *Area Universities*.

This selects the placeholder and positions the insertion point below the *Area Universities* heading.

13 Click the Paste button in the Clipboard group. If a blank line displays below *George Fox University*, press the Backspace key two times.

If a blank line displays below *George Fox University*, it means that the invisible paragraph symbol after the text was selected when copying.

14 Increase the indent of the universities' names by selecting the three names (*Portland State University*, *University of Portland*, and *George Fox University*) and then clicking the Increase List Level button in the Paragraph group on the Home tab.

15 Save **2-CVPVancouver.pptx**.

Check Your Work — Compare your work with the model answer to ensure that you have completed the activity correctly.

In Addition

Copying a Slide between Presentations

You can copy slides between presentations as well as within them. To copy a slide, click the slide you want to copy (either in Slide Sorter view or in the slide thumbnails pane in Normal view) and then click the Copy button in the Clipboard group on the Home tab. Open the presentation into which the slide is to be copied (in either Slide Sorter view or Normal view). Click in the location where you want the slide to be positioned and then click the Paste button. The copied slide will take on the formatting of the presentation into which it is pasted.

The Font group on the Home tab contains two rows of options and buttons. The top row contains options and buttons for changing the font and font size and a button for clearing formatting. The bottom row contains buttons for applying font effects such as bold, italic, underlining, text shadow, strikethrough, character spacing, and highlighting, as well as buttons for changing the case and/or font color of selected text.

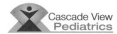
Cascade View Pediatrics

What You Will Do   As you continue working to improve the appearance of slides in the Vancouver presentation, you decide to apply font effects to specific text in the presentation.

Tutorial
Applying Font Formatting

1. With **2-CVPVancouver.pptx** open, display Slide 1 in the slide pane.

2. Select the text *Cascade View Pediatrics*, click the Bold button **B** in the Font group on the Home tab, and then click the Italic button **I**.

3. With the clinic name still selected, click the Decrease Font Size button **A** in the Font group.

4. Select the subtitle *Vancouver Clinic*, click the Bold button, and then click the Italic button.

5. With the subtitle still selected, click the Increase Font Size button **A** in the Font group two times.

6. Make Slide 2 active, select *161,791*, and then click the Underline button **U** in the Font group.

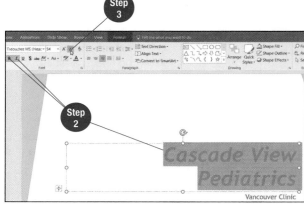

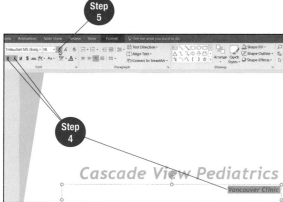

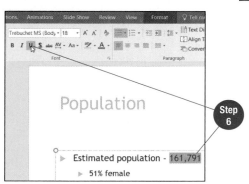

In Brief

Apply Font Effects with Font Group
1. Select text.
2. Click appropriate button in Font group.

Change Font
1. Select text or placeholder.
2. Click *Font* option box arrow.
3. Click font option.

Change Font Size
1. Select text or placeholder.
2. Click *Font Size* option box arrow.
3. Click font size option.

7 Make Slide 1 active and then select the text *Cascade View Pediatrics*.

8 Click the *Font* option box arrow in the Font group, scroll down the drop-down gallery (fonts display in alphabetical order), and then click *Cambria*.

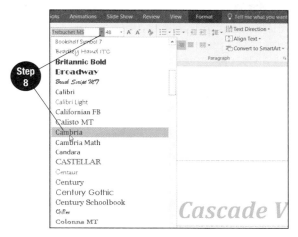

9 With the clinic name still selected, click the *Font Size* option box arrow and then click *54* at the drop-down gallery.

10 Select the subtitle *Vancouver Clinic*, click the *Font* option box arrow, and then click *Cambria* at the drop-down gallery.

> The drop-down gallery displays the most recently used fonts at the top.

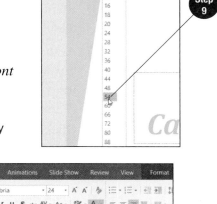

11 With the subtitle still selected, click the Font Color button arrow and then click the *Blue, Accent 2, Darker 25%* option at the drop-down gallery (sixth column, fifth row in the *Theme Colors* section).

12 Print Slide 1.

13 Save **2-CVPVancouver.pptx**.

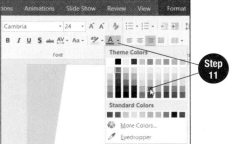

Check Your Work — Compare your work with the model answer to ensure that you have completed the activity correctly.

In Addition

Choosing Fonts

A **typeface** is a set of characters with a common design and shape. PowerPoint refers to a typeface as a **font**. Fonts can be decorative or plain and are either monospaced or proportional. A monospaced font allots the same amount of horizontal space for each character, while a proportional font allots a different amount of space for each character. Proportional fonts are divided into two main categories: serif and sans serif. A serif is a small line at the end of a character stroke. Consider using a serif font for text-intensive slides because the serifs help move the reader's eyes across the text. Use a sans serif font for titles, subtitles, headings, and short lines of text.

Activity 2.4 Applying Font Formatting at the Font Dialog Box; Replacing Fonts

In addition to using the buttons in the Font group on the Home tab, you can apply font formatting with options at the Font dialog box. Use options at this dialog box to change the font, as well as its style, size and color, and apply formatting such as underlining, strikethrough, superscript, subscript, small caps, and all caps. If you decide to change the font for all slides in a presentation, use the Replace Font dialog box to replace all occurrences of a specific font in the presentation.

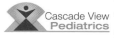

What You Will Do   As you are still not satisfied with the font in the Vancouver presentation, you decide to change the font for the title and subtitle and replace the Trebuchet MS font on the remaining slides.

Tutorial
Applying Font Formatting at the Font Dialog Box

Tutorial
Replacing Fonts

1. With **2-CVPVancouver.pptx** open, make sure Slide 1 is the active slide.

2. Select the text *Cascade View Pediatrics*.

3. Display the Font dialog box by clicking the Font group dialog box launcher on the Home tab.

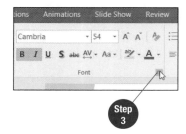

4. At the Font dialog box, click the *Latin text font* option box arrow and then click *Constantia* at the drop-down list. (You will need to scroll down the drop-down list to display *Constantia*.)

5. Click the *Font style* option box arrow and then click *Bold* at the drop-down list.

6. Select the current measurement in the *Size* measurement box and then type 50.

7. Click the Font color button in the *All text* section and then click the *Dark Blue* option (ninth option from the left in the *Standard Colors* section).

8. Click OK to close the Font dialog box.

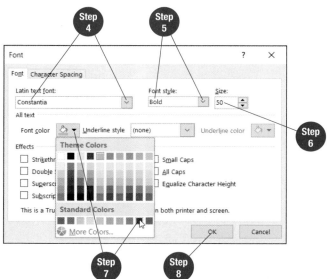

9. Select the subtitle *Vancouver Clinic*.

10. Click the Font group dialog box launcher.

In Brief

Change Font at Font Dialog Box
1. Select text.
2. Click Font group dialog box launcher.
3. Click options at Font dialog box.
4. Click OK.

Change All Occurrences of Font
1. Click Replace button arrow.
2. Click *Replace Fonts*.
3. Click *Replace* text box arrow.
4. Click font to replace.
5. Press Tab.
6. Click *With* option box arrow.
7. Click new font.
8. Click Replace button.
9. Click Close button.

11 At the Font dialog box, click the *Latin text font* option box arrow and then click *Constantia* at the drop-down list. (You will need to scroll down the drop-down list to display *Constantia*.)

12 Click the *Font style* option box arrow and then click *Bold* at the drop-down list.

13 Select the current measurement in the *Size* measurement box and then type 32.

14 Click OK to close the Font dialog box.

15 Make Slide 2 active.

16 You decide to replace all occurrences of the Trebuchet MS font with the Constantia font. To begin, click the Replace button arrow in the Editing group on the Home tab and then click *Replace Fonts* at the drop-down list.

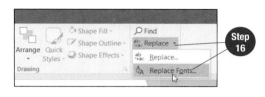

17 At the Replace Font dialog box, click the *Replace* option box and then click *Trebuchet MS* at the drop-down list.

18 Click the *With* option box arrow and then click *Constantia* at the drop-down list. (You will need to scroll down the drop-down list to display *Constantia*.)

19 Click the Replace button and then click the Close button.

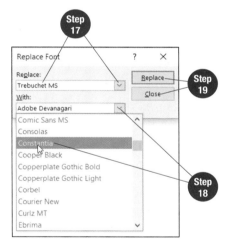

20 Save **2-CVPVancouver.pptx**.

Check Your Work — Compare your work with the model answer to ensure that you have completed the activity correctly.

In Addition

Choosing Presentation Fonts

Choose a font for a presentation based on the tone and message you want the presentation to convey. For example, choose a more serious font, such as Constantia or Cambria, for a conservative audience, and choose a less formal font, such as Comic Sans MS, Lucida Handwriting, or Mistral, for a more informal or lighthearted audience. For text-intensive slides, choose a serif font, such as Cambria, Constantia, Garamond, or Bookman Old Style. For titles, subtitles, headings, and short text items, consider a sans serif font such as Calibri, Candara, Arial, or Trebuchet MS. Use no more than two or three different fonts in each presentation. To ensure text readability in a slide, choose a font color that contrasts with the slide background.

Use the Format Painter feature to apply the same formatting in more than one location in a slide or slides. To use Format Painter, apply formatting to text, position the insertion point anywhere in the formatted text, and then double-click the Format Painter button in the Clipboard group on the Home tab. Using the mouse, select the additional text to which you want to apply the formatting. After applying the formatting in the desired locations, click the Format Painter button to deactivate it. If you only need to apply formatting in one other location, click the Format Painter button just one time. The first time you click or select text, the formatting will be applied and the Format Painter button will be deactivated.

Cascade View Pediatrics

What You Will Do Improve the appearance of slides in the Vancouver presentation by applying a font and then using Format Painter to apply the formatting to other text.

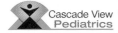
Tutorial
Formatting with
Format Painter

1. With **2-CVPVancouver.pptx** open, make sure Slide 2 is the active slide.

2. Select the title *Population*.

3. Click the Font group dialog box launcher.

4. At the Font dialog box, click the *Latin text font* option box arrow and then click *Cambria* at the drop-down list.

5. Click the *Font style* option box arrow and then click *Bold* at the drop-down list.

6. Click the Font color button in the *All text* section and then click the *Blue, Accent 2, Darker 25%* option (sixth column, fifth row in the *Theme Colors* section).

7. Click the *Small Caps* check box in the *Effects* section to insert a check mark.

8. Click OK to close the Font dialog box.

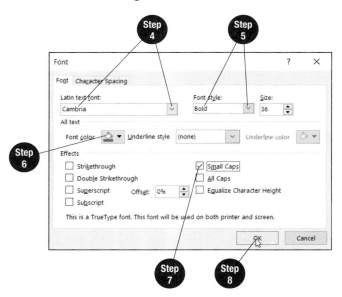

9. Deselect the text by clicking in the slide in the slide pane.

In Brief

Use Format Painter
1. Click in formatted text.
2. Double-click Format Painter button.
3. Click in or select text to be formatted.
4. Click Format Painter button.

10 Click anywhere in the title *POPULATION*.

11 Double-click the Format Painter button in the Clipboard group on the Home tab.

The mouse pointer displays with a paintbrush attached. This indicates that the Format Painter feature is active.

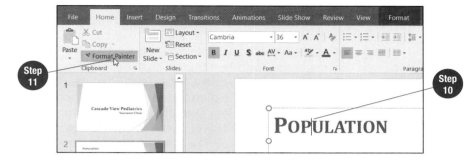

12 Click the Next Slide button to display Slide 3.

13 Using the mouse, select the words *Commercial Property*.

You can also apply the formatting by clicking individual words in the title, but doing so will not format the spaces within titles that consist of more than one word. If the paintbrush is no longer attached to the mouse pointer, Format Painter has been turned off. Turn it back on by clicking in a slide title with the desired formatting and then double-clicking the Format Painter button.

14 Click the Next Slide button to display Slide 4.

15 Click any character in the title *Statistics*.

16 Click the Next Slide button to display Slide 5.

17 Click any character in the title *Employment*.

18 Apply formatting to the titles in the remaining three slides.

19 When formatting has been applied to all slide titles, click the Format Painter button in the Clipboard group on the Home tab.

Clicking the Format Painter button turns off the feature.

20 Save **2-CVPVancouver.pptx**.

Check Your Work Compare your work with the model answer to ensure that you have completed the activity correctly.

In Addition

Choosing a Custom Color

Click the Font color button at the Font dialog box and a palette of color choices displays. Click the *More Colors* option and the Colors dialog box displays with the Standard tab selected, showing a honeycomb of color options. Click the Custom tab and the dialog box displays as shown at the right. Use options at this tab to mix your own color. Click the desired color in the *Colors* palette or enter values for the color in the *Red*, *Green*, and *Blue* measurement boxes. Adjust the luminosity of the current color by dragging the slider at the right side of the color palette.

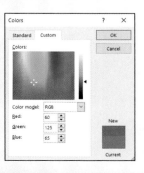

Changing Alignment and Line and Paragraph Spacing; Drawing a Text Box and Shape

The slide design template generally determines the horizontal and vertical alignment of text in placeholders. Text may be left-aligned, center-aligned, right-aligned, or justified-aligned in a placeholder, as well as aligned at the top, middle, or bottom of the placeholder. You can change the alignment of specific text with buttons in the Paragraph group on the Home tab or with options at the Align Text button drop-down gallery. Use options at the Line Spacing button drop-down list or the *Line Spacing* option at the Paragraph dialog box to change line spacing. The Paragraph dialog box also contains options for changing text alignment, indentation, and spacing before and after text. If you want to add text to a slide but do not want to use the Title and Text layout, draw a text box in a slide and then type text inside the box. Use the Shapes button on the Home tab or Insert tab to draw shapes in a slide, such as squares, circles, block arrows, callouts, stars, and banners. Use options on the Drawing Tools Format tab to format and customize a text box or a shape.

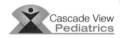
Cascade View Pediatrics

What You Will Do   Change the alignment of specific text in slides and improve the appearance of text in slides by adjusting the vertical alignment and paragraph spacing. Dr. Severin has also asked you to insert a slide containing a description of Vancouver.

Tutorial
Changing Alignment

Tutorial
Changing Line Spacing

Tutorial
Changing Paragraph Spacing

Tutorial
Inserting and Formatting Text Boxes

Tutorial
Inserting, Sizing, and Positioning a Shape

Tutorial
Formatting Shapes

1. With **2-CVPVancouver.pptx** open, make Slide 1 active.

2. Click anywhere in the text *Cascade View Pediatrics* and then click the Center button in the Paragraph group on the Home tab.

   You can also change text alignment with the keyboard shortcuts shown in Table P2.2.

3. Select the subtitle *Vancouver Clinic* and then click the Center button in the Paragraph group.

4. Click the Align Text button in the Paragraph group and then click *Middle* at the drop-down gallery.

5. With Slide 1 active, click the New Slide button arrow and then click *Title Only* at the drop-down list.

6. Click in the *Click to add title* placeholder and then type About Vancouver.

7. Make Slide 3 active, click any character in the title *POPULATION*, and then click the Format Painter button in the Clipboard group.

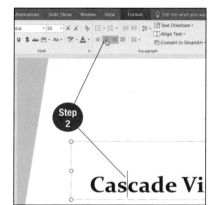

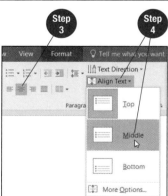

Table P2.2 Keyboard Shortcuts for Changing Alignment

Alignment	Keyboard Shortcut
left-align	Ctrl + L
center-align	Ctrl + E
right-align	Ctrl + R
justify-align	Ctrl + J

8 Make Slide 2 active and then select the title *About Vancouver*.

Format Painter applies the formatting and then deactivates automatically.

9 Draw a text box in the slide. Begin by clicking the Insert tab and then clicking the Text Box button ⃞ in the Text group.

10 Using the mouse, draw a box that is approximately the size shown below.

To draw a text box, click and hold down the mouse button as you drag in the slide.

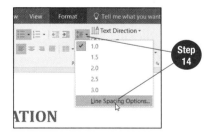

11 Type the text shown in Figure P2.1. Do not press the Enter key after typing the web address. If you do so accidentally, immediately click the Undo button.

12 Select all of the text in the text box and then change the font to 24-point Constantia.

13 Justify-align the text by clicking the Justify button ▤ in the Paragraph group.

14 Make Slide 3 active, select the bulleted text, click the Line Spacing button ⌷ in the Paragraph group, and then click *Line Spacing Options* at the drop-down gallery.

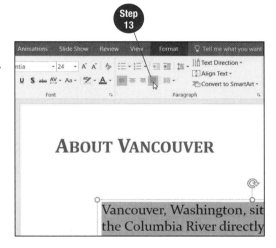

Figure P2.1 Step 11

Vancouver, Washington, sits on the north bank of the Columbia River directly across from Portland, Oregon. The Pacific Coast is less than 90 miles to the west. The Cascade Mountain Range rises on the east. Mount St. Helens National Volcanic Monument and Mt. Hood are less than two hours away. The spectacular Columbia River Gorge National Scenic Area lies 30 minutes to the east. (www.cityofvancouver.us)

15 At the Paragraph dialog box, click the *After* measurement box up arrow in the *Spacing* section.

> This displays *6 pt* in the *After* measurement box.

16 Click OK to close the dialog box.

17 Make Slide 4 active (contains the title *COMMERCIAL PROPERTY*) and then select the bulleted text.

18 Click the Line Spacing button and then click *1.5* at the drop-down gallery.

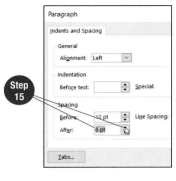

19 Make Slide 5 active, select the text from the second bullet through the fourth bullet, click the Line Spacing button, and then click *Line Spacing Options* at the drop-down gallery.

20 At the Paragraph dialog box, click the *Before* measurement box up arrow in the *Spacing* section two times (this displays *18 pt* in the measurement box) and then click OK.

21 Make Slide 6 active and then follow steps similar to those in Steps 19 and 20 to change the *Before* spacing to *18 pt*.

22 Make Slide 8 active and then select text from the second bullet through the eighth bullet. Display the Paragraph dialog box, change the *Before* spacing to *0 pt*, and then click OK to close the dialog box.

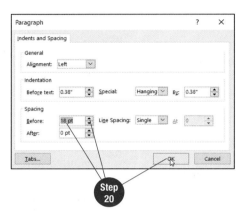

23 Make Slide 9 active and then insert a new blank slide by clicking the New Slide button arrow and then clicking *Blank* at the drop-down list.

24 Draw a shape in the slide. Begin by clicking the Insert tab, clicking the Shapes button in the Illustrations group, and then clicking the bevel shape in the first column, third row in the *Basic Shapes* section.

> Shape options are also available in the Drawing group on the Home tab.

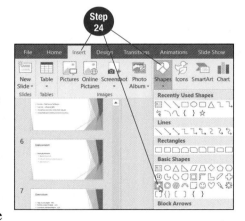

25 Position the mouse pointer in the slide, click and hold down the left mouse button, drag to create the shape shown below, and then release the mouse button.

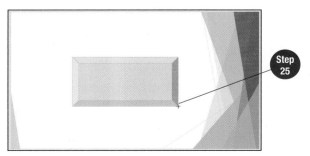

In Brief

Change Horizontal Text Alignment
1. Select text or click in paragraph.
2. Click alignment button in Paragraph group.

Change Vertical Text Alignment
1. Select text or click in paragraph.
2. Click Align Text button.
3. Click alignment option.

Change Line Spacing
1. Select text or click in placeholder.
2. Click Line Spacing button.
3. Click spacing option.
OR
1. Select text or click in placeholder.
2. Click Line Spacing button.
3. Click *Line Spacing Options*.
4. At Paragraph dialog box, specify spacing.
5. Click OK.

Insert Text Box
1. Click Insert tab.
2. Click Text Box button.
3. Click or drag in slide to create text box.

Draw Shape
1. Click Insert tab.
2. Click Shapes button.
3. Click shape option.
4. Click or drag in slide to draw shape.

26 With the shape selected, click in the *Shape Height* measurement box in the Size group on the Drawing Tools Format tab and then type 3.2. Click in the *Shape Width* measurement box, type 6.5, and then press the Enter key.

27 With the shape still selected, type the text To schedule a tour of our clinic, please call (503) 555-7700.

> When a shape is selected, text you type will automatically appear inside it.

28 Click the More Shape Styles button at the right of the shape style thumbnails in the Shape Styles group on the Drawing Tools Format tab and then click the blue style in the third column, fourth row in the *Theme Styles* section.

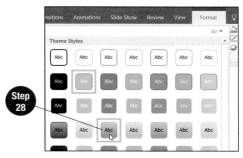

29 Click the Shape Outline button arrow in the Shape Styles group and then click the *Dark Blue* option in the *Standard Colors* section.

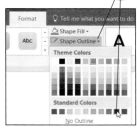

30 Select the text in the shape, click the Home tab, change the font to 40-point Candara, and then change the font color to *Blue, Accent 2, Darker 50%* (sixth column, last row in the *Theme Colors* section).

31 With the text still selected, click the Drawing Tools Format tab, click the Text Effects button in the WordArt Styles group, point to *Glow*, and then click the blue option in the second column, second row in the *Glow Variations* section.

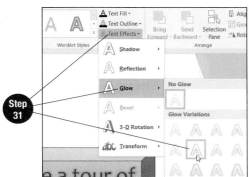

32 Print Slide 2 and Slide 10.

33 Save **2-CVPVancouver.pptx**.

Check Your Work — Compare your work with the model answer to ensure that you have completed the activity correctly.

In Addition

Inserting a New Line

When creating bulleted text in a slide, pressing the Enter key causes the insertion point to move to the next line, inserting another bullet. Situations may occur wherein you want to create a blank line between bulleted items without creating another bullet. One method for doing this is to use the New Line command, Shift + Enter. Pressing Shift + Enter inserts a new line that is considered part of the previous paragraph.

Activity 2.7   Inserting Headers and Footers

Insert information you want to appear at the top or bottom of individual slides or at the top or bottom of individual printed notes or handout pages using options at the Header and Footer dialog box. If you want the same types of information to appear on all slides, display the Header and Footer dialog box with the Slide tab selected. With options at this dialog box, you can insert the date and time, the slide number, and a footer. To insert header or footer elements you want to print on all notes or handouts pages, choose options at the Header and Footer dialog box with the Notes and Handouts tab selected.

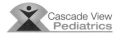
Cascade View Pediatrics

What You Will Do   You decide to insert the current date and slide number in the Vancouver presentation and create a header for notes pages.

> **Tutorial**
> Inserting Headers and Footers

1. With **2-CVPVancouver.pptx** open, display Slide 1 in the slide pane.

2. Insert a footer that prints at the bottom of each slide. To begin, click the Insert tab and then click the Header & Footer button ⬚ in the Text group.

3. At the Header and Footer dialog box with the Slide tab selected, click the *Date and time* check box to insert a check mark. If it is not already selected, click the *Update automatically* option to select it.

4. Click the *Slide number* check box to insert a check mark.

5. Click the *Footer* check box and then type Vancouver Clinic in the *Footer* text box.

6. Click the Apply to All button.

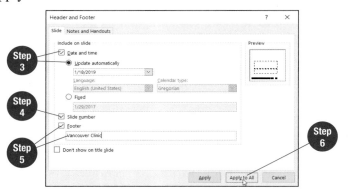

7. Make Slide 4 active.

8. Display the notes pane by clicking the Notes button on the Status bar.

9. Click in the notes pane and then type Contact two commercial real estate companies about available office space.

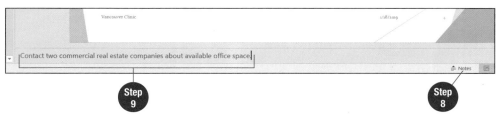

10. Insert a header and footer that will print on notes and handouts pages by clicking the Header & Footer button in the Text group on the Insert tab.

In Brief

Insert Header/Footer on Slide
1. Click Insert tab.
2. Click Header & Footer button.
3. At Header and Footer dialog box with Slide tab selected, choose options.
4. Click Apply to All button.

Insert Header/Footer in Notes and Handouts
1. Click Insert tab.
2. Click Header & Footer button.
3. At Header and Footer dialog box, click Notes and Handouts tab.
4. Choose options.
5. Click Apply to All button.

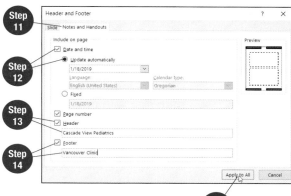

11 At the Header and Footer dialog box, click the Notes and Handouts tab.

12 Click the *Date and time* check box to insert a check mark and then, if necessary, click the *Update automatically* option to select it.

13 Click the *Header* check box and then type Cascade View Pediatrics.

14 Click the *Footer* check box and then type Vancouver Clinic.

15 Click the Apply to All button.

16 Print the presentation as handouts with six slides displayed horizontally per page.

17 Print Slide 4 as a notes page. To do this, click the File tab, click the *Print* option, click the second gallery in the *Settings* category (contains the text *6 Slides Horizontal*), and then click *Notes Pages* in the *Print Layout* section.

18 Click in the *Slides* text box (below the first gallery in the *Settings* category) and then type 4.

19 Click the Print button.

20 Remove the footer that displays on each slide. Begin by clicking the Insert tab and then clicking the Header & Footer button in the Text group.

21 With the Slide tab selected, click the *Date and time* check box, the *Slide number* check box, and the *Footer* check box to remove the check marks.

22 Click the Apply to All button.

23 Click the Notes button on the Status bar to close the notes pane.

24 Save **2-CVPVancouver.pptx**.

Check Your Work — Compare your work with the model answer to ensure that you have completed the activity correctly.

In Addition

Using the Package for CD Feature

The safest way to transport a PowerPoint presentation to another computer is to use the Package for CD feature. With this feature, you can copy a presentation onto a CD or to a folder or network location and include all of the linked files, fonts, and the PowerPoint Viewer program in case the destination computer does not have PowerPoint installed on it. To use the Package for CD feature, click the File tab, click the *Export* option, click the *Package Presentation for CD* option, and then click the Package for CD button. At the Package for CD dialog box, type a name for the CD and then click the Copy to CD button.

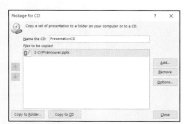

By default, the slide size in PowerPoint 2016 is Widescreen (16:9), but you can change the slide size with options at the Slide Size button drop-down list in the Customize group on the Design tab. Change the design theme applied to slides in a presentation or change the colors, fonts, effects, or background style of a theme with options on the Design tab. Click the More Variants button in the Variants group on the Design tab to display options for changing the theme colors, fonts, effects, and background styles.

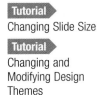

Cascade View
Pediatrics

What You Will Do   You are not pleased with the design theme for the Vancouver presentation, so you decide to apply a different theme and then change the colors and fonts for the theme.

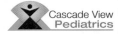
Tutorial

Changing Slide Size

Tutorial

Changing and
Modifying Design
Themes

1 With **2-CVPVancouver.pptx** open, click the Design tab.

2 Click the Slide Size button ▢ in the Customize group and then click *Standard (4:3)* at the drop-down list.

3 At the Microsoft PowerPoint dialog box, click the Ensure Fit button.

> Clicking the Ensure Fit button scales down the contents of the slide to fit within the new slide size. Click the Maximize button to maximize the size of the content on the new slide.

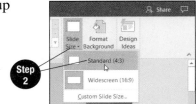

4 Run the slide show beginning with Slide 1 and notice any changes to the layout of the slides.

5 Click the Undo button on the Quick Access Toolbar to return the presentation to the original slide size (Widescreen).

6 Click the More Themes button in the Themes group and then click the *Dividend* option at the drop-down gallery.

7 Click the More Variants button in the Variants group, point to *Colors*, and then click *Blue Green* at the side menu.

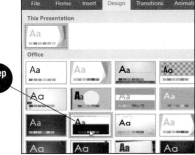

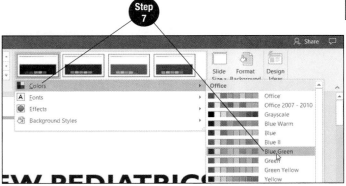

8 Click the More Variants button in the Variants group, point to *Fonts*, scroll down the side menu, and then click *Consolas-Verdana*.

In Brief

Change Slide Size
1. Click Design tab.
2. Click Slide Size button.
3. Click slide size.
4. Click Maximize or Ensure Fit button.

Change Theme
1. Click Design tab.
2. Click More Themes button.
3. Click theme.

Change Theme Colors
1. Click Design tab.
2. Click More Variants button.
3. Point to *Colors*.
4. Click color option.

Change Theme Fonts
1. Click Design tab.
2. Click More Variants button.
3. Point to *Fonts*.
4. Click font option.

Change Slide Background
1. Click Design tab.
2. Click More Variants button.
3. Point to *Background Styles*.
4. Click background option.

9. Apply a background style by clicking the More Variants button in the Variants group, pointing to *Background Styles*, and then clicking the option in the second column, third row.

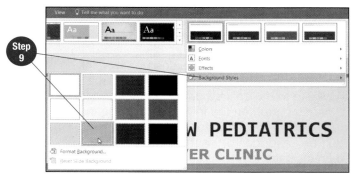

10. With Slide 1 active, change the font of the title and subtitle to *Constantia*.

11. Make Slide 2 active. Notice that the title of the slide is difficult to see. Select the title *ABOUT VANCOUVER*, click the Home tab, click the Font Color button arrow in the Font group, and then click the *Dark Blue* option at the drop-down gallery (ninth option from the left in the *Standard Colors* section).

12. Click in the title *ABOUT VANCOUVER*, double-click the Format Painter button in the Clipboard group on the Home tab, make Slide 3 active in the slide pane, and then select the title *POPULATION*. Apply the Dark Blue font color to the titles in Slides 4 through 9. Click the Format Painter button to turn off the feature.

13. Run the slide show beginning with Slide 1.

14. After running the slide show, remove the background style by clicking the Design tab, clicking the More Variants button in the Variants group, pointing to *Background Styles*, and then clicking the option in the first column, first row.

15. Make Slide 2 active and then move the text box placeholder so it is positioned in the center of the slide.

16. Make Slide 10 active and then move the shape so it is positioned in the center of the slide.

17. Save **2-CVPVancouver.pptx**.

Check Your Work Compare your work with the model answer to ensure that you have completed the activity correctly.

In Addition

Customizing Theme Colors

Theme colors consist of four text colors, six accent colors, and two hyperlink colors. You can customize these theme colors with options at the Create New Theme Colors dialog box, shown at the right. Display this dialog box by clicking the More Variants button in the Variants group on the Design tab, pointing to *Colors*, and then clicking *Customize Colors* at the side menu. Change a color by clicking the desired color option button in the *Theme colors* section and then clicking the desired color at the color palette. Changes made to colors display in the *Sample* section of the dialog box. You can name a custom color theme with the *Name* option in the dialog box. Click the Reset button to return the colors to the default theme colors.

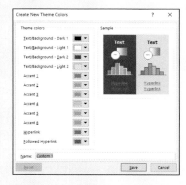

Inserting, Sizing, Moving, and Formatting an Image

Add visual interest to a presentation by inserting an image such as a logo, picture, or clip art in a slide. Insert an image from a drive or folder with the Insert Picture dialog box. Display the Insert Picture dialog box by clicking the Pictures button in the Images group on the Insert tab or by clicking the picture image in the content placeholder. At this dialog box, navigate to the desired drive or folder and then double-click the image. Click the Online Pictures button on the Insert tab and the Insert Pictures window displays. Use options in this window to search for images using Bing. At the window, type a category in the search text box and then press the Enter key. In the list of images that displays, click an image and then click the Insert button. The image is inserted in the slide and the Picture Tools Format tab is selected. Use buttons on the Picture Tools Format tab to recolor the image, apply a picture style, arrange the image in the slide, and size the image. You can also size an image using the sizing handles that display around the selected image and move the image using the mouse.

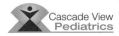

What You Will Do   Dr. Severin has asked you to insert the clinic logo on the first slide and enhance the visual appeal of some of the slides by inserting and formatting images.

Tutorial
Inserting, Sizing, and Moving an Image

Tutorial
Formatting an Image

1. With **2-CVPVancouver.pptx** open, make sure Slide 1 is active.

2. Insert the clinic logo in the slide. To begin, click the Insert tab and then click the Pictures button [icon] in the Images group.

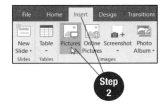

Step 2

3. At the Insert Picture dialog box, navigate to the PowerPointMedS2 folder on your storage medium and then double-click *CVPLogo.jpg*.

   The image is inserted in the slide, selection handles display around the image, and the Picture Tools Format tab is selected.

4. Decrease the size of the logo by clicking in the *Shape Height* measurement box in the Size group on the Picture Tools Format tab, typing 0.5, and then pressing the Enter key.

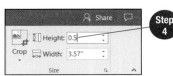

Step 4

   When you change the height of the logo, the width automatically changes to maintain the proportions of the logo. You can also size an image using the sizing handles that display around the selected image. Use the middle sizing handles to increase or decrease the width of an image, use the top and bottom handles to increase or decrease the height, and use the corner sizing handles to increase or decrease both the width and height of the image at the same time.

5. Move the logo so it is positioned in the lower right corner of the slide (within the teal background). To do this, position the mouse pointer on the image until the pointer displays with a four-headed arrow attached, click and hold down the left mouse button, drag the image to the lower right corner, and then release the mouse button.

6. With the image selected, click the *Drop Shadow Rectangle* option in the Picture Styles group (fourth option from the left).

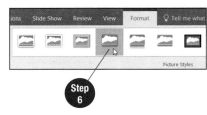

Step 6

7 Make Slide 4 active and then insert an online image. Begin by clicking the Insert tab and then clicking the Online Pictures button 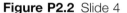 in the Images group.

8 At the Insert Pictures window, click in the search text box, type office building, and then press the Enter key.

9 Click the image shown below and in Figure P2.2 and then click the Insert button.

> If the building image shown below and in Figure P2.2 is not available, insert **building.png** from the PowerPointMedS2 folder on your storage medium.

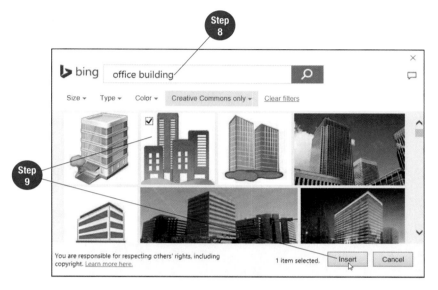

10 With the image selected, decrease the size by clicking in the *Shape Height* measurement box, typing 4, and then pressing the Enter key.

11 Move the image so it is positioned as shown in Figure P2.2.

12 Make Slide 8 active, click the Insert tab, and then click the Pictures button.

13 At the Insert Picture dialog box, navigate to the PowerPointMedS2 folder and then double-click *college.png*.

14 Click in the *Shape Height* measurement box in the Size group on the Picture Tools Format tab, type 3.7, and then press the Enter key.

Figure P2.2 Slide 4

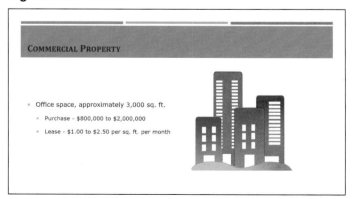

15 Change the color of the image so it complements the color scheme of the presentation. To do this, click the Color button 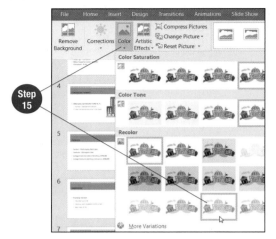 in the Adjust group and then click the aqua option in the third column, third row in the *Recolor* section.

16 Click the Corrections button 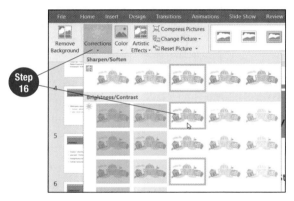 in the Adjust group and then click the option in the third column, first row in the *Brightness/Contrast* section.

17 Using the mouse, drag the image so it is positioned as shown in Figure P2.3.

18 Make Slide 2 active, click the Insert tab, and then click the Pictures button.

19 At the Insert Picture dialog box, navigate to the PowerPointMedS2 folder and then double-click *mountains.png*.

20 Click in the *Shape Height* measurement box, type 4.8, and then press the Enter key.

Figure P2.3 Slide 8

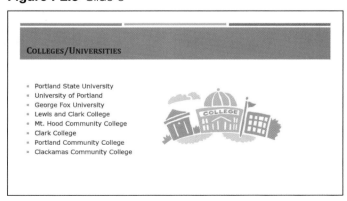

21 Format the image as a watermark by clicking the Color button in the Adjust group on the Picture Tools Format tab and then clicking the color option in the fourth column, first row in the *Recolor* section.

22 Click the Send Backward button arrow 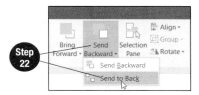 in the Arrange group on the Picture Tools Format tab and then click *Send to Back* at the drop-down list.

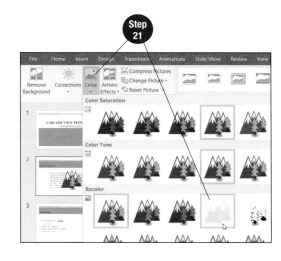

23 Using the mouse, drag the image so it is positioned as shown in Figure P2.4.

24 Save **2-CVPVancouver.pptx**.

Figure P2.4 Slide 2

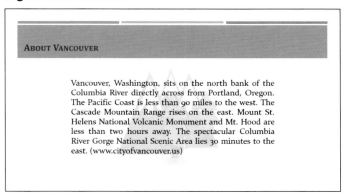

Check Your Work Compare your work with the model answer to ensure that you have completed the activity correctly.

In Addition

Formatting with Buttons on the Picture Tools Format Tab

Format images in a slide with buttons and options on the Picture Tools Format tab, shown below. Use buttons in the Adjust group to adjust the brightness and contrast of the image; change the image color or change to a different image; reset the image to its original size, position, and color; and compress the image. (Compress an image to reduce the resolution or discard extra information to save room on a hard drive or reduce download time.) Use buttons in the Picture Styles group to apply a predesigned style, insert a picture border, or apply a picture effect. The Arrange group contains buttons for positioning the image and aligning and rotating the image. Use options in the Size group to crop the image and specify the height and width of the image.

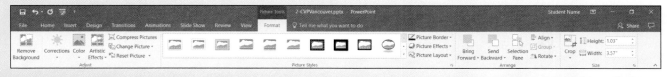

Activity 2.10　Inserting and Formatting WordArt

Use the WordArt feature to create text with special formatting that makes it stand out. You can format WordArt in a variety of ways, including conforming it to a shape. To insert WordArt, click the Insert tab, click the WordArt button in the Text group, and then click a WordArt style at the drop-down list. When WordArt is selected, the Drawing Tools Format tab displays. Use options and buttons on this tab to modify and customize WordArt.

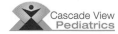
Cascade View Pediatrics

What You Will Do　To complete the presentation, Dr. Severin has asked you to insert a WordArt image containing the proposed opening date of the Vancouver clinic.

Tutorial
Inserting and Formatting WordArt

1　With **2-CVPVancouver.pptx** open, make Slide 9 active.

2　Click the New Slide button in the Slides group on the Home tab.

3　Click the Layout button in the Slides group and then click the *Blank* option.

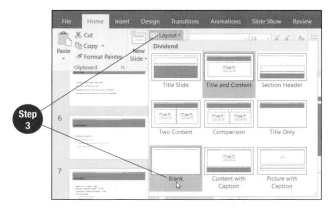

4　Insert WordArt by clicking the Insert tab, clicking the WordArt button 𝒜 in the Text group, and then clicking the aqua option in the third column, first row in the drop-down list.

> This inserts a text box containing the words *Your text here* and also makes active the Drawing Tools Format tab.

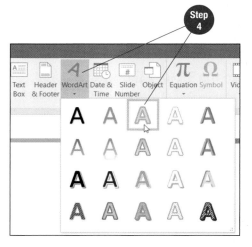

5　Type Opening, press the Enter key, and then type September 2019.

In Brief

Insert WordArt
1. Click Insert tab.
2. Click WordArt button.
3. Click WordArt option.
4. Type WordArt text.
5. Apply formatting.

6 Select the text *Opening September 2019*, click the Text Effects button 🅰 in the WordArt Styles group, point to *Transform* at the drop-down list, and then click the option in the second column, sixth row in the *Warp* section.

7 Click the Text Effects button, point to *Glow* at the drop-down list, and then click the aqua option in the first column, second row in the *Glow Variations* section.

8 Click in the *Shape Height* measurement box in the Size group, type 4, and then press the Enter key.

9 Click in the *Shape Width* measurement box in the Size group, type 10, and then press the Enter key.

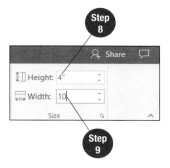

10 Drag the WordArt text so it is centered on the slide, as shown in Figure P2.5.

11 Save **2-CVPVancouver.pptx**.

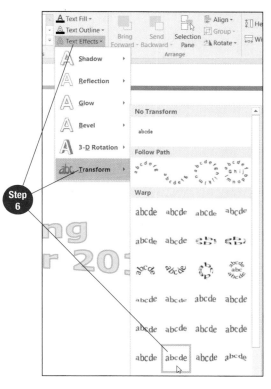

Figure P2.5 Slide 10

[Figure showing "Opening September 2019" WordArt on a slide]

Check Your Work — Compare your work with the model answer to ensure that you have completed the activity correctly.

In Addition

Using Buttons and Options on the Drawing Tools Format Tab

When WordArt is selected in a slide, the Drawing Tools Format tab displays as shown below. You can draw a shape or text box with buttons in the Insert Shapes group. Apply a style, fill, outline, and/or effects to the WordArt text box with options in the Shape Styles group. Change the style of the WordArt text with options in the WordArt Styles group, specify the layering of the WordArt text with options in the Arrange group, and identify the height and width of the WordArt text box with measurement boxes in the Size group.

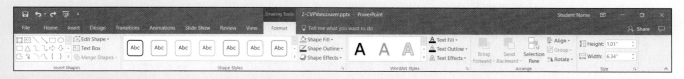

Inserting and Formatting an Organizational Chart with SmartArt

Use the SmartArt feature to create a variety of graphic diagrams, including process, cycle, relationship, matrix, and pyramid diagrams. You can also use SmartArt to visually illustrate hierarchical data. To display a menu of SmartArt choices, click the Insert tab and then click the SmartArt button in the Illustrations group. This displays the Choose a SmartArt Graphic dialog box. At this dialog box, click the type of organization chart or graphic in the left panel and then double-click the graphic in the middle panel. This inserts the chart or graphic in the slide. Most SmartArt graphics are designed to include text. Type text in a graphic shape by selecting the shape and then typing text in the shape. Use buttons on the SmartArt Tools Design tab and the SmartArt Tools Format tab to customize a graphic.

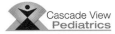 Cascade View Pediatrics

What You Will Do   As part of the presentation, Dr. Severin has asked you to insert an organizational chart identifying project personnel and a graphic diagram identifying the major steps in the new clinic project.

Tutorial
Inserting, Sizing, and Moving SmartArt

Tutorial
Formatting SmartArt

1 With **2-CVPVancouver.pptx** open, make Slide 9 active and then click the New Slide button in the Slides group on the Home tab.

2 Create the organizational chart shown in Figure P2.6. To begin, click the Insert tab and then click the SmartArt button 📇 in the Illustrations group.

> You can also click the Insert SmartArt Graphic option in the content placeholder.

3 At the Choose a SmartArt Graphic dialog box, click *Hierarchy* in the left panel and then double-click the first option in the middle panel, *Organization Chart*.

> This displays the organizational chart in the slide with the SmartArt Tools Design tab selected. Use buttons on this tab to add additional boxes, change the order of the boxes, choose a different layout, apply formatting with a SmartArt style, and reset the formatting of the organizational chart.

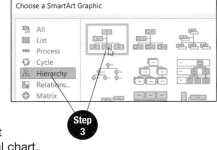

4 If the pane that reads *Type your text here* displays at the left side of the organizational chart, close it by clicking the Text Pane button 🔲 in the Create Graphic group.

> You can also close the pane by clicking the Close button in the upper right corner of the pane.

5 Delete one of the boxes in the organizational chart by clicking the border of the first box from the left in the bottom row and then pressing the Delete key.

> Make sure that the selection border that surrounds the box is a solid line and not a dashed line. If a dashed line displays, click the box border again. This should change it to a solid line.

6 With the bottom left box selected, click the Add Shape button arrow 🔳 in the Create Graphic group on the SmartArt Tools Design tab and then click *Add Shape Below* at the drop-down list.

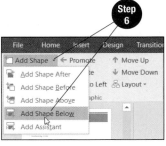

> This inserts a box below the selected box. Your organizational chart should contain the same boxes as shown in Figure P2.6.

7 Click *[Text]* in the top box, type Dr. Severin, press the Enter key, and then type Project Leader. Click in each of the remaining boxes and type the text as shown in Figure P2.6.

8 Click the Change Colors button in the SmartArt Styles group on the SmartArt Tools Design tab and then click the second option in the *Colorful* section.

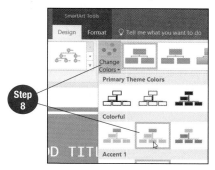

9 Click the More SmartArt Styles button at the right side of the SmartArt Styles group.

10 Click the *Polished* option at the drop-down gallery (first column, first row in the *3-D* section).

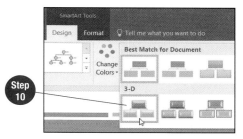

11 Click the SmartArt Tools Format tab.

12 Click inside the SmartArt graphic border but outside the SmartArt shapes.

13 Click in the *Shape Height* measurement box in the Size group, type 4.9, and then press the Enter key.

Figure P2.6 SmartArt Organizational Chart

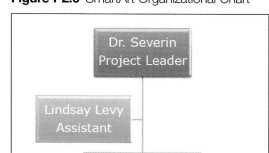

14 Click the *CLICK TO ADD TITLE* placeholder and then type Project Personnel.

15 Make Slide 9 active and then click the Home tab.

16 Click any character in the title *TOP EMPLOYERS* and then click the Format Painter button in the Clipboard group.

17 Make Slide 10 active and then select the title *Project Personnel*.

> This changes the font to 28-point Cambria, applies bold and small caps formatting, and changes the font color to Dark Blue.

18 With Slide 10 the active slide, click the New Slide button arrow in the Slides group on the Home tab, and then click the *Blank* option at the drop-down list.

19 Create the SmartArt graphic shown in Figure P2.7. To begin, click the Insert tab and then click the SmartArt button in the Illustrations group.

20 At the Choose a SmartArt Graphic dialog box, click *Relationship* in the left panel of the dialog box and then double-click the *Converging Radial* option in the middle panel.

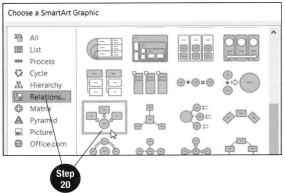

21 If necessary, close the pane that displays as *Type your text here* by clicking the Close button in the upper right corner of the pane.

22 Click the Add Shape button in the Create Graphic group on the SmartArt Tools Design tab.

23 Click in each of the shapes and type the text shown in Figure P2.7.

24 Click the Change Colors button in the SmartArt Styles group and then click the first option in the *Colorful* section.

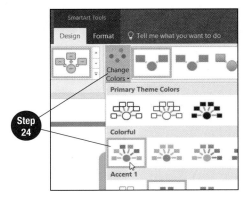

25 Click the More SmartArt Styles button in the SmartArt Styles group.

26 Click the *Inset* option at the drop-down gallery (second column, first row in the *3-D* section).

27 Click the SmartArt Tools Format tab.

28 Click inside the SmartArt graphic border but outside the SmartArt shapes.

> This deselects the shapes but keeps the graphic selected.

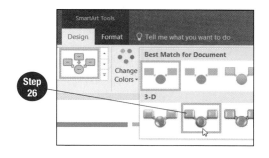

29 Click the More WordArt Styles button in the WordArt Styles group and then click the light blue outline option in the fourth column, third row.

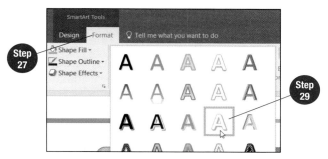

30 Position the arrow pointer on the SmartArt graphic border until the pointer displays with a four-headed arrow attached, click and hold down the left mouse button, and then drag the SmartArt graphic down so it is positioned as shown in Figure P2.7.

31 Save **2-CVPVancouver.pptx**.

Figure P2.7 SmartArt Relationship Graphic

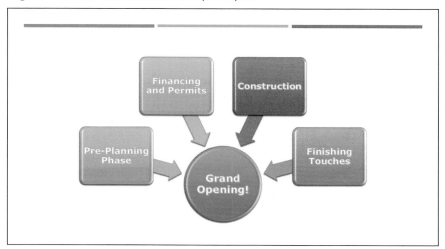

Check Your Work Compare your work with the model answer to ensure that you have completed the activity correctly.

In Addition

Inserting Text in the Type Your Text Here Pane

Enter text in a SmartArt shape by clicking in the shape and then typing the text. You can also insert text in a SmartArt shape by typing text in the pane that displays *Type your text here*. Display this pane by clicking the Text Pane button in the Create Graphic group on the SmartArt Tools Design tab.

Activity 2.12 Applying Animation to Objects and Text

Animate individual objects and text in a slide with options on the Animations tab. Click the Animations tab to display a variety of animation styles and options for customizing and applying times to animations in a presentation. Click the More Animations button at the right side of the gallery in the Animation group to display a drop-down gallery of animation styles that you can apply to objects and text as they enter a slide, exit a slide, and/or follow a motion path. You can also apply animations to emphasize objects in a slide. If you want the same animation applied to other objects in a presentation, use the Animation Painter button in the Advanced Animation group on the Animations tab.

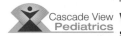
Cascade View Pediatrics

What You Will Do   Dr. Severin has asked you to apply animation effects to some of the slides in the presentation.

Tutorial
Applying and
Removing Animations

Tutorial
Modifying Animations

1. With **2-CVPVancouver.pptx** open, make sure Slide 11 is the active slide and that the SmartArt graphic is selected.

2. Click the Animations tab and then click the *Fly In* option in the Animation group.

3. Click the Effect Options button ⬆ in the Animation group and then click *One by One* at the drop-down list.

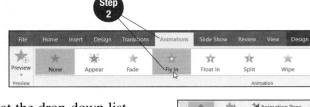

4. Click the *Duration* measurement box up arrow in the Timing group two times.

   This displays *01.00* in the measurement box.

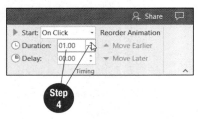

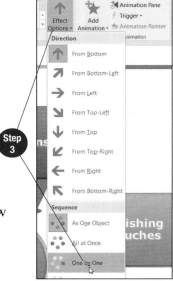

5. Click the Preview button ⭐ in the Preview group to view the animation applied to the SmartArt graphic.

6. Make Slide 10 active and then click the organizational chart to select it.

7. Click the More Animations button at the right of the Animation gallery and then click the *Grow & Turn* option in the *Entrance* section of the drop-down list.

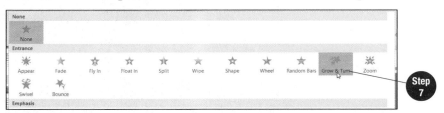

8. Click the Effect Options button in the Animation group and then click *One by One* at the drop-down list.

9 Click Slide 3 to make it active and then click the bulleted text to select the placeholder.

10 Click the *Fly In* option in the Animation group.

Applying this animation creates a build for the bulleted items. A build displays important points in a slide one point at a time and is useful for keeping the audience's attention focused on the point being presented rather than allowing them to read ahead.

11 Click the *Duration* measurement box up arrow in the Timing group two times.

This displays *01.00* in the measurement box.

12 Apply the same animation to the bulleted text in Slides 4 through 8. To begin, click anywhere in the bulleted text to select the placeholder and then double-click the Animation Painter button in the Advanced Animation group.

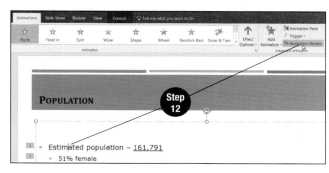

13 Make Slide 4 active and then click anywhere in the bulleted text. (This selects the placeholder and applies the Fly In animation and the duration time.)

14 Make Slide 5 active and then click anywhere in the bulleted text.

15 Make Slide 6 active and then click in the bulleted text. Make Slide 7 active and then click in the bulleted text. Make Slide 8 active and then click in the bulleted text.

16 Click the Animation Painter button to turn off the feature.

17 Delete Slide 9.

The presentation should now contain 12 slides.

18 Make Slide 1 active and then run the slide show. Click the left mouse button to advance slides and to display the individual organizational chart boxes, bulleted items, and SmartArt graphic boxes.

19 Print the presentation as handouts with six slides displayed horizontally per page. To do this, click the File tab and then click the *Print* option.

20 At the Print backstage area, click the second gallery in the *Settings* category (contains the text *Notes Pages* or *Full Page Slides*) and then click *6 Slides Horizontal* at the drop-down list.

21 Click the Print button.

22 Save and then close **2-CVPVancouver.pptx**.

Check Your Work ▶ Compare your work with the model answer to ensure that you have completed the activity correctly.

In Addition

Applying a Custom Animation

Apply custom animation to selected objects in a slide by clicking the Animation Pane button in the Advanced Animation group on the Animations tab. This displays the Animation task pane at the right side of the screen.

Use options in this task pane to control the order in which objects appear on a slide, choose animation direction and speed, and specify how objects will appear in the slide.

Features Summary

Feature	Ribbon Tab, Group	Button	Keyboard Shortcut
align left	Home, Paragraph		Ctrl + L
align right	Home, Paragraph		Ctrl + R
align vertically	Home, Paragraph		
animation effect options	Animations, Animation		
bold	Home, Font	B	Ctrl + B
center	Home, Paragraph		Ctrl + E
copy selected text	Home, Clipboard		Ctrl + C
cut selected text	Home, Clipboard		Ctrl + X
decrease font size	Home, Font		Ctrl + Shift + <
decrease list level	Home, Paragraph		Shift + Tab
font	Home, Font		
font color	Home, Font		
Font dialog box	Home, Font		Ctrl + Shift + F
font size	Home, Font		
Format Painter	Home, Clipboard		
header and footer	Insert, Text		
increase font size	Home, Font		Ctrl + Shift + >
increase list level	Home, Paragraph		Tab
italic	Home, Font	I	Ctrl + I
justify	Home, Paragraph		Ctrl + J
line spacing	Home, Paragraph		
online image	Insert, Images		
paste selected text	Home, Clipboard		Ctrl + V
picture	Insert, Images		
preview animation	Animations, Preview		
replace font	Home, Editing		Ctrl + H
shape	Insert, Illustrations OR Home, Drawing		
SmartArt	Insert, Illustrations		

continues...

Feature	Ribbon Tab, Group	Button	Keyboard Shortcut
text box	Insert, Text		
theme	Design, Themes		
underline	Home, Font	U	Ctrl + U
WordArt	Insert, Text		

Workbook Section study tools and assessment activities are available in the Workbook pages of the ebook. These resources are designed to help you further develop and demonstrate mastery of the skills learned in this section.

Integrating Programs

Word, Excel, and PowerPoint

Data Files Before beginning section work, copy the IntegratingMed2 folder to your storage medium and then make IntegratingMed2 the active folder.

Skills

- Export a PowerPoint presentation to a Word document
- Export a Word outline document to a PowerPoint presentation
- Link an Excel chart with a Word document and a PowerPoint presentation
- Edit a linked object
- Embed a Word table in a PowerPoint presentation
- Edit an embedded object

Precheck Check your current skills to help focus your study of the skills taught in this section.

Activities Overview

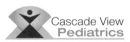

Create and format a Word document containing information on opening a clinic in Vancouver.

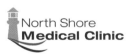

Prepare a presentation for the quarterly staff meeting using a Word outline; copy and link an Excel chart to the staff meeting presentation and to a Word document and then edit the linked chart; copy a Word table containing data on new patients, embed it in the staff meeting presentation, and then update the table; and copy a Word table containing information on quarterly equipment purchases and embed it in the staff meeting presentation.

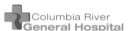

Export a PowerPoint presentation containing information on the Community Commitment plan to a Word document; copy and link an Excel chart containing information on class enrollments to an Education Department presentation and then edit the chart; and embed and edit a table containing information on department contacts into the Education Department presentation.

Model Answers Preview the model answers for an overview of the activities you will complete in each section.

299

One of the benefits of a suite like Microsoft Office is that you can send data in one program to another program. For example, send Word content to a PowerPoint presentation and PowerPoint content to a Word document. To send presentation content to a document, click the File tab, click the *Export* option, click the *Create Handouts* option, and then click the Create Handouts button. At the Send to Microsoft Word dialog box, specify the layout of the content in the Word document and whether you want to paste or paste the link of the content and then click OK. One of the advantages to sending PowerPoint presentation content to a Word document is that you can have greater control over the formatting of the content in Word.

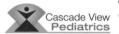

What You Will Do   Dr. Severin has asked you to export the information from his presentation on opening a clinic in Vancouver to Word as a handout.

1️⃣ Open PowerPoint and then open **CVPVancouver.pptx**.

2️⃣ Save the presentation with the name **2-CVPVancouver**.

3️⃣ Click the File tab, click the *Export* option, click the *Create Handouts* option, and then click the Create Handouts button.

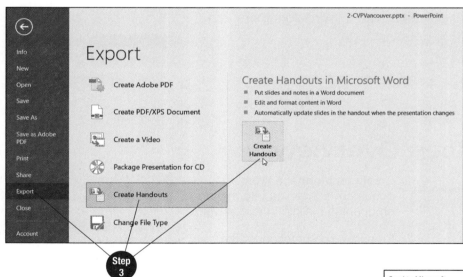

4️⃣ At the Send to Microsoft Word dialog box, click the *Blank lines next to slides* option.

5️⃣ Click the *Paste link* option at the bottom of the dialog box and then click OK.

> Click the *Paste link* option if you plan to update data in a PowerPoint presentation and want the data to update automatically in the Word document.

6️⃣ Click the Word button on the taskbar.

> The slides display in a Word document as thumbnails followed by blank lines.

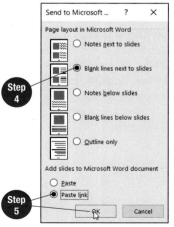

7 Save the Word document in the IntegratingMed2 folder on your storage medium and name it **2-CVPVanHandout**.

8 Print and then close **2-CVPVanHandout.docx**.

9 Click the PowerPoint button on the taskbar.

10 Make Slide 2 active and then change *8.5%* to *9.6%*.

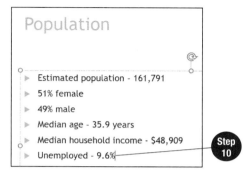

Population

- Estimated population - 161,791
- 51% female
- 49% male
- Median age - 35.9 years
- Median household income - $48,909
- Unemployed - 9.6%

Step 10

11 Make Slide 4 active, change *$199,300* to *$207,000*, and then change *$208,000* to *$216,800*.

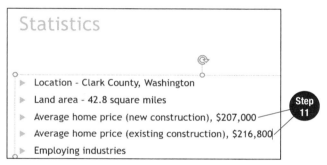

Statistics

- Location - Clark County, Washington
- Land area - 42.8 square miles
- Average home price (new construction), $207,000
- Average home price (existing construction), $216,800
- Employing industries

Step 11

12 Save **2-CVPVancouver.pptx**.

13 Make Word the active program and then open **2-CVPVanHandout.docx**. At the message asking if you want to update the document with the data from the linked files, click the Yes button.

14 Scroll through the document and notice that the percentage in Slide 2 and prices in Slide 4 reflect the changes you made in the PowerPoint presentation.

15 Save, print, and then close **2-CVPVanHandout.docx**.

16 Make PowerPoint active and then close **2-CVPVancouver.pptx**.

Check Your Work — Compare your work with the model answer to ensure that you have completed the activity correctly.

In Addition

Pasting and Linking Data

The *Paste* option at the Send to Microsoft Word dialog box is selected by default and is available for all of the page layout options. With this option selected, the data inserted in Word is not connected or linked to the original data in the PowerPoint presentation. If you plan to update the data in the PowerPoint presentation and want the data to be updated in the Word document as well, select the *Paste link* option at the Send to Microsoft Word dialog box. This option is available for all of the page layout options except the *Outline only* option.

As you learned in the previous activity, the Microsoft Office suite allows you to send content in one program to another program. For example, you can send Word content to a PowerPoint presentation and content in a PowerPoint presentation to a Word document. You can create text for slides in a Word outline and then export that outline to PowerPoint. PowerPoint creates new slides based on the heading styles used in the Word outline. Text formatted with the Heading 1 style becomes the slide titles. Heading 2 text becomes first-level bulleted text, Heading 3 text becomes second-level bulleted text, and so on. If styles are not applied to outline text in Word, PowerPoint uses tabs or indents to place the text on slides. To export a Word document to a PowerPoint presentation, you need to insert the Send to Microsoft PowerPoint button on the Quick Access Toolbar.

North Shore Medical Clinic

What You Will Do   Lee Elliott has asked you to take the outline for the quarterly staff meeting and convert it to a PowerPoint presentation.

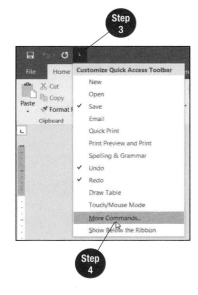

Step 3

Step 4

1 Make sure both Word and PowerPoint are open.

2 With Word active, open **NSMCOutline.docx**.

Text in this document has been formatted with the Heading 1 and Heading 2 styles.

3 Add the Send to Microsoft PowerPoint button to the Quick Access Toolbar. Begin by clicking the Customize Quick Access Toolbar button ⬛ at the right side of the Quick Access Toolbar.

4 Click *More Commands* at the drop-down list.

5 At the Word Options dialog box, click the *Choose commands from* option box arrow and then click *All Commands* at the drop-down list.

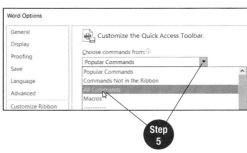

Step 5

6 Scroll down the list box that displays below the *Choose commands from* option box and then double-click *Send to Microsoft PowerPoint*.

Items in the list box display in alphabetical order.

7 Click OK to close the Word Options dialog box.

8 Send the outline to PowerPoint by clicking the Send to Microsoft PowerPoint button ⬛ on the Quick Access Toolbar.

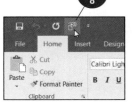

Step 8

9 When the presentation displays on the screen, click the Enable Editing button below the ribbon.

The presentation is created with a blank design template.

10 Change the layout of Slide 1 by clicking the Layout button [icon] in the Slides group on the Home tab and then clicking *Title Slide* at the drop-down list.

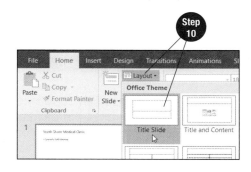

11 Make Slide 4 active and then change the layout to *Title Only*. Make Slide 9 active and then change the layout to *Title Only*. Make Slide 10 active and then change the layout to *Title Only*.

12 Apply a theme by clicking the Design tab, clicking the More Themes button [icon] at the right side of the theme thumbnails in the Themes group, and then clicking the *Parallax* option at the drop-down gallery.

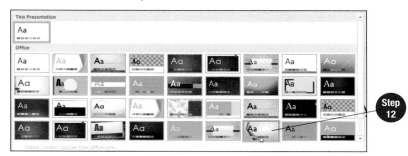

13 Save the presentation in the IntegratingMed2 folder on your storage medium and name it **2-NSMCMeeting**.

14 Close **2-NSMCMeeting.pptx**.

15 Click the Word button on the taskbar.

16 Right-click the Send to Microsoft PowerPoint button on the Quick Access Toolbar and then click *Remove from Quick Access Toolbar* at the shortcut menu.

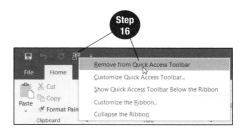

17 Close **NSMCOutline.docx** without saving the changes.

> **Check Your Work** Compare your work with the model answer to ensure that you have completed the activity correctly.

In Addition

Applying a Style in Word

If you create an outline in Word that you want to export to PowerPoint, apply styles using options in the Styles group on the Home tab. A Word document contains a number of predesigned formats grouped into style sets. Click the Design tab to display the available style sets in the Document Formatting group. Choose a style set and the styles visible in the Styles group on the Home tab change to reflect your selection. To display additional available styles, click the More Styles button (contains a horizontal line and a down-pointing triangle) at the right side of the gallery in the Styles group on the Home tab. To apply a heading style, position the insertion point in the desired text, click the More Styles button, and then click the specific style at the drop-down gallery.

Activity 2.3

Linking an Excel Chart with a Word Document and a PowerPoint Presentation

You can copy and link an object such as a table or chart to files created in other programs. For example, you can copy an Excel chart and link it to a Word document and/or a PowerPoint presentation. The advantage to copying and linking over copying and pasting is that when you edit the object in the originating program, called the source program, the object is automatically updated in the linked file in the other program, called the destination program. When an object is linked, it exists in the source program but not as a separate object in the destination program. Since the object is located only in the source program, changes made to the object in the source program will be reflected in the destination program. An object can be linked to more than one destination program or file.

North Shore Medical Clinic

What You Will Do To improve the readability of data, you will link an Excel chart to the quarterly staff meeting presentation and to a Word document.

1. Open Word, Excel, and PowerPoint.

2. Make Word active and then open **NSMCQtrlyEx.docx**. Save the document with the name **2-NSMCQtrlyEx**.

3. Make PowerPoint active, open **2-NSMCMeeting.pptx**, and then make Slide 10 active.

4. Make Excel active and then open **NSMCChart.xlsx**. Save the workbook with the name **2-NSMCChart**.

5. Copy and link the Excel chart to the Word document and the PowerPoint presentation. Begin by clicking once in the chart to select it.

   Make sure you select the entire chart and not a specific chart element. Try selecting the chart by clicking just inside the chart border.

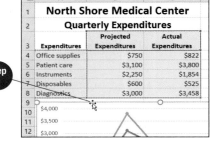

6. With the chart selected, click the Copy button in the Clipboard group on the Home tab.

7. Click the Word button on the taskbar.

8. Press Ctrl + End to move the insertion point to the end of the document.

9. Click the Paste button arrow and then click *Paste Special* at the drop-down list.

10. At the Paste Special dialog box, click the *Paste link* option, click *Microsoft Excel Chart Object* in the *As* list box, and then click OK.

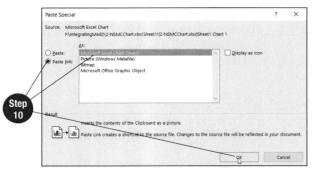

⑪ Save, print, and then close **2-NSMCQtrlyEx.docx**.

⑫ Click the PowerPoint button on the taskbar.

⑬ With Slide 10 the active slide, make sure the Home tab is selected, click the Paste button arrow, and then click *Paste Special*.

⑭ At the Paste Special dialog box, click the *Paste link* option, make sure *Microsoft Excel Chart Object* is selected in the *As* list box, and then click OK.

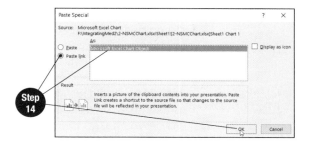

⑮ Increase the size of the chart so it better fills the slide and then move the chart so it is centered on the slide below the title.

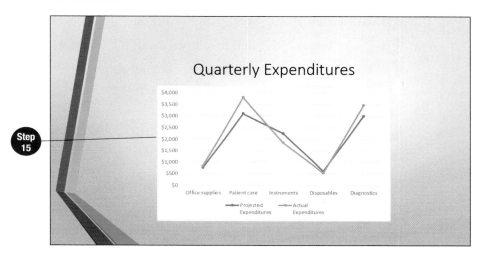

⑯ Click outside the chart to deselect it.

⑰ Save the presentation with the same name (**2-NSMCMeeting.pptx**), print only Slide 10, and then close **2-NSMCMeeting.pptx**.

⑱ Click the Excel button on the taskbar.

⑲ Click outside the chart to deselect it.

⑳ Save and then close **2-NSMCChart.xlsx**.

Check Your Work — Compare your work with the model answer to ensure that you have completed the activity correctly.

In Addition

Linking Data or an Object within a Program

In this section, you learned to link an object between programs using the Paste Special dialog box. You can also link an object in Word using options at the Object dialog box. To do this, click the Insert tab and then click the Object button in the Text group. At the Object dialog box, click the Create from File tab. At the dialog box, type the file name in the *File name* text box or click the Browse button and then select the file from the appropriate folder. Click the *Link to file* check box to insert a check mark and then click OK.

The advantage to linking an object over simply copying it is that editing the object in the source program will automatically update the object in the destination program(s) as well. To edit a linked object, open the file containing the object in the source program, make edits, and then save the file. The next time the document, workbook, or presentation is opened in the destination program, the object will be updated.

North Shore Medical Clinic

What You Will Do   As you are proofreading the text in the quarterly staff meeting presentation, you realize that you left out a category in the quarterly expenditures chart. Since you linked the Excel chart to the presentation and to a Word document, you decide to edit the chart in Excel. The charts in the Word document and PowerPoint presentation will update automatically.

1. Make sure Word, Excel, and PowerPoint are open.

2. Make Excel active and then open **2-NSMCChart.xlsx**.

3. Add a row to the worksheet by clicking cell A6 to make it the active cell. Click the Insert button arrow in the Cells group on the Home tab and then click *Insert Sheet Rows* at the drop-down list.

4. Insert the following data in the specified cells:

   A6: Respiratory
   B6: 925
   C6: 1200

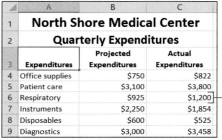

5. Click in cell A3.

6. Save, print, and then close **2-NSMCChart.xlsx**.

7. Make Word active and then open **2-NSMCQtrlyEx.docx**. At the message asking if you want to update the linked file, click the Yes button.

8. Notice how the linked chart is automatically updated to reflect the changes you made to the chart in Excel.

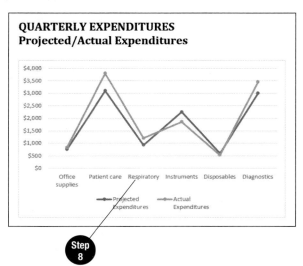

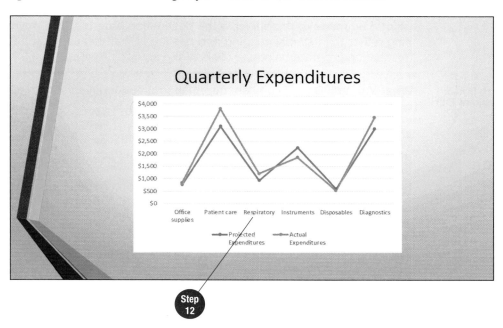

In Brief

Edit Linked Object
1. Open source file.
2. Make changes to object.
3. Save and then close source file.
4. Open destination file(s) to check if linked object updated.

9 Save, print, and then close **2-NSMCQtrlyEx.docx**.

10 Make PowerPoint active and then open **2-NSMCMeeting.pptx**.

11 At the message telling you that the presentation contains links, click the Update Links button.

12 Make Slide 10 the active slide and then notice how the linked chart is automatically updated to reflect the changes you made to the chart in Excel.

13 Save the presentation and then print only Slide 10.

14 Close **2-NSMCMeeting.pptx**.

Check Your Work Compare your work with the model answer to ensure that you have completed the activity correctly.

In Addition

Updating a Link Manually

You can choose to update a link manually in the destination program. To do this, open a Word document containing a linked object. Right-click the object, point to *Linked (type of object) Object*, and then click *Links*. At the Links dialog box, click the *Manual update* option and then click OK. With *Manual update* selected, the link will only be updated when you right-click the linked object and then click *Update Link* or when you display the Links dialog box, click the link in the list box, and then click the Update Now button.

Copy and paste, copy and link, or copy and embed an object from one file into another. A linked object resides in the source program but not as a separate object in the destination program. An embedded object resides in the source program as well as in the destination program. If a change is made to an embedded object in the source program, the change will not be made to the object in the destination program. The main advantage to embedding rather than simply copying and pasting is that you can edit an embedded object in the destination program using the tools of the source program.

North Shore
Medical Clinic

What You Will Do   To present information on new patients seen at the clinic, you decide to create a table in Word and then embed it in a slide in the staff meeting presentation.

1 Make sure Word and PowerPoint are open.

2 Make PowerPoint active and then open **2-NSMCMeeting.pptx**.

3 At the message telling you the presentation contains links, click the Update Links button.

4 Make Slide 4 the active slide.

5 Make Word active and then open **NSMCTable01.docx**.

6 Click in a cell in the table and then select the table. To do this, click the Table Tools Layout tab, click the Select button in the Table group, and then click *Select Table* at the drop-down list.

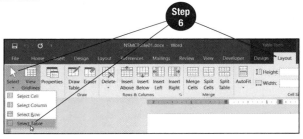

7 With the table selected, click the Home tab and then click the Copy button in the Clipboard group.

8 Click the PowerPoint button on the taskbar.

9 With Slide 4 the active slide, click the Paste button arrow and then click *Paste Special* at the drop-down list.

10 At the Paste Special dialog box, click *Microsoft Word Document Object* in the *As* list box and then click OK.

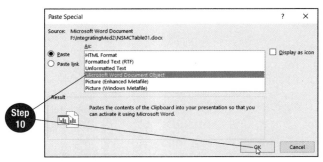

11 With the table selected in the slide, use the sizing handles to increase the size and change the position of the table as shown below.

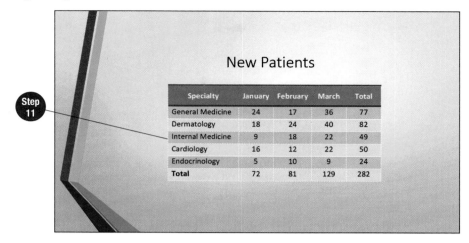

Step 11

New Patients

Specialty	January	February	March	Total
General Medicine	24	17	36	77
Dermatology	18	24	40	82
Internal Medicine	9	18	22	49
Cardiology	16	12	22	50
Endocrinology	5	10	9	24
Total	72	81	129	282

12 Click outside the table to deselect it.

13 Save **2-NSMCMeeting.pptx** and then print only Slide 4.

14 Make Slide 9 the active slide.

15 Click the Word button on the taskbar and then close the document.

16 With Word active, open **NSMCTable02.docx**.

17 Click in a cell in the table and then select all cells in the table by clicking the table move handle in the upper left corner of the table (a square with a four-headed arrow inside).

18 Click the Home tab and then click the Copy button in the Clipboard group.

19 Click the PowerPoint button on the taskbar.

20 With Slide 9 the active slide, click the Paste button arrow and then click *Paste Special* at the drop-down list.

21 At the Paste Special dialog box, click *Microsoft Word Document Object* in the *As* list box and then click OK.

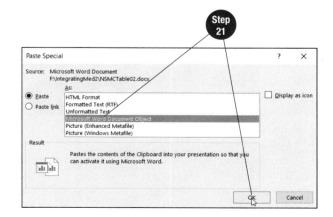

Step 21

22 Increase the size and change the position of the table in the slide so it displays as shown at the right.

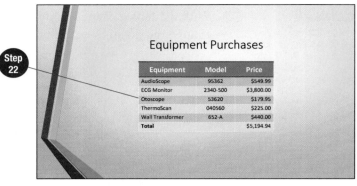

Step 22

23 As you look over the slide, you realize that the price of the otoscope is incorrect. Double-click the table to edit the amount.

> Double-clicking the table displays the Word tabs and ribbon at the top of the screen. Horizontal and vertical rulers also display around the table.

24 Using the mouse, select *$179.95* and then type $299.99.

25 Recalculate the total by selecting *$5,194.94* and then pressing F9.

> F9 is the keyboard shortcut to update a field. You could also update the formula by selecting the amount, clicking the Table Tools Layout tab, clicking the Formula button in the Data group, and then clicking OK at the Formula dialog box.

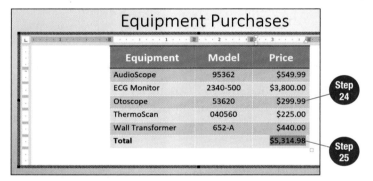

Step 24

Step 25

26 Click outside the table to deselect it.

> Clicking outside the table also removes the Word tabs.

27 Print Slide 9 of the presentation.

28 Apply a transition and transition sound of your choosing to all slides in the presentation and then run the slide show.

29 Save and then close **2-NSMCMeeting.pptx**.

30 Click the Word button on the taskbar and then close **NSMCTable02.docx**.

Check Your Work — Compare your work with the model answer to ensure that you have completed the activity correctly.

In Addition

Working with a Cropped Object

Some embedded or linked objects may appear cropped on the right or bottom side even if enough room is available to fit the image on the page or slide. A large embedded or linked object may appear cropped because Word converts the object into a Windows metafile (.wmf), which has a maximum height and width. If the embedded or linked object exceeds this maximum size, it appears cropped. To prevent an object from appearing cropped, consider reducing the size of the data by reducing the font size, column size, line spacing, and so on.

Word

A

Account option, 7
Add Field dialog box, 96
Address Block button, 98
Align Bottom Center button, 113
Align Center button, 112
aligning
    methods for changing, 41
    paragraphs, 40–41
    text, 40–41
Align Left button, 45
Alignment button, 50
Align Right button, 41
Arrange All button, 21
AutoCorrect, using, 5, 16–17
automatic numbers/bulleting, turning off, 47

B

background, customizing page, 74–75
backstage area, 6, 27
    options, 7
Blank document template, 4
blank page, inserting, 75
Blank Page button, 75
Bold button, 34
borders
    adding to tables, 114
    adding to text, 52–53
    applying to page, 74–75
    changing options, 74
Borders and Shading dialog box, 52–53
Borders button, 52
boxes, enclosing text within, 86–87
Breaks button, 78
Building Blocks Organizer dialog box
    inserting building blocks, 57–59
    sorting data in, 59
bullets
    inserting, 46–47
    turning off automatic, 47
Bullets button, 47

C

cells
    changing size, 112–113
changing width, 112–113
creating, 110–113
customizing size, 117
described, 110
keyboard shortcuts for selecting, 113
moving insertion point, 110
selecting all, 111
Center button, 40
center tab symbol, 50
Change Case button, 34
characters, inserting special, 48–49
Check Box Content Control button, 120
Check Box Content Control properties, customizing, 122
Clear All button, 51
Clear All Formatting button, 35
Clip Art, inserting, sizing and moving, 80–83
Clipboard group, 68–69
Clipboard task pane
    choosing options, 71
    using, 70–71
Close button, 9
Close option, 7, 9
closing document, 8, 9
Collapse the Ribbon button, 4, 5, 23
color
    adding in WordArt, 85
    changing theme color, 55, 73
    customizing page, 74–75
    in tables, 114–115
Color button, 81
columns
    changing size, 112–113
    changing width, 79, 112–113
    creating, 110–111
    customizing, 117
    formatting text in, 112–113
    newspaper, 78–79
Columns button, 78
Columns dialog box, 79
company logos, creating and modifying using WordArt, 84–85
Content Control Properties dialog box, 126
    customizing check box, 123
customizing plain text content, 123
inserting drop-down list content, 125–126
continuous section breaks, inserting, 78
Copy button, 68
copying text, 68–69
cover page, inserting, 75
Cover Page button, 75
Customize Address List dialog box, 96
Customize Columns button, 96
Cut button, 68
cutting text, 68–69

D

data, sorting in building Blocks Organizer dialog box, 59
data source file
    described, 96
    editing, 100–103
    filtering records in, 106–107
    inserting new field, 102
    for mail merge, 96
    sorting records in, 104–105
date
    inserting, 56–57
    keyboard shortcut for insert current, 41
    updating automatically, 56
decimal tab, setting, 51
Decrease Indent button, 45
default document formatting
    changing, 54–55
    elements, 7
Delete button, 111
deleting
    tabs, 51
    text, 10–13
Design tab, 54, 73
Developer tab, 118–120
dictionary, downloading, 17
directory, preparing using Mail Merge feature, 109
display percentage, changing, 20–21
document icon, 30
documents. *See also* text
    changing
        default formatting, 54–55
        display percentage, 20–21
        line and paragraph spacing, 44–45
views, 18–19
closing, 8, 9
creating, 4–7
creating using template, 28–29
default formatting, 7
formatting with Font group and Mini toolbar, 34–35
forms
    creating and saving as template, 118–121
    creating for handwritten entries, 116–117
    creating with Legacy Tools, 127
    defining group, 120
    editing form template, 124–125
    filling in and printing, 122–123
    inserting drop-down list content control, 125–127
insert one document into another, 78–79
main, 96
merging with envelopes, 96–99
naming, 9
navigating in, 12–13
opening, 10–11
previewing, 26
printing, 6–7, 25–27
readability, 78
resuming reading or editing, 13
saving, 6, 8–9
    in different format, 30–31
scrolling in, 12–13
section break, 78–79
spelling and grammar check, 14–15
viewing multiple, 21
Draft button, 18, 78
Draft view, 18
Drawing Tools Format tab, 85
Drop-down list
    inserting content control, 125–127
    selecting option in, 127
Drop-Down List Content Control button, 125

print area, 152
Print option, 134
Save as button, 134
bar chart
creating, 198–199
modifying, 202–203
Bold button, 169
bold italic typeface, 168
bold typeface, 168
borders
adding, 176–177
creating custom, 177
Bottom Border button arrow, 176

C

calculations, performing using formulas, 142–143
Cancel button, 137
cell address, 132
including in formula, 142
cell pointer, 132, 133
cells, 132
active, 132, 133, 136
aligning data in, 148–149, 172–174
cell address, 132
changing font size, style, and color, 168–169
clearing, 160–161
copying, 164–165
deleting, 163
editing, 160–161
entering data, 133, 136–137
entering formulas into, 142–143
fill options, 140–141
formatting numeric, 170–171
formatting options, 148–149
going to specific, 138
indentation changes, 172–173
inserting, 163
inserting line break, 137
keyboard movement commands, 136
linking, 164–165
moving, 164–165
range, 136, 137
range name, 194–195
selecting, 136–137
sorting, 148, 149
undo and redo, 170–171
cell styles
applying, 178–179
creating new, 179
described, 178

Cell Styles button, 178
Center button, 172
chart elements, 200, 203
Chart Elements button, 200
charts
bar, 198–199, 203
chart elements, 200, 203
creating
column, 198–199
pie, 200–201
modifying and formatting, 202–203
Recommended Charts button, 199
Sparklines group, 201
Chart Styles button, 201
Clear button, 160
clip art, inserting, moving and resizing, 158–159
clipboard, 146, 147, 164–165
Close button, 135
Collapse the Ribbon button, 132, 133
color
adding shading, 176–177
adding to cells, 176–177
fill, 176–177
font, 168–169
Colors button, 179
column chart
creating, 198–199
modifying, 202–203
columns
adjusting width of, 166–167
deleting, 162–163
inserting, 162–163
letters for, 132
printing column headings, 153
printing headings on multiple pages, 207
sorting, 148, 149
sorting table by single or multiple columns, 214–215
width default setting, 166
width of, 166–167
Column Width dialog box, 166
comma style, 170
Comma Style button, 170
comments
described, 172
inserting, 174–175
printing, 175
Content pane, 134
Convert to Range button, 213

copy and paste
cells, 164–165
copying formulas, 146–147
versus fill handle, 147
linking cells, 164–165
Copy button, 146
copying
cells, 164–165
formats, 176–177
formulas, 1460147
relative, 146
COUNTA function, 191
COUNTBLANK function, 191
COUNT function, 190–191
currency style, 170
Current Date button, 209
custom borders, creating, 177
cut and paste, cells, 164–165
Cut button, 164

D

data
alignment of, in cells, 172–174
editing, 160–161
entering into cell, 133, 136–137
filtering data not formatted in table, 217
formatting in table, 210–213
Date and Time button, 192
date functions, 192–193
decimals, adjusting, 170–171
Decrease Decimal button, 171
Decrease Indent button, 173
default font, 168
Delete button arrow, 163
deleting
cells, 163
columns, 162–163
rows, 162–163
destination cell, 146
copy and paste cell contents, 164–165
dialog box launcher, 132, 133
division (/), 142, 143
dollar symbol ($), 184
drag and drop, 164, 165
drawing shapes, 204–205

E

editing
cells, 160–161
proofing tools, 160–161
undo and redo, 170–171
Enter button, 137, 140

equals sign, 142, 143
Excel Options dialog box, displaying formulas at, 149
exponentiation (^), 142, 143

F

File Name button, 209
File name text box, 134
files, naming, 134
File tab, 132, 133
Fill button, 141
Fill Color button arrow, 169
fill handle
Copy and Paste versus, 147
copying formulas, 146–147
to enter pattern, 141
using, 140–141
filter
data not formatted in table, 217
removing, 217
Filter arrow button, 216
filter icon, 216
filtering, table, 216–217
Find and Replace, 180–181
Find feature, 180–181
Find Next button, 180–181
Find & Select button, 138, 180
Font Color button arrow, 169
fonts
attributes, 168–169
changing size of, 168–169
color, 168–169
default, 168
size, 168–169
style, 168
Fonts button, 179
footers, inserting, 208–209
Format as Table button, 210
Format button, 166
Format Cells dialog box, 169
Format Painter, copying formats with, 176–177
Format Painter button, 177
formatting
charts, 202–203
copying with Format Painter, 176–177
data in table, 210–213
numeric cells, 170–171
replacing formats, 181
Formula Auditing group, 149
Formula bar, 132, 133
formulas
copying, 146–147

creating, with absolute
addressing, 184–185
with date functions and
dates, 192–193
displaying, 148–149
elements of, 142
entering in cell, 142–143
function formula structure,
190
including cell address in,
142
order of operations, 143
performing calculations
using, 142–143
with relative addressing,
184
Freeze Panes button, 182
Freeze Panes options,
182–183
Function Arguments dialog
box, 197
functions
AVERAGE, 190–191
COUNT, 190–191
COUNTA, 191
COUNTBLANK, 191
date, 192–193
described, 144
IF, 196–197
logical, 196–197
MAX, 190–191
MEDIAN, 191
MIN, 190–191
NOW, 192–193
statistical, 190–191
SUM function, 144–145
time, 192–193
TODAY, 192–193

G

General format, 170
Go To dialog box, 138
Go to Footer button, 209
gridlines, printing, 153
group, 132, 133

H

hard copy, 152
headers, inserting, 208–209
Help task pane
opening, 150
using, 150–151
horizontal alignment,
changing, 172–173
horizontal scroll bar, 132,
133, 139

I

IF function, 196–197
arguments for, 197

illustrations, inserting, moving
and resizing, 158–159
images, inserting, moving
and resizing, 158–159
Increase Decimal button, 171
Increase Indent button, 173
indentation
changing for cells,
172–173
increasing, 173
Insert button arrow, 162
Insert Column Chart button,
198
inserting
cells, 163
columns, 162–163
comments, 174–175
headers and footers,
208–209
images, 158–159
rows, 162–163
shapes, 204–205
text box, 204–205
Insert Pie or Doughnut Chart
button, 200
invoice, creating from
template, 154–155
italic typeface, 168

K

keyboard shortcut
display formula, 148, 149
inserting line break, 137
movement commands,
136, 138
opening Help task pane,
150
Scroll Lock mode, 139
selecting multiple cells,
137

L

labels
alignment of, 148–149
entering, 136, 137
finding, 180–181
replacing, 180–181
landscape orientation, 153
line break, inserting in cell,
137
linking
cells, 164–165
copy and paste, 164–165
Live Preview, 168
Logical button, 196
logical functions, 196–197
logical test, 196

M

margins
changing, 206–207

default, 206
Margins button, 207
marquee, 143
moving, 144, 146
mathematical operations,
142, 143
MAX function, 190–191
MEDIAN function, 191
Merge & Center button, 148
Middle Align button, 174
MIN function, 190–191
mixed referencing, 184–185
More Cell Styles button, 178
More Chart Styles button, 199
mouse, adjusting column
width and row height,
166
mouse wheel, 138, 139
Move Chart button, 199
movement commands, 136,
138
moving
cells, 164–165
images, 158–159
moving marquee, 144, 146
multiplication (*), 142, 143

N

name
creating and using range,
194–195
files, 134
managing range, 195
Name box, 132, 133, 139, 194
Name Manager button, 195
navigating, in worksheet,
138–139
New button, 175
New Cell Style option, 179
New Comment button, 174
New sheet button, 132, 133
NOW function, 192–193
Number Format options, 171
numerical values, 198
numeric cells, formatting,
170–171
numeric formats, 170–171

O

Online Pictures button, 158
order of operations, 143
orientation
landscape, 153
portrait, 153
Orientation button, 207
Outside Borders button, 176

P

Page Layout options,
changing, 206–207
Page Layout tab, 206, 207

Page Layout view, 208–209
pages
changing margins,
206–207
changing orientation, 153
inserting headers and
footers, 208–209
printing column or row
headings on multiple,
207
Page Setup dialog box,
printing comments, 175
panes, freezing, 182–183
paste
copy and paste, 164–165
cut and paste, 164–165
drag and drop, 164, 165
Paste button, 146, 164
Paste Options button, 146
Paste Options gallery, 165
pattern, fill handle to enter,
141
percents (%), 143
percent style, 170
pictures, inserting, moving
and resizing, 158–159
Pictures button, 158–159
Picture Tools Format tab, 159
pie charts, creating, 200–201
pinning, template, 155
points, 168
portrait orientation, 153
Previous button, 175
printing
column or row headings
on multiple pages, 207
comments, 175
gridlines, 153
row and column heading,
153
workbook, 134
worksheet, 152–153
proofing tools, using,
160–161

Q

Quick Access Toolbar, 132,
133, 170
Quick Layout button, 199

R

range, 144
range name
creating, 194–195
managing, 195
range of cells, 136, 137
Recommended Charts button,
199
redo, 170
relative addressing, 146, 184

Drawing Tools Format tab, using buttons and options on, 289

E

editing, while checking spelling, 253–254
Effect Options button, 260

F

File tab, 237, 239
Font Color button arrow, 271
Font dialog box, changing fonts at, 272–273
font effects, applying, 270–271
fonts
  applying formatting, 270–271
  changing
    all occurrences of, 273
    at Font Dialog box, 272–273
    theme, 282–283
  defined, 271
  replacing, 272–273
Font Size button, 270
footers, inserting, 280–281
Format Painter, formatting with, 274–275
formatting
  with buttons in Picture Tools Format tab, 287
  with font effects, 270–271
  with Format Painter, 274–275
  SmartArt graphic, 290–293
  WordArt, 288–289
From Beginning button, 251

H

Header & Footer button, 280
headers, inserting, 280–281
Help feature, using, 252–253
Hide Slide button, 251
hiding
  mouse pointer, 259
  slides, 250–251
highlighting, 270
Home tab, 239
horizontal text alignment, changing, 276–278

I

I-beam pointer, 237
images
  compress, 287
  formatting with buttons in Picture Tools Format tab, 287

inserting, 284–287
moving, 284–287
sizing, 284–287
Increase List Level button, 266
indents
  decreasing, 266–267
  increasing, 266–267
Ink Tools, using during presentation, 259
Ink to Shape button, 259
inserting
  headers and footers, 280–281
  image, 284–287
  new line, 279
  slides into presentation, 240–243
  SmartArt graphic, 290–293
  text into slides, 240–243
  WordArt, 288–289
insertion point, 237
  movement commands for, 242
Italic button, 270
italic typeface, 270

J

Justify button, 277

K

keyboard shortcuts
  changing alignment, 276
  displaying blank presentation, 240
  Help task pane, displaying, 252
  insertion point movement commands, 242
  for navigating presentation, 247

L

laser pointer, using during presentation, 258
Layout button, 248
lines
  changing line spacing, 276–278
  inserting new, 279
Line Spacing button, 277
live preview, 240

M

monospaced typeface, 271
More Shape Styles button, 279
More Themes button, 240
mouse pointer
  hiding/displaying, 259

rearranging slides with, 250–251
rearranging text in Outline View, 267
moving
  image, 284–287
  placeholder, 248–249
  slides, 250–251

N

navigating, in presentation, 244–245, 247
New Slide button, 241
Next Slide button, 244
Normal button, 247
Normal view, 246–247
Notes Page button, 246
Notes Page view, 246–247

O

objects, applying animation to, 294–295
Online Pictures button, 285
Open dialog box, 244
opening, presentation, 236, 244, 245
organizational chart, inserting and formatting in SmartArt, 290–293
Outline View, 246–247
Outline View button, 246

P

Package for CD feature, 281
paragraph, changing spacing, 276–278
Paste button, 268
pasting, text, 268–269
pen, using during presentation, 256–259
Pen button, 259
pictures
  compress, 287
  formatting with buttons in Picture Tools Format tab, 287
  inserting, sizing and moving, 284–287
  insert in slide background, 283
Pictures button, 284
Picture Tools Format tab, formatting with buttons in, 287
placeholder, 237, 241
  AutoFit Options button, 249
  selecting and moving, 248–249
  sizing, 249

PowerPoint
  closing, 239
  opening, 236–239
  window elements in, 237
presentation
  blank presentation, 240
  choosing typeface for, 273
  closing, 243
  copying slides within, 251
  creating with installed template, 236–239
  design theme, choosing, 240–243
  editing, 253–254
  inserting slides in, 240–243
  keyboard for navigating, 247
  main purpose of, 243
  navigating in, 244–245, 247
  opening, 244, 245
  planning, 243
  previewing, 262–263
  printing, 262–263
  running, 256–259
    automatically, 260–261
    from current slide, 256–259
  saving, 243
  sound, 260–261
  transitions, 260–261
  using Ink Tools during, 259
  using pen during, 256–259
presentation cycle, completing, 236–239
Preview button, 294
previewing, presentation, 262–263
Previous Slide button, 244
Print backstage area, 262–263
printing
  determining needs for, 243
  presentation, 262–263
  presentation in outline layout, 239
proportional typeface, 271

Q

Quick Access toolbar, 237

R

Reading view, 246, 247
Reading View button, 247
rearranging
  slides, 250–251
  text in Outline View, 267

Recent option list, opening
    presentation from, 245
Replace Font dialog box, 273
replacing, fonts, 272–273
ribbon, 237, 239
running, presentation,
    256–259, 261

S

san serif typeface, 271
Save As dialog box, 238
Save button, 238
saving, presentation, 243
ScreenTip, 239
scroll bar, vertical, 237, 244
Send Backward button arrow,
    286
serif typeface, 271
Shape Outline button arrow,
    279
shapes, drawing, 278–279
Shapes button, 278
sizing
    image, 284–287
    placeholder, 249
slide design, maintaining
    consistent, 243
slide layout
    changing, 248–249
    choosing, 244–245
slide orientation, 263
slide pane, 237, 240
slides
    adding, 241–243
    changing orientation, 263
    changing size, 282–283
    copying
        within presentation, 251
        between presentations,
            269
    creating, 240–243
    deleting, 250–251
    formatting background,
        282–283
    headers and footers in,
        280–281
    hiding, 250–251
    increasing and decreasing
        indent, 266–267
    inserting, 240–245
    keeping easy to read, 243
    moving, 250–251
    navigating through,
        244–245
    new, 241–243
    one idea per slide, 243
    picture in background, 283
    rearranging, 250–251
    running from current,
        256–259

slide show, running, 256–259
    automatically, 236, 261
    manually, 256
Slide Show toolbar, 256
Slide Size button, 282
Slide Size dialog box, 263
Slide Sorter button, 247
Slide Sorter View, 246, 247
slide thumbnails, 240
slide thumbnails pane, 237
SmartArt button, 293
SmartArt graphic
    formatting, 290–293
    inserting, 290–293
    inserting text, 293
    organizational chart in,
        290–293
SmartArt graphic dialog box,
    290–292
spacing, changing line and
    paragraph, 276–278
spelling
    buttons on spelling task
        pane, 254
    editing while checking,
        254
    options in, 255
Spelling button, 253
spelling checker, 253–254
Spelling task pane, 253–254
Start From the Beginning
    button, 236
Start Inking button, 259
Status bar, 237
strikethrough typeface, 270
synonyms, 254

T

tabs, 237
    using, 239
Tell Me feature, 237
    using, 252–253
template, creating
    presentation with
    installed, 236–239
text
    applying animation to,
        294–295
    copying, 268–269
    creating bulleted, 277–278
    cutting, 268–269
    horizontal text alignment,
        276–278
    increasing and decreasing
        indent, 266–267
    inserting
        into slides, 240–243
        in SmartArt graphic,
            293
    pasting, 268–269

rearranging, in Outline
    View, 267
selecting, 268–269
vertical text alignment,
    276–278
text box, drawing, 277–278
Text Box button, 277
Text Effects button, 279, 289
text pane, inserting text in,
    293
Text Pane button, 290, 293
text shadow, 270
theme color
    changing, 282–283
    customizing, 283
theme font, changing,
    282–283
thesaurus, 254–255
Thesaurus button, 254
Title bar, 237
transitions, adding, 260–261
typefaces
    choosing, 271, 273
    defined, 271
    monospaced, 271
    proportional, 271
    san serif, 271
    serif, 271

U

Underline button, 270
underline typeface, 270

V

vertical scroll bar, 237, 244
vertical text alignment,
    changing, 276–278
view area, 237
views, changing, 246–247
View tab, 246

W

WordArt, inserting and
    formatting, 288–289
WordArt button, 288

Z

Zoom button, 247
Zoom dialog box, 247
Zoom In button, 247
Zoom Out button, 247
Zoom slider bar, 247
Zoom to Page button, 262

Integrating

A

AutoSum button, 221

B

Break Link button, 225

C

Center button, 226
charts, linking Excel, with
    Word document,
    226–227
Copy button, 220, 304
copying, Word data into
    worksheet, 220–221
cropped objects, 310
cycling between open
    programs, 221

D

data
    copying and pasting Word
        data into worksheet,
        220–221
    editing linked data,
        224–225
    linking
        within program, 223,
            305
        between programs,
            222–223
    pasting and linking, 301
destination program, 220,
    304, 306, 308
document, linking Excel
    worksheet with Word
    document, 222–223

E

editing
    embedded objects,
        230–231, 310
    linked data, 224–225
    linked object, 306–307
    Word table in PowerPoint
        slide, 308–310
embedded objects, 228
    editing, 310
    inserting, from existing
        file, 229
embedding
    editing embedded
        worksheet, 230–231
    Excel worksheet into Word
        document, 228–229
    troubleshooting problems,
        231
    Word table in PowerPoint
        slide, 308–310
Excel, linking chart with
    Word document and
    PowerPoint presentation,
    304–305
exporting
    PowerPoint presentation to
        Word, 300–301

Word outline to
PowerPoint
presentation, 302–303

F

files, inserting embedded
object from existing file,
229

I

icons, displaying linked
objects as, 224, 225
images, working with
cropped objects, 310
Insert button arrow, 306
Insert Function button, 222
inserting, embedded object,
from existing file, 229

K

keyboard shortcuts, cycling
between open programs,
221

L

Layout button, 303
link(s)
breaking, 225
customizing, 227
updating manually, 307
viewing, 224–225
linked data
editing, 224
updating, 224–225
linked object, 228
displaying, as an icon,
224, 225
editing, 306–307
updating, 227
linking
data, 301
within program, 305
data within program, 223
Excel chart with Word
document, 226–227

Excel chart with
Word document
and PowerPoint
presentation, 304–305
Excel worksheet with
Word document,
222–223
objects
between programs, 305
within programs, 305
troubleshooting problems,
231
Links dialog box, 225, 227

M

manual updating of link, 307
Microsoft Office, advantages
of, 300
More Themes button, 303

O

Object dialog box, 229
objects
cropped objects, 310
editing linked, 306–307
embedded, editing, 310
linking
within program, 305
between programs, 305
open programs, cycling
between, 221
outline, exporting Word, to
PowerPoint presentation,
302–303

P

paste, Word data into
worksheet, 220–221
Paste button, 221
pasting data, 301
PowerPoint
embedding and editing
Word table in slide in,
308–310

exporting presentation to
Word, 300–301
exporting Word outline to
presentation, 302–303
linking Excel chart with
Word document and
presentation in, 304–305
presentation
exporting to Word,
300–301
exporting Word outline to
PowerPoint, 302–303
linking Excel chart with
Word document and
PowerPoint, 304–305
programs
cycling between, 221
linking data within, 223

Q

Quick Access Toolbar button,
302

S

Select button, 308
Send to Microsoft Word
dialog box, 300, 301
Send to PowerPoint button,
302
source program, 220, 304,
306, 308
styles, applying in Word, 303
suite program, advantages
of, 300

T

tables, embedding and
editing Word table
in PowerPoint slide,
308–310

U

updating
linked data, 224–225
link manually, 307

V

viewing a link, 224–225

W

Word
applying styles in, 303
embedding and editing
table in PowerPoint
slide, 308–310
exporting outline
to PowerPoint
presentation, 302–303
exporting PowerPoint
presentation to,
300–301
linking Excel chart
with document in,
and PowerPoint
presentation, 304–305
Word document
copying and pasting data
into Excel worksheet,
220–221
embedding Excel
worksheet into,
228–229
linking Excel chart with,
226–227
linking Excel worksheet
with, 222–223
worksheets
copying and pasting Word
data into, 220–221
editing embedded
worksheet, 230–231
embedding, into Word
document, 228–229
linking, with Word
document, 222–223